TRANSFORMING PUBLIC HEALTH PRACTICE

TRANSFORMING PUBLIC HEALTH PRACTICE

Leadership and Management Essentials

BERNARD J. HEALEY
CHERYLL D. LESNESKI

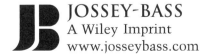

JOSSEY-BASS
A Wiley Imprint
www.josseybass.com

Published by Jossey-Bass
A Wiley Imprint
989 Market Street, San Francisco, CA 94103-1741—www.josseybass.com

Jossey-Bass books and products are available through most bookstores. To contact Jossey-Bass directly call our Customer Care Department within the U.S. at 800-956-7739, outside the U.S. at 317-572-3986, or fax 317-572-4002.

Wiley also publishes its books in a variety of electronic formats and by print-on-demand. Not all content that is available in standard print versions of this book may appear or be packaged in all book formats. If you have purchased a version of this book that did not include media that is referenced by or accompanies a standard print version, you may request this media by visiting http://booksupport.wiley .com. For more information about Wiley products, visit us at www.wiley.com.

Library of Congress Cataloging-in-Publication Data

Healey, Bernard J., 1947–
  Transforming public health practice : leadership and management essentials / Bernard J. Healey, Cheryll D. Lesneski.—1st ed.
      p. cm.
  Includes bibliographical references and index.
  ISBN 978-0-470-50895-4 (pbk.); 978-1-118-08993-4 (ebk.); 978-1-118-08994-1 (ebk.); 978-1-118-08995-8 (ebk.)
  1. Public health administration. I. Lesneski, Cheryll D., 1949– II. Title.
  RA425H383 2011
  362.1–dc23

                                                                                          2011021315

Printed in the United States of America
FIRST EDITION
PB Printing   10 9 8 7 6 5 4 3 2 1

CONTENTS

Case Studies

To Kathy, my wife of forty years, my two wonderful children, Alison and Bryan, and my two-year-old grandson, John.

Bernard J. Healey

To the memory of my parents, Melton Harold and Clara Eva Smith, for their wonderful love and support for me throughout our lives together.

Cheryll D. Lesneski

IN THE EARLY YEARS of the last century the life expectancy of most Americans was approximately forty-five years of age. The length of life has increased for men and women in this country by over thirty years since then. A large portion of this longevity is the direct result of public health activities associated with immunizations, health education programs, and various prevention programs developed by state and local public health departments. This represents a success story for public health in the United States.

The activities of public health departments, which focus on the prevention of health problems before they occur, make up one of the most important components for achieving better population health in every community in the United States. If we are ever to improve the health of the population, there is a very real need for public health interventions within every community population. This will not happen until the public health system's infrastructure is rebuilt, an endeavor that must include leadership training for those placed in charge of this area of health care services delivery in our country.

Improvement of the Health of the Population

When we think about the U.S. health care system, the process of curing and treating diseases is usually the only idea that pervades our thought process. Turnock (2009) points out that activities dedicated to maintaining and promoting health are not usually considered health services by our current medical care system, which has always left the prevention and promotion of health to public health agencies primarily funded by the government. Over time, however, the interest in and funding for these public health activities have been reduced, and it seems that public health activities only become visible in times of crisis.

According to Mays et al. (2004), the public health system in the United States has been receiving growing attention because of emerging health dangers, trends in health policy, and developments in the health care marketplace. In recent years, primarily due to threats of bioterrorism, the epidemic of obesity, and type 2 diabetes, a great deal of attention has been given to the role of prevention in our health care system. The new health care reform bill, signed by President Obama in April 2010, mentions the need to prevent chronic diseases and their complications. Prevention is the major responsibility of public health departments, so a great deal of attention has recently been given to the potential role of public health as our health care system is being reformed.

According to the April 2010 issue of the Nation's Health ("Q&A with Surgeon General Benjamin"), the eighteenth surgeon general of the United States, Regina Benjamin, wants to "transform our sick care system into a wellness system." Benjamin believes that although the public health system is the cornerstone of the U.S. population's health, it has not received the resources that it deserves. She advocates reversing this trend, pointing out that Congress has appropriated $1 billion for prevention and wellness programs as part of the American Recovery and Reinvestment Act. This money will be used to increase the number of public health workers and continue the expansion of prevention and wellness efforts in U.S. communities.

The increase in life expectancy in the United States can in large part be directly attributed to the many public health accomplishments that were made possible by dedicated workers. Work directed toward reduction of tobacco use, efforts to encourage better nutrition and more physical activity, proper immunizations, and health education programs are just a few of the services that public health departments developed and implemented during the last twenty years. These accomplishments in the area of preventive health care occurred despite the depleted public health infrastructure.

Chronic diseases—such as heart disease, cancer, and diabetes—are the leading causes of death and disability in the United States. As the burden of chronic diseases in the United States continues to increase, public health departments should make greater efforts to identify and implement interventions that successfully reduce disease risk, especially in the workplace. According to the Florida Department of Health (2011), these diseases account for seven of every ten deaths and affect the quality of life of ninety million Americans. Although chronic diseases are among the most common and costly health problems, however, they are also among the most preventable.

The public health challenge has moved way beyond defeating organisms that cause communicable diseases and into the new world of preventing community populations from developing chronic diseases that cannot be cured. These chronic diseases are caused by high-risk health behaviors that result from lifestyle choices that can be changed. Altering lifestyle behaviors may very well serve to increase longevity as well as quality of life in older years. In order to meet this challenge, public health departments need strong leadership and empowered followership to unite the community.

Opportunities for Public Health Departments

The primary role of public health is to prevent illness or disease from ever occurring. Because practitioners in this field prevent things from happening, public health has never been given the respect that it deserves—we are often unable to understand the value of something that did not happen. Because most of medical care encompasses very visible efforts to cure disease, most of the credit for medicine success usually is reserved for the medical care system. This is unfortunate because the increase in the length of life since the early 1900s resulted from such public health services as immunizations and health education programs.

Hemenway (2010) argues that public health is constantly underfunded due to the fact that the benefits of public health activities usually show visible results in the future rather than the present. Unfortunately, most people do not seek medical care until they have become very ill, whereas public health is performing its magic before illness occurs. This is the main reason why the leaders of public health departments need to spend more time communicating what they do and why they do it. Public health has always been one of the best-kept secrets of our health care system. It is time for public health leaders to spend less of their time fighting undeserved budget cuts and more time publicizing their success stories. It is time to raise public health to the stature that it has earned with its various triumphs over the years.

Health care services delivery in this country is undergoing rapid change in structure, process, and required outcomes. The recently enacted health care reform bill has included $500 million a year to be allocated to "comparative effectiveness research," which is designed to reduce the cost of health care by requiring the health care system to become more efficient in its use of resources. It is becoming the norm to compare various treatment options in order to ascertain the least expensive method of producing the required outcome without sacrificing quality. It is indeed a time of change for the delivery of health care in the United States.

This change will also produce great opportunities for the improvement of Americans' health, as the nation slowly begins to realize the necessity of preventing very expensive health problems from occurring in the first place. This reform in our health care system is producing a great opportunity for public health departments to increase their relevancy in the delivery of health care services to millions of Americans. According to Beerel (2009), relevancy is engaged power that can be used to achieve goals. This is clearly the opportunity that has presented itself to public health departments in our country. Americans are starting to realize the relevancy of population-based medicine, health promotion, and disease prevention—especially in relation to the current epidemic of chronic diseases.

Even though they have high costs at the start, chronic disease and injury prevention programs do very well when cost-benefit analysis is applied to the outcomes associated with their implementation. Public health departments need to expand their success with identifying the causes of chronic diseases into an effort to prevent the occurrence of these diseases or, at the very least, to postpone the onset of their complications until later in life.

We wrote this book in order to discuss the need for new skill development for our public health workforce, leadership training for those responsible for public health programs, along with empowerment of public health employees to expand prevention efforts for the population. Among the skills that public health workers require are change management and conflict management techniques, culture-building abilities, quality improvement skills, communication skills, and team-building and collaboration skills.

There is no question that developing a strong public health infrastructure is one of the most important things we can do to improve the health of our population. It is also critical to note that this infrastructure needs strong leaders dedicated to the achievement of public health goals, which must focus on pursuing outcomes rather than activities that are not producing measurable results. This is going to require profound change in the way public health departments are organized and led.

ACKNOWLEDGMENTS

W<small>E WOULD LIKE</small> to begin by acknowledging the dedicated people who work in public health and who, despite limited resources, have accomplished so much in making the United States a better place to lead a healthy life. This is really a book about how to help public health departments achieve even greater success stories in the future through better leadership. Those who work in public health departments throughout this country have so much more to contribute if only allowed to do their work. This can only be accomplished through leadership, worker empowerment, and increased resources.

During the process of writing this book we met many dedicated people who demanded professionalism in everything they tried to accomplish. A number of individuals, to whom we are truly indebted, helped us with the writing of particular chapters. They are the wonderful individuals who work at Prevention Institute, a nonprofit national center dedicated to improving community health and equity through effective primary prevention: Larry Cohen, Rachel Davis, Anthony Iton, and Sharon Murriguez.

A number of additional individuals contributed case studies in public health, including Julia Joh Elligers and Lisa Jacobs from the National Association of County and City Health Officials; Ted Kross from the Wilkes-Barre City Health Department; Jill D. Morrow-Gorton, who is a developmental pediatrician serving as the medical director of the Office of Developmental Programs in the Commonwealth of Pennsylvania's Department of Public Welfare; and Marc C. Marchese, a professor at King's College in Wilkes-Barre, Pennsylvania.

Three more individuals to whom we are truly indebted helped us with the review of this new public health text. They are Celeste Torio, Michele Shade and Helda Pinzon Perez. They helped us sharpen our ideas to make this book a much better addition to the literature concerning public health practice.

During the entire research and writing process for this book we were surrounded by intelligent, caring individuals who cared only about making our ideas better. We are very fortunate individuals to have had the opportunity to write a book for a national publisher, but we are equally fortunate to have been able to work with such talent.

Bernard J. Healey is a professor of health care administration at King's College in Wilkes-Barre, Pennsylvania, and is currently the director of the King's College graduate program in health care administration. He began his career in 1971 as an epidemiologist for the Pennsylvania Department of Health, retiring from that position in 1995. During his tenure with the government he completed advanced degrees in business administration and public administration, and in 1990 he finished his doctoral work at the University of Pennsylvania. Dr. Healey has been teaching undergraduate and graduate courses in business, public health, and health care administration at several colleges since 1974.

Dr. Healey has published over one hundred articles about public health, health policy, leadership, marketing, and health care partnerships. He has also written and published two books, one about health promotion and one about occupational safety and health in public health practice.

Dr. Healey is a member of the American Association of Public Health and the Association of University Programs in Health Care Administration. He is also a part-time consultant in epidemiology for the Wilkes-Barre City Health Department and a consultant for numerous public health projects in Pennsylvania.

Cheryll D. Lesneski teaches courses in public health practice and community health improvement as an assistant professor in the Public Health Leadership Program at the University of North Carolina at Chapel Hill's Gillings School of Global Public Health. She also works for the U.S. Department of Health and Human Services, promoting sound financial management of public health organizations within a continuous quality improvement framework. In 2005 Dr. Lesneski received a doctorate in public health in the Department of Health Policy and Administration at the Gillings School. Her dissertation, Developing Performance Measurement Systems for Local Public Health Agencies Using the Balanced Scorecard, was published by VDM in 2009. Dr. Lesneski has been a public health practitioner for over twenty years, serving as a local public health agency director for ten years in the Florida Department of Health. She continues to work with the Florida Department of Health to promote continuous quality improvement techniques in learning collaborative settings. Dr. Lesneski also served as an improvement adviser and evaluator with the North Carolina Center for Children's Healthcare Improvement and the National Initiative for Children's Healthcare Quality.

Larry Cohen MSW, is founder and executive director of Prevention Institute, a nonprofit national center dedicated to improving community health and equity through effective primary prevention—taking action to build resilience and to prevent illness and injury before they occur. With an emphasis on health equity, Mr. Cohen has led many successful public health efforts at the local, state, and federal levels concerning injury and violence prevention, mental health, transportation and health, and chronic disease prevention as it relates to diet and physical activity. Mr. Cohen has advanced a deeper understanding of how social determinants shape health outcomes, and Prevention Institute provides resources, conceptual frameworks, and tools to help communities address the underlying causes of health inequities. Prevention Institute has also successfully led state and national efforts to incorporate a focus on and investment in primary prevention as a significant part of health care reform and stimulus funding for communities.

Rachel Davis MSW, is managing director at Prevention Institute. Mrs. Davis oversees Prevention Institute's work in the areas of health equity, community health, violence prevention, mental health, and children and youth. She develops tools for advancing primary prevention, provides consulting and training for various community and government organizations, and advances the conceptual work of the organization. With funding from the federal Office of Minority Health (OMH), Mrs. Davis developed and piloted THRIVE (Tool for Health and Resilience in Vulnerable Environments), a community resilience assessment tool that helps communities bolster factors that will improve health outcomes and reduce disparities experienced by racial and ethnic minorities. An article written by Mrs. Davis on the tool and its initial pilot testing was published in the American Journal of Public Health. She is currently overseeing an OMH-funded project to disseminate THRIVE.

Anthony Iton MD, JD, MPH, was in October 2009 appointed as senior vice president of healthy communities at The California Endowment. Prior to his appointment, Dr. Iton served from 2003 as both the director and county health officer for the Alameda County Public Health Department. In that role he oversaw the creation of an innovative public health practice designed to eliminate health disparities by tackling the root causes of poor health that limit quality of life and life span in many of California's low-income communities. Dr. Iton, who has been published in numerous public health and medical publications, is a regular public health lecturer and keynote speaker at conferences across the nation. He earned his BS in neurophysiology, with honors, from McGill University, in Montreal, Quebec; his JD and MPH at the University of California, Berkeley; and his MD from Johns Hopkins University School of Medicine. Dr. Iton has served on the Board of Directors of Prevention Institute.

Lisa M. Jacobs is currently a full-time MSW candidate at the University of Pennsylvania in Philadelphia. Prior to beginning her graduate studies, Ms. Jacobs served as the Mobilizing for Action through Planning and Partnerships (MAPP) Program Associate at the National Association of County and City Health Officials (NACCHO) in Washington DC. As program associate, Ms. Jacobs supported the MAPP program and National Public Health Performance Standards Program (NPHPSP) by developing and posting Web content, communicating with local health department staff in regard to MAPP and NPHPSP activities, developing fact sheets and guidance documents, and planning and cofacilitating MAPP trainings in communities throughout the United States. While at NACCHO, Ms. Jacobs also served as a member of several organization-wide initiatives including the Health Equity and Social Justice Team. Prior to joining NACCHO, Ms. Jacobs participated in the National Women's Health Network's Helen Rodriguez-Trias Women's Health Leadership Internship. Ms. Jacobs received her BA from Scripps College of the Claremont Colleges Consortium in Claremont, California.

Julia Joh Elligers, MPH, is a senior analyst at NACCHO. She provides technical assistance and training to local communities, implementing a strategic planning process for community health improvement called Mobilizing for Action through Planning and Partnerships (MAPP). She also provides assistance to communities using the National Public Health Performance Standards (NPHPS); NPHPS helps local public health systems assess their capacity to deliver the ten essential public health services.

Ted Kross is director of the Wilkes-Barre City Health Department. He graduated from Pittston Hospital School of Nursing (as a registered nurse with a diploma in nursing) in spring 1982. He was hired as a staff nurse at the NPW Medical Center in 1982 with an interest in critical care nursing. He began working in emergency medicine in 1983 and continued in various leadership positions at several different institutions through 2008. In 1995 he graduated from King's College in Wilkes-Barre, Pennsylvania, with a BS in health care administration (HCA), and he continued in school at King's College and graduated with honors in 2005 with an MS in HCA. He managed the emergency department from 1997 through 2007 at Geisinger Wyoming Valley Medical Center in Wilkes-Barre, and has worked as a prehospital registered nurse (health professional) on life flight interfacility transfers and emergency medical services (EMS) on several ground advance life support (ALS) units up to the present. He wanted to expand his professional career and pursued a director position at Calvert Memorial Hospital just south of Washington DC in 2007. He has been married to a registered nurse for twenty-three years with four children ages thirteen to twenty.

Marc C. Marchese, PhD, received his doctoral degree in industrial-organizational psychology from Iowa State University in 1992. For the past seventeen years he has been a faculty member at King's College in Wilkes-Barre, Pennsylvania. He is currently a professor of human resources management and health care administration. He has also published numerous articles in academic journals. Some recent examples include "Tobacco: The Trigger to Other High Risk Health Behaviors" in the Academy of Health Care Management Journal; "Mentor and Protégé Predictors and Outcomes in a Formal Mentoring Program" in the Journal of Vocational Behavior; and "The Use of Marketing Tools to Increase Participation in Worksite Wellness Programs" in the Academy of Health Care Management Journal.

Jill D. Morrow-Gorton, MD, MBA, is a developmental pediatrician serving as the medical director of the Office of Developmental Programs in the Commonwealth of Pennsylvania's Department of Public Welfare. She graduated from the University of Pennsylvania School of Medicine and did her pediatric internship and residency at Tufts New England Medical Center at the Boston Floating Hospital. She completed a developmental pediatric fellowship at St. Louis University at the Knights of Columbus Developmental Center at Cardinal Glennon Children's Hospital. She is board certified in both pediatrics and developmental and behavioral pediatrics. In 2004 she completed an MBA at Lebanon Valley Hospital in Annville, Pennsylvania.

Sharon Murriguez (formerly Sharon Rodriquez), BA, worked as a program assistant at Prevention Institute from 2007 to 2009. While at Prevention Institute, Mrs. Murriguez focused her efforts on developing training tools and strategies aimed at eliminating health disparities and promoting health equity and community health. She was instrumental in designing and delivering a health disparities training series for grantees of The California Endowment. She also worked on Advancing Public Health Advocacy to Eliminate Health Disparities, a national effort funded by the Robert Wood Johnson Foundation to strengthen public health capacity through policy. A key component of this effort was to develop, pilot, and disseminate a Web-based tool to provide policy and prevention training to assist public health professionals and local elected and appointed officials in eliminating health disparities and improving health outcomes within their communities.

TRANSFORMING PUBLIC HEALTH PRACTICE

ISSUES AND METHODS OF PUBLIC HEALTH PRACTICE

CHAPTER 1

THE NEED FOR CHANGE IN THE PRACTICE OF PUBLIC HEALTH

LEARNING OBJECTIVES

- Explain the primary mission of public health
- Define health
- Define primary prevention
- Describe population health
- Discuss the history of public health and its impact on current public health services
- Identify the characteristics of quality in the field of public health

Mission and Services of Public Health

Public health organizations, particularly government agencies, are pulled in many directions, and have had difficulty in both addressing the multiple determinants of health and providing population-centered services to improve community health outcomes. **Determinants of health** are the factors in the personal, social, economic, and environmental areas of life that affect the health status of individuals and populations.

The challenges facing modern-day societies require interventions and services that move beyond the traditional local public health offerings of personal health care, communicable disease control, and enforcement of environmental health laws. Public health organizations are now expected to understand and address the many factors affecting health produced by the environment, social relationships, communities, and institutions—while in the process forming multiple partnerships to improve health around the globe.

Mission of Public Health

The definition of **mission of public health** has undergone transformation over time. The earliest mission of public health involved the control of communicable diseases, such as cholera, smallpox, tuberculosis, and yellow fever, that inevitably led to epidemics. The most recent definition originated from the Institute of Medicine (IOM) in 2002 and is much broader. The IOM declared that the new mission of public health encompasses the organized efforts of society toward assuring conditions in which people can be healthy. Society has a dual interest in reducing communities' exposure to risk factors known to negatively affect health and in promoting healthy conditions that create and sustain health in the social and environmental spheres of everyday life.

Society's interest stems from the concept of health as a primary public good that promotes the many goals of a society, including the ability of humans to work, to enter into social relationships, and to participate in a political process. As a result of this broad interest, public health practitioners are expected to focus primarily on the health of community populations as opposed to expending their resources on the treatment of individuals for health problems that are usually addressed by physicians or hospitals providing medical services.

Population-Centered Health Services

A public health organization is expected to provide **primary prevention** services to a population. Primary prevention approaches to improving the health status of populations seek to inhibit the occurrence of disease and injuries by reducing exposure to risk factors that cause health problems. In other words, public health services intended to fulfill the mission of public health address the fundamental causes of disease and help foster or sustain conditions that contribute to health, with the goal of preventing undesirable health outcomes (Public Health Leadership Society, 2002). Public health's role also extends to health promotion and helping people gain control of their life and the determinants of health, creating healthier community populations.

What is a population-centered service? To answer this question, we must define the terms *population* and *health*. A **population** is a group of people with shared characteristics, such as location, race, ethnicity, occupation, or age. *Community* is a word that is often used interchangeably with the term *population*. Students in a school system, migrant and seasonal farmworkers, employees of the automobile industry, and county residents and visitors are all examples of populations or communities on which public health organizations may choose to focus and in which they might plan services designed to improve overall health outcomes, such as by reducing obesity or cancer rates.

A **population-centered** service organization seeks to improve health across multiple individuals over a period of time. Healthy People 2010 and 2020 are national initiatives to promote health and prevent disease by setting and monitoring national health objectives (Centers for Disease Control and Prevention [CDC], 1999a, 2009d). Proponents of these initiatives work collaboratively with partners to realize the goal of healthy people in healthy communities, a population-centered approach to improving the nation's health. Two examples of the proposed population-centered goals for Healthy People 2020 are increasing the quality and years of healthy life for individuals of all ages and eliminating health disparities among segments of the population that experience poorer health due to gender, race, ethnicity, education, income, disabilities, geographic location, or sexual orientation—the social determinants of health (U.S. Department of Health and Human Services [HHS], 2011). Population-centered health services designed to increase rates of physical activity across communities are examples of public health interventions that incorporate evidence, are population-centered, and promote health. The application of evidence-based practices increases the likelihood of achieving improved community health outcomes. **Evidence-based public health practice** is the use of the best available scientific evidence to make informed decisions about public health services (Brownson, Fielding, and Maylahn, 2009).

Defining and Modeling Health

A current and popular definition of **health** was first presented by the World Health Organization (WHO) in its constitution in 1946, when health was defined as the state of complete physical, mental, and social well-being, and not just the absence of disease (WHO, 1947). This definition of health points to the intersecting domains of life (biological, social, political, cultural, and environmental) that work together in complex ways to produce the health of individuals who form populations. Models of health, such as the Healthy People 2010 determinants of health (see Figure 1.1), present the multiple parts of the system of health and help us understand the interrelationships among those parts. With models of health we can consider and address the various factors influencing the health of individuals and groups. Broadly understanding how communities maintain or promote health will assist us in adopting the public health interventions that are most likely to reduce or eliminate community populations' exposure to risks and improve their overall health status.

In the Healthy People model of the determinants of health, it is clear that health is contingent on more than individual biology or behavior. Current efforts to reform the health care system center on the issues of health care access,

FIGURE 1.1   Healthy People in Healthy Communities—A Systematic Approach to Health Improvement

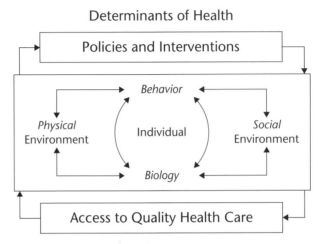

Source: HHS, 2010a, p. 6.

quality, and cost. However, physical and social environments are also important determinants of health, including the educational and income-earning potential of individuals. The policies implemented through legislation and the interventions to achieve policy goals that public health agency leaders and their staff select are also key in determining the health status of populations. Failure to enact the policies and interventions with the greatest likelihood of improving population health, evidence-based practices, can have dire consequences for communities if health outcomes decline as a result. A population-centered approach to health aims to improve health for all members of a population and reduce health disparities among segments of that group. Many experts and practitioners in public health are concerned about the lack of emphasis on population-centered policies and initiatives to promote health and reduce risks, such as laws that mandate the use of seat belts and control tobacco, and about the perpetuation of a system of personal health care services that are overly disease focused.

Intersectoral Public Health

The 2002 IOM definition of public health states that an organized effort is deemed essential for reducing risk and promoting healthy conditions in which people can experience improved quality of life. The absence of an organized societal effort to address identified risk factors that are connected to poor health is a barrier to progress on the front lines of improving the health of communities. Tobacco use, inadequate physical activity, poor diet, and excessive alcohol use cause many of the illnesses, disabilities, and early deaths attributed to chronic diseases. These are great challenges for a local public health system that is in disarray, and in which efforts to improve population health in a community or region show little signs of coordination across the various practitioners of public health. Relatively little coordination occurs across the various sectors working on public health to address the major health issues of our time—chronic and infectious diseases, tobacco use, poverty, environmental pollution, and man-made and natural disasters. Minimal integration of the delivery of personal health care, community health services, and environmental health services by a local public health agency reduces the effectiveness of that agency in preventing risk factors that contribute to common health problems, such as chronic illnesses. Recent assessments of the performance of some local public health systems revealed a number of serious deficiencies and indicated that little progress had been made over recent decades to provide the essential public health services (Brooks, R., Beitsch, L., Street P., Chukmaitov, A., 2009; Smith, T., Minyard, K., Parker, C. Valkenburg, R., and Shoemaker, J., 2007; FL DOH, 2005). Gaps continue to be found across local public health systems in the performance of the essential public health services, and the Centers for Disease Control and Prevention (CDC, 2008b) report that no state is completely prepared to respond to a major public health threat. A National Association of County and City Health Officer's (2010) profile study of over 80 percent of **local public health agencies (LPHAs)** in the USA revealed that from 2005 to 2008, immunizations were the most stable service category in LPHAs and population-based primary prevention services were the least stable service group.

The complex health problems on which public health systems are focused require interactions across the multiple sectors of society contributing to health outcomes. Public health experts and practitioners have worked together to identify the main sectors of society that have a role in promoting health—governmental public health, mass media, academia, business, communities, and health care institutions (IOM, 2002). Together these multiple players and disciplines form **local public health systems,** which have the potential to coordinate services and have a powerful impact on the challenging health problems in the world today.

Local public health agencies, also known as local health departments, are located in most counties or regions in the United States and are the primary government entities with the statutory responsibility for protecting and promoting populations' health. Local public health agency workers help form the backbone of a local public health system and are skilled in multiple disciplines, including epidemiology, surveillance, laboratory testing, health education, environmental health, and medicine. State public health offices or departments exist in every state in the nation. The national arm of public health is present in the Department of Health and Human Services, which houses the CDC, along with the Health Services Research Agency, the Office of the

Assistant Secretary for Preparedness and Response, the U.S. Food and Drug Administration, and the National Institutes of Health.

As mentioned already, health care providers are important partners in promoting the public's health. For decades, the Internal Revenue Service has required nonprofit hospitals to report community benefit expenditures that improve community health status and reduce the burden for individuals of diseases and injuries that increase health care costs (Barnett, 2009). **Community benefit** was defined in a 1983 ruling by the Internal Revenue Service as the promotion of health for "a class of persons sufficiently large so that the community as a whole benefits." The ruling called for nonprofit hospitals to be more proactive in improving health at the community level—a population-centered approach—and legislators and policy experts are now requesting that nonprofit hospitals play a more strategic role in allocating resources for improving health in local communities (Barnett). Beginning in 2010, new Internal Revenue Service requirements for nonprofit hospitals have led to major revisions in the form used to account for tax-exempt status and charitable activities.

The Public Health Institute and a diverse group of hospitals have developed uniform standards for community benefit programming and reporting, promoting charitable activities beyond the traditional emergency room and in-hospital charitable care widely reported by tax-exempt health care organizations. The Association for Community Health Improvement, part of the Public Health Institute, is working with seventy hospitals to develop standards and guidelines for accomplishing community health improvement (Association for Community Health Improvement, 2006). The initiative is focused on three goals:

1. Reducing health disparities
2. Reducing health care costs
3. Enhancing communities' problem-solving capacity for addressing health issues

A myriad of other national and local organizations also provide public health services to promote and improve the health of populations. The American Cancer Society, the American Heart Association, the American Diabetes Association, the Public Health Foundation, the American Public Health Association, community health care providers, and local community churches and civic groups are all examples of organizations that provide some level of public health services and contribute to the mission of public health. Evidence is accumulating concerning the important contributions to the public's health that such private organizations make. However, determining these contributions' effect on public health services and outcomes requires further examination of the nature and intensity of these relationships (Mays et al., 2009).

Although the U.S. public health system has multiple organizations working fairly independently to achieve better health for their own constituents, there are notable examples of partners in the system working together successfully to address population health issues. For example, local, state, and national public health organizations, in partnership with the American Cancer Society, community groups, and other government agencies, successfully reduced tobacco use in California, Massachusetts, Florida, and elsewhere through policy changes, social marketing, and tobacco cessation services. Further, the number of tuberculosis cases in the United States sharply decreased by an average of 7 percent each year from 1993 to 2000, in part due to private and public partnerships among government entities; the National Heart, Lung and Blood Institute; the Robert Wood Johnson Foundation; and the American Thoracic Society. Such examples demonstrate the power of an effective public health system in which public health services are coordinated across multiple organizations to improve community health outcomes.

Public Health Services

Many public health leaders have accepted and promoted the 2002 IOM definition of public health as the official mission of public health; however, public health organizations, stakeholders, and community groups are still unclear about the type and scope of services public health organizations should be performing to improve the nation's health. The IOM's earlier report (1988) on local public health systems named the following **core functions** of public health: assessment, policy development, and assurance. The core functions were further described in terms of the ten essential public health services (see Figure 1.2). Assessment embodies the important services of monitoring health status to identify health problems, and diagnosing and investigating health problems and hazards in a community. Policy development includes informing, educating, and empowering people about health and potential actions they can take to stay healthy; mobilizing and organizing communities to identify and address health issues; and finally developing policies or procedures to support healthy communities. The function of assurance entails enforcing public health laws and regulations that protect the community's health; linking people to needed health services; making sure there is a competent workforce for the delivery of public health services; evaluating the effectiveness and quality of public health programs and activities; and conducting the necessary research to build a better, more responsive, and effective public health system.

Within the local public health agencies, the essential services are posted on walls, but public health leaders continue to openly question how they can market these core functions to their stakeholders. The underlying issue is how to implement the ten essential services when principal funding to local public

FIGURE 1.2   Core Functions and the Ten Essential Public
Health Services

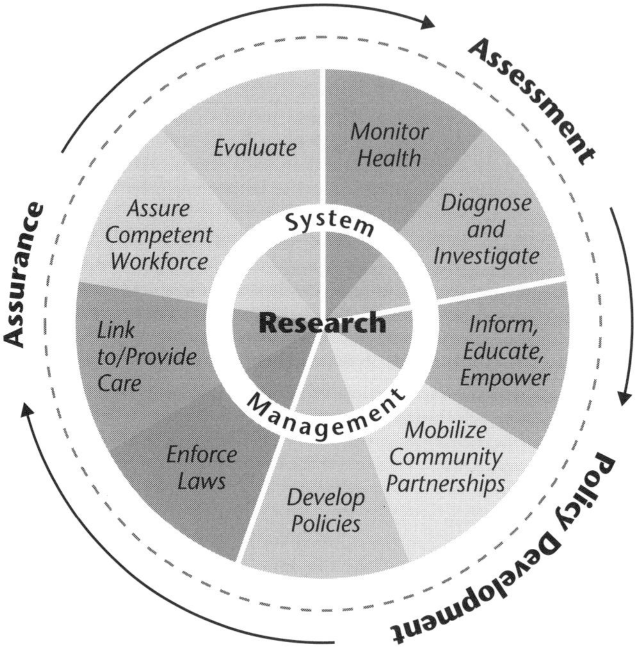

Source: CDC, n.d., p. 2.

health agencies is not designated for core functions that are so broad in scope. The revenues local public health agencies receive are primarily categorical, and are designed to support such separate programs as family planning, maternal and child health, immunizations, tuberculosis screening, and water safety. Improving the competencies of the public health workforce in the areas of assessment, assurance, or policy development has been hampered by funding streams designed to support more specific services, such as tuberculosis screening and treatment or maternal services.

Public Health's History and Its Impact on Current Services

A brief history of public health in the United States provides some insights into the evolution of the mission of public health and the ever-changing scope of services delivered by government public health agencies, primarily in response to the many demands from various sectors of society. This historical review can help us understand the context in which the mission of public health has been defined over the past 150 years and the lingering uncertainty about the purpose and services of public health organizations as part of the larger U.S. public health system. Understanding the historic roles and services of public health entities will provide a foundation for considering the transformations public health organizations must make to deal with old and new risk factors affecting the current health of the U.S. population.

Among the earliest pioneers in assuring conditions that would keep the public healthy was John Snow, an Englishman who linked an outbreak of cholera in London in 1854 to well water drawn from a public pump. His historic work in detecting the root causes of the disease was instrumental in controlling the spread of cholera and protected hundreds of people from the fatal disease. As one of the earliest practitioners of public health, Snow defined a role for public health in the identification and control of potentially fatal communicable diseases. Louis Pasteur's discovery of pathogenic bacteria in France in the 1860s, along with Robert Koch's work in Germany in the 1870s, led to the birth of the new science of microbiology. Further, the study of parasites and the development of immunology gave public health professionals the tools they needed to understand the spread of disease and how to prevent it using vaccines. What is more, the advent of biomedical science was particularly important to the ongoing colonization and economic development of the tropical world by Europeans: guided by the principles of microbiology, they were able to partially or completely control the insect vectors of such debilitating diseases as yellow fever and malaria.

Public health professionals today offer services that include promoting safer sources and distribution of water and foods through inspection and enforcement programs; developing and providing immunizations; and surveying and controlling dangerous infectious diseases, such as malaria, tuberculosis, syphilis, HIV/AIDS, hepatitis, influenza, and SARS. The public by and large attributes the success of disease control to the health care treatments that evolved from the biomedical sciences. The services of a public health agency to prevent diseases in the first place or identify and control emerging diseases through systems of surveillance, inspection, enforcement, and quarantine or isolation are not widely known to—or understood by—the general public. Visits to the doctor or to the local public health agency to receive care that restores an individual's health after the onset of disease or injury are more familiar to the average community resident. We have observed, however, that awareness of the role of local public health systems to prevent disease increases during times of large outbreaks or pandemics, like the 2009 H1N1 pandemic.

Following in Snow's footsteps, Edwin Chadwick led a sanitary movement at the end of the nineteenth century in England that created an official role for the government in maintaining sanitary conditions, thereby protecting the public from disease. Lemuel Shattuck's *Report of the Sanitary Commission* extended Chadwick's ideas and proposed a system of state and local public health agencies that would contend with communicable diseases, conduct sanitary inspections of foods and water systems, collect and provide information on births and deaths, and offer services to children (Turnock, 2009).

Charles-Edward A. Winslow, a public health leader during the early twentieth century, defined public health as the "science and the art of preventing disease, prolonging life, and promoting physical health and efficiency through organized community efforts for the sanitation of the environment, the control of community infections, the education of the individual in principles of personal hygiene, the organization of medical and nursing services for the early diagnosis and preventive treatment of disease, and the development of the social machinery which will ensure to every individual in the community a standard of living adequate for the maintenance of health" (quoted in Turnock, 2009, p. 10). Winslow's definition incorporates much of what public health agencies now provide as services to their communities each day, through environmental health programs; disease identification and control; health education in clinical and community settings; and provision of medical services to prevent, diagnose, and treat primarily communicable diseases. When public health agencies become the medical homes for uninsured people, as do a number of organizations throughout the United States, they also engage in the delivery of chronic disease services that include diagnostics, prevention, and treatment. The development of a "social machinery" to ensure a health-promoting quality of life is an area in which public health practitioners require additional skills and funding. The ten essential services contain elements of the "social machinery" Winslow addresses—mobilizing communities; educating, informing, and empowering individuals and their neighborhoods; and developing policy that promotes the overall health of communities.

In the twentieth century public health services expanded to address the appalling rates of infant mortality in the United States. Local and state public health agencies developed children's programs with a focus on nutrition, health care, and school inspections to lower these mortality rates and improve the living conditions associated with social and environmental determinants of health. By the 1950s the primary services of public health agencies encompassed communicable disease control; sanitary environmental inspection and enforcement; maternal and child health services, including limited nutritional support for mothers and children; vital statistics; health education primarily associated with maternal and child health and communicable diseases; and medical care. In the United States the provision of medical care through public health agencies is confined to indigent or uninsured families (primarily women and children) and populations with certain health conditions, such as HIV/AIDS, syphilis, and tuberculosis. Many public health agencies experienced an infusion of federal primary care funds during the 1980s. They billed Medicaid along with other third-party insurers, and they successfully pursued contracts with health mainte- nance organizations (HMOs) contracted by state governments to manage care and costs of low-income and indigent populations covered by state Medicaid funds. Public health agencies, suffering from inadequate funding, believed that the influx of Medicaid funds would help support public health efforts and expand a safety net for uninsured families of women and children, affording them access to primary care services.

Many community residents today are familiar with the role public health agencies have played in ensuring the sanitation of the environment by inspecting restaurants and assigning sanitation scores for public review on restaurant walls. Others have dealt with their local and state public health agencies' environmental health sanitarians and engineers when installing private septic or small wastewater systems to treat and test wastewater from their homes, and have sought recommendations for systems that guarantee safe drinking water. The expansion of public health programs for women and children in the first half of the twentieth century continues today as major public health services funded by federal, state, and local revenues. Women, Infants, and Children (WIC), the federal program to provide nutritional services and food coupons to pregnant mothers and their newborns, can be found in many public health agencies in the nation. Further, many local public health agencies provide prenatal care services to indigent families to promote healthier birth outcomes. For families—primarily women and children—with little or no access to care or an inability to find a health care provider willing to accept Medicaid and lower reimbursement rates, the local public health agency has become the primary health care provider.

Gap Between Mission and Current Public Health Practice

The mission of public health of assuring conditions in which the population can be healthy is possible through a population-based primary prevention and health promotion framework. Public health services that address such conditions include community health assessments and collaborative community health improvement initiatives. In addition, national public health priorities, such as the Healthy People 2020 promotion of healthy weight for community members and reduction of health disparities, are opportunities to work locally on national initiatives to create healthy conditions. According to a national self-assessment survey of local health departments (LHDs) conducted by the National Association of County and City Health Officials (NACCHO, 2008, p. 2):

- 63 percent of LHDs had completed a community health assessment in the last three years.
- 49 percent of LHDs had participated in community health improvement planning in the last three years.
- 58 percent of LHDs supported community efforts to address health disparities.

Community health assessments examine determinants of health and health outcomes and report on the overall health status of a community. Quality community health improvement processes incorporate the assessment information into strategic plans to implement evidence-based public health services that improve identified priority health issues, such as obesity or tobacco use. Community health improvement is an effective tool for collaborating with stakeholders on a vision and plan to improve community health (IOM, 1997). The 2008 NACCHO survey demonstrates that LHDs must do more to comprehensively assess and monitor the health of the population using community health data. In addition, more work is needed by LHDs to conduct comprehensive and strategic community health improvement.

Primary Care and Primary Prevention in Local Public Health

Researchers find it very challenging to analyze the performance of local public health systems and their governmental arm, local public health agencies, given the complexity of the implementation of public health programs. There is also an absence of clarity in regard to what types of government activities constitute public health services (Sensenig, 2007). An emerging body of evidence points to the wide variation in the availability and quality of public health services across many communities (Mays et al., 2006). Researchers in Georgia, for example, found that public health services were not aligned with the essential services and core functions of public health, after examining an extensive body of literature on the practice of public health and conducting a case study on the core business of public health in the state of Georgia (Smith et al., 2007).

A growing number of public health experts have expressed concern about the focus on primary care services and treatment of medical conditions by local public health agencies. A recent study on the Florida Department of Health found that local public health agency expenditures on clinical services exceeded substantially the expenditures attributed to the provision of the core functions and essential services included in the mission of public health (Brooks, Beitsch,

Street, and Chukmaitov, 2009). Since the 1950s, the public has considered the provision of medical services to indigent or low-income community residents to be a primary function of the local public health agency. At the same time, the public has only a limited understanding of the role of a local public health agency in the delivery of primary prevention services to promote population health. We can understand the basis for this public perception if we consider the programs that have received consistent funding from federal and state governments for more than fifty years: maternal and child health, screening for and treatment of sexually transmitted diseases, family planning, immunizations, and tuberculosis screening. A number of public health programs have a clinical and community focus; but the emphasis, both in the financing and staffing, is primarily clinical or medical. As discussed earlier, across the United States over the past twenty years, local public health agencies have sought new sources of funding by billing Medicaid, Medicare, and third-party insurers—further indication of the growth of medical services in the practice of public health. Evidence of similar efforts on the part of local public health agencies to secure funds for the provision of preventive health services can be found in pockets around the nation, but these attempts have not resulted in revenues and expenditures equal to those for medical services. Explanations for the disparate funding include the emphasis on medical care in the United States as well as the absence of leadership in public health agencies to advocate and secure necessary funding for the appropriate levels of public health services. Total funding for health care services and medical research dwarfs the funding for federal public health programs. Gaps in the provision of the ten essential public health services and the lack of primary prevention and health promotion activities in LPHAs are not surprising when we realize the large disparity in funding between medical and public health services.

Preparedness

Following the 2001 terrorist attacks in New York City, public health agencies received substantial increases in preparedness revenues, thereby improving their capacity to prepare for bioterrorist or chemical attacks as well as natural disasters. Beginning in 2008, however, funding for local public health agencies' preparedness programs have been declining, and their ability to respond effectively to a natural or man-made disaster, such as climate change, is doubtful. The U.S. General Accounting Office concluded in 2004 that "no State is fully prepared to respond to a major public health threat" (quoted in Kinner and Pelligrini, 2009, p. 1780). The CDC (2008b) recently came to the same conclusion.

Public health agencies in parts of the nation have been preparing and responding to natural disasters, including hurricanes, fires, and flooding, for at least two decades. The Florida Department of Health was commended for its 2004 responses to five major hurricanes that ripped across the peninsula. However, public health's lack of preparedness was front-page news in 2005 when Hurricane Katrina flooded New Orleans and devastated hundreds of communities along the coastal areas of Louisiana and Mississippi, killing over 1,800 people. This disaster clearly revealed that most aspects of the response, including the local public health system's actions, were inadequate, disorganized, and insensitive to the dangerous risk factors that people living in poverty, primarily African Americans, were facing. In New Orleans, thousands were stranded after the evacuation order. The risks from the heat, floodwaters, and other elements, combined with existing social disparities in health, contributed to an exacerbation of chronic health conditions and distrust of government agencies. More health risks evolved when thousands of people, evacuated from their homes, were exposed to dangerous chemicals in the trailers used to house the homeless, in which the indoor air tested positive for formaldehyde.

As we count the achievements in public health during the twentieth century, among them vaccinations, enhanced motor vehicle safety, control of infectious diseases, safer workplaces, safer food supply, family planning, and more, we must also assess the ways in which local public health systems and public health agencies can operate at levels of quality to achieve the mission of public health—ensuring the conditions in which people can live healthy and happy lives.

Future Public Health Services

People living in many countries throughout the world are healthier today than they were a century ago. Public health initiatives during the past one hundred years have been instrumental in improving living conditions in communities through cleaner water, food, and air; the use of sewage systems to safely handle wastewater; better nutrition; immunizations; and expanded education concerning the behaviors and risk factors that contribute to poorer health and preventable injuries. Public health practitioners now find themselves and their organizations faced with complex and seemingly insurmountable health problems, such as obesity and the effects of global climate change. Obesity, for example, will require new capacities and skills to reverse the increasing rates of early-onset diabetes and cardiovascular disease in young adults. In the meantime, what some believe is the failure of the U.S. public health system to prevent the obesity epidemic is actually an opportunity to learn from experience and begin applying public health practices with the greatest likelihood of improving health outcomes and reducing exposure to risks. By providing primary prevention services and attending to the social, environmental, and behavioral aspects of health, public health practitioners play an important role in reducing the occurrence of diseases and promoting healthy living conditions.

Joseph Juran, a twentieth-century quality management and improvement scholar and author of several books on quality, is well known for the axiom that every system is perfectly designed to achieve exactly the results it gets (cited in Berwick, James, and Coye, 2003). The phrase is powerful for leaders seeking improvement in public health, as it states the obvious fact that to attain a new level of performance, there must be a new system. A redesign of local public health systems would signal an intention to refocus on the mission of reducing risk through primary prevention strategies—in other words, directing the resources of the U.S. public health system on mitigating events that create risk and thereby reducing our exposure to those risks. What would be the characteristics of redesigned local public health systems, and what role would local public health agencies play in this system redesign?

Multiple conceptual guidelines or standards are available to direct the comprehensive redesign of the U.S. public health system. The CDC launched the National Public Health Performance Standards Program in 1998, and released the first assessment instruments in 2002 to assess local public health systems; state public health systems; and local boards of health, the governing bodies for many local public health systems in the United States (CDC, 2008c). The CDC designed the local public health system performance standards instruments to assess the performance of the ten essential services. The local public health system assessment was specifically developed to include the local public health agency, as well as other intersectoral partners in the community working on public health issues and contributing to the mission of public health. The latest reports from the CDC show that twenty-one states have completed the state public health assessment, ten states are actively using the local public health system instrument, and five states are using the local instrument at a moderate level (CDC, 2008c). Very little research is available on the impact of the use of these performance standards instruments on the implementation of local public health programs, or on whether conditions that promote the health of populations have improved. Because LPHAs are unable to account for either their work or their funding in terms of the ten essential services, the use of standards based on the ten essential services framework may not be feasible for LPHAs.

Ethical Practice of Public Health

The *Principles of the Ethical Practice of Public Health* (Public Health Leadership Society, 2002) makes explicit the ideals of the local public health institutions that serve communities and, if enforced, promotes accountability of those institutions to perform according to the principles outlined in this Public Health Code of Ethics (see Exhibit 1.1). The Code asserts the primary prevention mission of public health by explicitly stating that public health should address the "fundamental

EXHIBIT 1.1

PRINCIPLES OF THE ETHICAL PRACTICE OF PUBLIC HEALTH

1. Public health should address principally the fundamental causes of disease and requirements for health, aiming to prevent adverse health outcomes.

2. Public health should achieve community health in a way that respects the rights of individuals in the community.

3. Public health policies, programs, and priorities should be developed and evaluated through processes that assure an opportunity for input from community members.

4. Public health should advocate and work for the empowerment of disenfranchised community members, aiming to ensure that the basic resources and conditions necessary for health are accessible to all.

5. Public health should seek the information needed to implement effective policies and programs that protect and promote health.

6. Public health institutions should provide communities with the information they have that is needed for decisions on policies or programs and should obtain the community's consent for their implementation.

7. Public health institutions should act in a timely manner on the information they have within the resources and the mandate given to them by the public.

8. Public health programs and policies should incorporate a variety of approaches that anticipate and respect diverse values, beliefs, and cultures in the community.

9. Public health programs and policies should be implemented in a manner that most enhances the physical and social environment.

10. Public health institutions should protect the confidentiality of information that can bring harm to an individual or community if made public. Exceptions must be justified on the basis of the high likelihood of significant harm to the individual or others.

11. Public health institutions should ensure the professional competence of their employees.

12. Public health institutions and their employees should engage in collaborations and affiliations in ways that build the public's trust and the institution's effectiveness.

causes of disease and requirements for health." The Code emphasizes that the health of individuals is connected to their community life, and maintains that community health is to be achieved in a manner that respects individual rights, advocates for the empowerment of community members who are disenfranchised, and informs communities using the available and pertinent information they need to make decisions related to policy and program choices. Many working in public health are familiar with the Public Health Code of Ethics; however, its effect on public health system or agency performance has been minimal.

Definition of a Functional Local Public Health Agency

In 2005 a diverse group of public health practitioners and national public health organizations developed the "Operational Definition of a Functional Local Public Health Agency" (Lenihan, Welter, Chang, and Gorenflo, 2007). This attempt to clearly articulate the standards of achievement for the government entity of a local public health system—the local public health agency or local health department—was an offshoot of the CDC's National Public Health Performance Standards Program. Local public health officials wanted a set of standards that applied directly to their organization, considering the scope of the ten essential public health services to be quite broad and applicable to the wider array of community groups contributing to the mission of public health.

The operational definition is hailed by some as the next step in a chain of events over a twenty-year period to clearly define a shared understanding of what community members can expect from their local public health agency—no matter where they live (Lenihan et al., 2007). The definition is also based on the ten essential services and includes forty-five standards to help local public health practitioners define themselves in common terms and identify concrete areas for improvement of community health status. So far, little has been reported about local public health agencies' use of the operational definition. This initiative to drive changes in the practice of public health by LPHAs may experience the same relatively low level of use as the national performance standards, given the ten essential services framework on which the operational definition was based.

Accreditation

In 2007 the Robert Wood Johnson Foundation provided support for the establishment of the Public Health Accreditation Board (PHAB). PHAB works closely with national public health associations—the National Association of County and City Health Officials, the Association of State and Territorial Health Officials, and the National Association of Local Boards of Health—in the quest to accredit public health agencies. PHAB is a voluntary public health accreditation program, launched with the mission of advancing the quality and performance of local public health agencies. Beta testing of the state and local accreditation standards commenced in late 2009, with a planned implementation of a voluntary accreditation process in 2011. These standards were generated, in part, through a review of the "Operational Definition of a Functional Local Public Health Agency" and the CDC's National Public Health Performance Standards Program. The initial set of PHAB standards assesses the administrative capacity and governance of an agency, and the agency's ability to perform the ten essential services. Capacity, process, and outcome are all measured as part of the accreditation process. The Public Health Accreditation Board will award a local public health agency with accreditation based on its self-assessment using the standards instrument, a site visit report from the accreditation board, the agency's response to the site visit report, and the testimony of accreditation board staff (Public Health Accreditation Board, 2010).

Many in the field of public health are optimistic about the role of accreditation in bringing about needed changes to the practice of LPHAs. In this era of economic downturns, some experts in public health contend that accountability of LPHAs through an accreditation process will potentially bestow financial advantages for these agencies as they compete for shrinking resources with other government entities (Betisch and Corzo, 2009). Other public health professionals question the assertion that accreditation can lead to accountability and improved population health when the basis of accreditation centers on an agency's ability to perform core functions that are not clearly linked to health outcomes (Wholey, White, and Kader, 2009, p. 1546): "Currently most measures are process measures.... [Q]uality improvement efforts should demonstrate not only process improvement, but should also be linked to public health goals and overall improvements in population health outcomes." Little evidence exists to support a causal link between accreditation and population health outcomes, calling into question the push to spend limited public health resources on periodic accreditation programs. Helping public health agencies understand and implement population health services based on evidence through education programs and technical assistance is another area of weakness in the system that could be strengthened. Such efforts compete for limited public health resources. Clearly, the jury is still out on whether an accredited health department does better in improving health in the community it serves (Robert Wood Johnson Foundation, 2010).

Quality Characteristics of a Well-Functioning Local Public Health System

Local public health agencies and local public health systems are struggling to realize the mission of public health. New levels of performance are possible only through an extraordinary system-level redesign, achieving the goal of an idealized system that reaches new levels of improvement (Moen, 2002).

The U.S. Department of Health and Human Services in 2008 led an initiative to redefine quality in the practice of public health. This group of experts and experienced public health practitioners defined quality in public health practice to be "the degree to which policies, programs, services, and research for the population increase desired health outcomes and conditions in which the population can be healthy" (HHS, 2008). The group defined a set of quality characteristics of a well-performing local public health system, which are presented in Exhibit 1.2.

EXHIBIT 1.2
QUALITY CHARACTERISTICS TO GUIDE PUBLIC HEALTH PRACTICE

- **Population-centered**—protecting and promoting healthy conditions and the health for the entire population

- **Equitable**—working to achieve health equity

- **Proactive**—formulating policies and sustainable practices in a timely manner, while mobilizing rapidly to address new and emerging threats and vulnerabilities

- **Health promoting**—ensuring policies and strategies that advance safe practices by providers and the population and increase the probability of positive health behaviors and outcomes

- **Risk-reducing**—diminishing adverse environmental and social events by implementing policies and strategies to reduce the probability of preventable injuries and illness or other negative outcomes

- **Vigilant**—intensifying practices and enacting policies to support enhancements to surveillance activities (e.g., technology, standardization, systems thinking/modeling)

- **Transparent**—ensuring openness in the delivery of services and practices with particular emphasis on valid, reliable, accessible, timely, and meaningful data that is readily available to stakeholders, including the public

- **Effective**—justifying investments by utilizing evidence, science, and best practices to achieve optimal results in areas of greatest need

- **Efficient**—understanding costs and benefits of public health interventions and to facilitate the optimal utilization of resources to achieve desired outcomes

Source: HHS, 2008.

As we have already stated, ensuring conditions in which people can be healthy is the primary mission of public health. The overwhelming prevalence of preventable chronic diseases is in part a reflection on the choice organizations practicing public health have made to adopt a predominantly disease-focused approach, avoiding the less familiar areas of the social, policy, and environmental determinants of health. A quality public health organization, or any group with a public health focus, must be

- Population-centered
- Working on inequities that are attributed to a population's demographics, such as those pertaining to race or gender
- Promoting health and reducing exposure to risk factors that are known to cause disease or injury
- Delivering services or developing policies that are based on evidence or the best available knowledge in the field

The Guide to Community Preventive Services is a resource created by a task force of experts selected by the CDC that presents evidence-based recommendations and findings for public health services (Community Guide Branch, n.d.). The Community Guide is based on scientific reviews of studies that have demonstrated what does and does not work in reducing exposure to risk factors known to cause disease or injury, promoting protective factors that contribute to health, and improving health outcomes. Although the Community Guide is far from complete, it presents a good starting place for finding evidence-based, population-centered interventions to address such health issues as obesity, physical activity, tobacco use, nutrition, adolescent health, asthma, HIV/AIDS, motor vehicles, and more. For example, community-wide campaigns to increase physical activity are interventions that are recommended (Community Guide Branch).

Public health agencies conducting evaluation research in connection with current and future interventions are operating effectively and can make significant contributions to the growing body of evidence found in the Community Guide (Community Guide Branch, n.d.) and similar publications. Ongoing efforts by public health agencies to evaluate population-centered services will add momentum to the establishment of more evidence-based public health interventions that are aligned with the mission of public health. Conducting evaluation research and reporting on findings are characteristics of an efficiently functioning local public health system and local public health agency. Accountability and transparency must also define the local public health systems and agencies of the future. A quality local public health system measures and reports on performance to determine if strategies undertaken in the interest of community health actually led to improvement. Only by studying the effects of interventions to reduce risk and promote health in a variety of settings and across multiple public health organizations can we continue to build the public health evidence base and spread the knowledge of what works to improve population health.

Ecological Model to Improve the Quality of Public Health Services

Along with expanding our view of quality within the practice of public health, we must also concern ourselves with the shifts in our ecosystem, such as climate change, that are predicted to have devastating effects on populations worldwide. Newer models of health are emerging that incorporate ecosystems and the natural and built environments. Behind these newer models is the belief that sustainable use of finite resources is a major determinant of health (Griffiths, 2006). Reintegrating ecosystems within the models of health draws attention to the importance of ecosystems in connection with human well-being, health promotion, and disease prevention. Figure 1.3 presents an alternate ecological model of health, including domains similar to the determinants of health and well-being presented in Figure 1.1 and the additional domains of the global ecosystem and the built and natural environments.

The effects of the built environment and man-made pollution on the natural environment present new challenges that add to the burden of existing and unaddressed health problems facing the United States. The practice of public health must continue to evolve beyond the current state of personal health care, communicable disease control, and enforcement of environmental health laws. The field of public health must expand the delivery of population-centered health services and apply an ecological, population-centered focus when dealing with complex problems. Using an ecological, population-based approach to improving community health requires us to consider simultaneous changes in multiple dimensions of the ecological model of health shown in Figure 1.3. Healthier communities are possible when policies are enacted that reduce exposure to harmful risk factors, for example, increasing sales tax on tobacco purchases or requiring restaurants and school cafeterias to reduce unhealthy and nonnutritious ingredients in meals. Public health partnerships to reduce crime and discrimination and promote neighborhood recreational sites for social interaction and physical activity suggest further examples of public health services that address multiple components of the ecological model of health and possess the quality characteristics of being evidence-based and population-centered. Unhealthy choices, adverse environments, and increased exposure to risk factors that harm health work together to create unhealthy communities and perpetuate racial and socioeconomic inequities. Population health deteriorates when communities must live with contaminated water, air pollution, or food deserts in which the absence of grocers or fresh food markets seriously limits the quality of foods

FIGURE 1.3   Ecological Model of Health

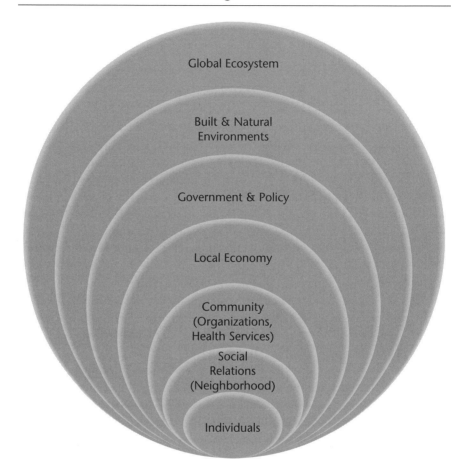

residents can purchase. The mission of public health to promote conditions in which people can be healthy is achievable when practitioners of public health work in all dimensions of the ecological model of health in partnership with others that have a stake in assuring healthy communities. Local public health agencies must redesign themselves to focus more on evidence-based, ecological, population-centered services and less on the clinical aspects of care in order to achieve community health improvement goals.

Summary

The current practice of public health in the United States remains in disarray, operating in a nonintegrated manner, and with a wide variation in the availability and quality of essential public health services. Multiple organizations contribute to the mission of public health; however, the primary focus continues to be detecting and controlling diseases, ignoring the wider determinants associated with the social and physical environments that improve or inhibit health. The public health organization of the future will help determine the health of a population by operating within and across the many organizations forming a local public health system, integrating the practice of public health into each domain of that system. At the same time, the intersectoral public health practitioner will promote and implement evidence-based, population-centered public health services with roots in the current ecological model of health, incorporating ecosystems and the natural and built environments. Increasing the capacity to perform public health services that are clearly linked to the mission of public health and to the quality characteristics is achievable by engaging multiple community partners, including health care organizations, with community health improvement goals and securing adequate resources to rebuild our U.S. public health agencies and system.

Key Terms

Community benefit

Core functions

Determinants of health

Evidence-based public health practice

Health

Local public health agency (LPHA)

Local public health system

Mission of public health

Population

Population-centered

Primary prevention

Discussion Questions

1. What types of services do public health organizations provide?
2. Explain why the provision of primary prevention services is critical to improving population health.
3. Describe the gap between the mission of public health and current public health practice.
4. What are the advantages of an intersectoral approach to addressing public health issues?

CHAPTER 2

THE SUCCESS OF PUBLIC HEALTH PROGRAMS: CRITICAL FACTORS

LEARNING OBJECTIVES

- Understand the major accomplishments of public health departments in the United States
- Become aware of the history and development of public health departments in this country
- Understand the value of health education programs in the prevention of disease
- Recognize the need for training and development of public health leadership

Most people have minimal awareness of the role public health departments, or agencies, play in maintaining the health and longevity of Americans. This is because these departments usually receive very little publicity unless there is a serious health problem. In fact, most Americans associate public health departments with their work to control outbreaks of disease among large numbers of people, such as in responding to the recent large outbreak of salmonellosis related to the consumption of peanut butter, or in issuing warnings about a possible pandemic of avian influenza or swine flu in the United States. It is unfortunate that our only knowledge of public health relates to emergencies, because we are then unaware of the day-to-day activities public health departments perform in order to keep people healthy. This perception of public health departments as primarily responders to health emergencies prevents health policy experts from understanding the contribution that these departments could make in solving the major health care problems in this country, which include issues of cost, access, health status, and quality of care. These departments do so many things to prevent disease that are never publicized and, therefore, are not known by the average person or policymakers. Scutchfield and Keck (2009) argue that public health departments have never received the credit they deserve for their many accomplishments, including articulating a vision of the possibilities for a healthy community.

The major problem found in our health care system today is the concentration of scarce health resources on the cure of disease rather than the prevention of disease. If we improve the health of the population through health education and health promotion, the other problems found in our health care system diminish in importance. Turnock (2009) points out that public health departments can also identify and address unacceptable realities that models of preventive health care can alleviate. Stallworth and Lennon (2003) argue that collaboration is required to improve the health of the population. The improvement of the health of a community requires all health agencies, including hospitals, to work together. This one statement summarizes the true success of public health departments: their ability to get people and communities to work together to improve the health of the population. Public health departments are the catalyst of preventive health programs.

The public health system in the United States is always working at making good health available for all individuals. It is usually seen as a very silent component of health services, demanding few resources and yet producing unbelievable value for our citizens in terms of better health for all. This system employs some of the most dedicated health professionals to be found in any part of this country's health care system. Although a large income is not usually associated with public health employment, public health work affords personnel a great sense of accomplishment. Public health employees are very special people who do extraordinary work because they like what they do. They enjoy helping people even though they receive very little recognition for their work.

The public health system should be considered one of the greatest success stories within the system of health care in our country. In fact, the public health system in the United States is responsible for most of the gains in long life Americans enjoy today. It is interesting to note that this system has actually increased its successes despite cuts in funding for many programs on an annual basis.

The public health system is more than a collection of government agencies; it is actually a **thick culture** of dedicated professionals whose very existence is dedicated to the effort to keep people healthy. This culture among public health employees is difficult to describe and even more difficult for others to understand. Many of those who work in public health look at their work as a calling to help others become healthier, and they feel rewarded when they accomplish even a small part of this goal. These talented and dedicated employees get a certain psychic income from being successful in helping others preserve or improve health. They claim that there is no better feeling than this.

The public health sector is usually supported with federal, state, and local funds and grants that are appropriated annually. It is a political entity, often led by political appointees who never quite understand the culture of the public health employees. These temporary administrators also do not appreciate the value of marketing what a public health department does on a daily basis. Therefore, very few people understand the value of public health, and the funding for these agencies is never enough for them to really do their job. It seems that public health departments are one of the best kept secrets in this country.

According to Novick, Morrow, and Mays (2008), the American Public Health Association made a statement in 1933 that outlined two major activities for public health agencies: controlling communicable diseases and promoting child health. This statement was signed by Haven Emerson and C.E.A. Winslow, among others. In 1945, Emerson expanded these two functions to include such additional functions as disease investigation and health education, which were not being performed by other government agencies and for which government funding was always set at a bare minimum. These official functions are all very important, but they also tend to limit the vision of what public health departments would be able to accomplish if they were given sufficient resources and better leadership and support.

According to the Centers for Disease Control and Prevention (CDC, 2006a), the life expectancy of Americans has increased by over thirty years since 1900. Much of this expanded longevity has resulted from a variety of public health programs. These programs are not a part of the health care system, but have come into being as a direct result of public health initiatives. Following are ten remarkable accomplishments of U.S. public health departments over a one-hundred-year history, from 1900 to 1999, which were achieved despite a very modest budget that was usually reduced rather than increased every year (CDC, 1999b):

- Mass vaccinations
- Increased motor-vehicle safety
- Safer workplaces
- Better control of infectious diseases
- A decline in deaths from coronary heart disease and stroke
- Safer and healthier foods
- Healthier mothers and babies
- Family planning initiatives
- Fluoridation of drinking water
- Recognition of tobacco use as a health hazard

The public health prevention initiatives that drove these admirable achievements today continue to protect the public from disease, allowing the majority of Americans to live longer, healthier lives. These prevention programs, which have been so successful in reducing communicable diseases, must now be modified and improved to deal with the epidemic of chronic diseases facing our country. The accomplishments listed above can be duplicated today, but public health departments need to employ different strategies. Unlike previous challenges the public health system has encountered, chronic diseases require a well-developed community approach, in which public health departments provide leadership and innovative ideas to educate every member of the U.S. population throughout his or her life span.

Despite the dedication of the public health workforce and previous successful public health initiatives, the public health departments in this country have not been able to achieve all of their goals. The Institute of Medicine (IOM) completed a very important study concerning public health in 1988. The resulting document, titled *The Future of Public Health,* looked at the mission of public health, the current state of public health, and the various barriers facing public health in this country. The report determined that there was widespread agreement on the mission of public health but that this mission was not being accomplished. In fact, the public health system in our country was not meeting its current objectives. Further, the report concluded with a very serious warning that the public health system was in total disarray. Public health, the IOM argued, was never allowed to develop into a strong sector with the resources necessary to continually improve the health of all Americans, primarily because many of the political appointees running local public health agencies allowed funding to be cut in order to keep their positions. It is very dangerous for political appointees in public health departments to question the budget decisions of the administrators who appointed them to their current position.

Definition of Public Health

As we have already stated, most people know very little about the organizations and services provided by public health departments in this country, and the valuable contributions public health professionals make year after year are largely taken for granted. We only look for guidance and answers from public health officials and the various government agencies they represent when an emergency threatens our health. Problems like E. coli in our food supply, anthrax in the mail, contaminated water, or drug-resistant tuberculosis bring public health to the forefront until the crisis subsides . . . and then the public health system seems to disappear until we need its help again.

In 1920 Charles-Edward A. Winslow defined public health as "the science and art of preventing disease, prolonging life and promoting health through the organized efforts and informed choices of society, organizations, public and private, communities and individuals" (quoted in Turnock, 2009, p. 10). McKenzie, Pinger, and Kotecki (2005) define public health as a field preserving the health status of members of the population through government action to promote, protect, and preserve their health. Novick et al. (2008) argue that public health involves a structured approach to improve the health of the population. Finally, Vetter and Matthews (1999) argue that public health includes the processes of promoting health, preventing disease, and prolonging and improving the quality of life through the organized efforts of society. These are definitions that support the use of public health expertise to solve many of the current health care problems in this country.

All of these definitions point to a science dedicated to the improvement of the health of a given population. The various definitions of public health also conjure up a vision of population-based medicine rather than health care that is centered on specific individuals. These definitions further emphasize the prevention of health problems rather than efforts to cure them. The tools of public health are exactly those required to solve many of the problems present in the U.S. system of health care.

According to the IOM (2002), the public health system needs to partner with the health care delivery sector to attain their shared population health goals. Public health agencies implement a large number of prevention programs very well, but they need to change some of the activities that they have continued for years and that have only a marginal impact on health outcomes.

Despite the success of public health strategies in improving the longevity and quality of life of the majority of Americans over the last one hundred years, resources for public health departments have been reduced. Making matters worse, these public health departments have been assigned new responsibilities, while at the same time losing many of their most experienced workers to retirement. There needs to be an expansion of public health programs, such as health education efforts, which have proven their worth in the reduction of high-risk health behaviors. These programs are crucial in dealing with problems of obesity, physical inactivity, and poor diet. Although public health departments have had wonderful accomplishments, it is time to move on to even greater success stories. They need to develop and use new tools to deal with the epidemic of chronic diseases that is so different from previous epidemics of communicable diseases.

Public Health Systems

The government-funded public health agencies in the United States are separated into three systems that work together in different ways to improve the health of the population. The government-funded public health departments operate at

EXHIBIT 2.1

U.S. DEPARTMENT OF HEALTH AND HUMAN SERVICES PRIMARY OPERATING DIVISIONS AND MISSIONS

Administration for Children and Families (ACF), www.acf.dhhs.gov

To promote the economic and social well-being of families, children, individuals, and communities

Agency for Healthcare Research and Quality (AHRQ), www.ahrq.gov

To support, conduct, and disseminate research that improves access to care and the outcomes, quality, cost, and use of health care services

Administration on Aging (AoA), www.aoa.gov

To promote the dignity and independence of older people and to help society prepare for an aging population

Agency for Toxic Substances and Disease Registry (ATSDR), www.atsdr.cdc.gov

To serve the public by using the best science, taking responsive public health actions, and providing trusted health information to prevent harmful exposures and diseases related to toxic substances

Centers for Disease Control and Prevention (CDC), www.cdc.gov

To promote health and quality of life by preventing and controlling disease, injury, and disability

Centers for Medicare & Medicaid Services (CMS), www.cms.hhs.gov

To ensure effective, up-to-date health care coverage and to promote quality care for beneficiaries

Food and Drug Administration (FDA), www.fda.gov

To rigorously assure the safety, efficacy, and security of human and veterinary drugs, biological products, and medical devices and assure the safety and security of the nation's food supply, cosmetics, and products that emit radiation

Health Resources and Services Administration (HRSA), www.hrsa.gov

To provide the national leadership, program resources, and services needed to improve access to culturally competent, quality health care.

Indian Health Service (IHS), www.ihs.gov

To raise the physical, mental, social, and spiritual health of American Indians and Alaska Natives to the highest level

National Institutes of Health (NIH), www.nih.gov

To employ science in pursuit of fundamental knowledge about the nature and behavior of living systems and the application of that knowledge to extend healthy life and reduce the burdens of illness and disability

Substance Abuse and Mental Health Services Administration (SAMHSA), www.samhsa.gov

To build resilience and facilitate recovery for people with or at risk for substance abuse and mental illness

Source: National Institutes of Health, n.d.

the federal, state, or local level. The people who work for each agency are usually government employees headed by a political appointee, and they are funded primarily by tax dollars.

Public Health at the Federal Level

Exhibit 2.1 lists some federal public health agencies that are responsible for addressing a large number of population-based health concerns. Several of these federal agencies are involved in formulating national objectives and policies that in turn help establish standards for both the provision of health services and the protection of the public's health. They are also responsible for the distribution of funding to state and local health department activities, including emergency preparedness initiatives. Several of the federal public health agencies, such as the Indian Health Service, also provide population-based health services to certain subgroups of the population.

Public Health at the State Level

Every state in the United States has a public health department that is empowered to protect the health and safety of its population. State health departments are responsible for gathering and interpreting various pieces of statistical data pertaining to population health and sharing this information with a number of federal health agencies. The states also offer laboratory testing and investigation services for a variety of communicable diseases that hospitals or other laboratories do not provide. Further, these agencies grant licenses to health care professionals and most medical facilities, and monitor their performance. They also finance and implement a number of health education programs.

Public Health at the Local Level

Local health departments are usually the responsibility of cities or counties that have decided to offer public health services through funding from state and federal sources. These departments are responsible for actually performing the public health activities that are legislated by the state and federal government. Their tasks include collecting health statistics, investigating communicable diseases, providing environmental sanitation services, implementing maternal and child health programs, and disseminating health education information.

Community Health Workers

The community health worker (CHW) has become a critical player in public health activities around the world. This classification of public health occupation began to develop in the 1960s. According to the U.S. Department of Health and Human Services (HHS, 2007), this type of worker has been used in cost containment and cost-effective strategies designed to provide health care to the underserved populations throughout the world. **Community health workers** are formally defined as "lay members of communities who work either for pay or as volunteers in association with the local health care system in both urban and rural environments and usually share ethnicity, language, socioeconomic status and life experiences with the community members they serve. They have been identified by many titles such as community health advisors, lay health advocates, 'promotores(as),' outreach educators, community health representatives, peer health promoters, and peer health educators" (HHS, pp. iii–iv).

CHWs work in for-profit and nonprofit agencies, such as schools, universities, clinics, hospitals, physicians' offices, individual-family-child services, and education programs. There were approximately eighty-six thousand individuals working in this field in 2000 in the United States, with approximately 67 percent being paid and 33 percent working on a volunteer basis.

The majority of CHWs are females between the ages of thirty and fifty, and are usually Hispanic or African American. They work for very low wages or volunteer, and they serve all ethnic and racial groups. The volunteers are usually employed by faith-based organizations or as part of outreach and health education efforts designed by university researchers and local health care providers. The most frequent issues that CHWs handle are women's health and nutrition, prenatal and pregnancy care as well as children's health, immunizations, and high-risk sexual behavior. The vast majority of CHWs' work in these areas involves health education and health promotion activities. These individuals are a necessary adjunct to public health departments, especially at the local level, and are most useful in the provision of health education programs, especially for underserved populations. They also provide informal counseling, which helps individuals make basic decisions in regard to healthy or unhealthy behavioral choices.

The study conducted by HHS (2007) identified roles that CHWs may assume:

- *Member of the care delivery team.* In this role the CHW works with a lead provider of care, typically a physician, nurse, or social worker.
- *Navigator.* This role requires greater emphasis on the capabilities for assisting individuals and families in negotiating increasingly complex service systems and for helping clients build confidence when dealing with providers of care.
- *Screening and health education provider.* This role has been one of the more common, and has been included in many categorically funded initiatives on specific health conditions, such as asthma and diabetes.
- *Outreach-enrolling-informing agent.* This role involves reaching individuals and families eligible for benefits or services and persuading them to apply for help or to come to a provider of care's location.
- *Organizer.* In this role, a volunteer CHW becomes active in a community over a specific health issue, promoting self-directed change and community development.

It is evident that CHWs are a vital component of any form of population-based medicine a given community might use. These individuals are dedicated community members who have developed collaboration skills and are motivated to improve the health of their community.

Population-Based Medicine

The health care system in our country revolves around individual patients, with an emphasis on curing diseases or other ailments. In recent years, however, managed care insurance has been moving from a focus on payment for health care to a focus on keeping the population healthy. Practicing **population-based medicine** is a mass strategy of which the prevention of common diseases of the population is the primary goal (Webb, Bain, and Pirozzo, 2005). Those implementing population-based medicine recognize that many diseases originate in the behavior and circumstances of members of the population, and place emphasis on the reduction of risk factors for that population. This has always been the focus of public health departments, which have long been concerned with the prevention of illness and disease in the entire population. This strategy can only be accomplished through well-developed health education programs, along with some regulation of high-risk health behaviors.

The Association of American Medical Colleges (1998) argues that population-based medicine usually involves

- The assessment of the health needs of the entire population being served
- The implementation and evaluation of specific interventions that are designed to improve the health of that specific population
- The provision of care for individual patients while considering the culture, health status, and health needs of the specific population being served

The overall goal of this approach to medicine is to reduce specific high-risk behaviors in a given population in order to improve its health.

Problems in Our Health Care System

According to McKenzie, Pinger, and Kotecki (2005), health care delivery in the United States is the greatest challenge to public health in the twenty-first century. The health care system has become extremely large and complex, and those responsible for the system seem to be more interested in money and enormous profits than in keeping people healthy. These groups and individuals seem baffled by the need to prevent illness, as opposed to using the scarce resources to repair damages to people's health after they become ill. It is up to public health agencies to help clear up this confusion, but this will require leadership.

The American health care system is receiving over 17 percent, or more than $2 trillion, of gross domestic product (GDP) each year to keep people healthy. These expenditures for health services are expected to continue rising into the foreseeable future. Despite this massive spending, however, comparisons of various health indices suggests that the United States is not doing as well as most other industrialized countries. There is now a sense of urgency in this country surrounding the question of how to cut health care costs, give access to care to millions who are without health insurance, and at the same time keep people healthy. This cannot happen if we fail in our effort to stop the epidemic of chronic diseases and the incurable complications that usually result from them.

According to McGinnis (2006), the health care system has developed resentment toward public health over the years. On the one hand, public health departments have been seen as meddling in the practice of medicine and providing health services to individuals who should be going to their family doctor. On the other hand, public health departments have seemed arrogant and often too busy to deal with the average physician. This lack of collaboration must stop, and a true partnership needs to begin between medicine and public health. These sectors need to work on common problems that require the expansion of partnerships in order to be solved.

There is now a growing body of evidence that enlightened leadership from the medicine and public health sectors is expanding collaboration, including partnerships in preventive health services. There are many examples from recent years of successful collaboration that has resulted in immunizations, treatment and investigation of sexually transmitted diseases, injury-prevention efforts, and diabetes initiatives. These partnerships need to be expanded in order to successfully pursue the prevention of chronic diseases.

It is ironic that public health departments must forge partnerships with the very individuals who make the most money from an unhealthy population. In fact, the self-interest of our medical complex is threatened by a country that practices healthy behaviors. The field of public health is undergoing a major change as the system of health care delivery is very slowly moving toward a model of prevention, away from the old curative model. The key player in health care, the physician, receives very little training in preventive care while in medical school and virtually no continuing education in this area after graduating. It is an absolute necessity that public health departments and physicians partner in the improvement of community health. The lack of cooperation between physicians and the public health sector must end.

These partnerships must flourish if our country is ever going to improve the health of the public. To this end, there must be public health education in medical schools, financial incentives from insurance companies to keep people healthy, and strong leadership from the medical care and public health systems.

Tilson and Berkowitz (2006) argue that public health agencies have an obligation to develop a better relationship with medical care providers in order to make preventive care the norm in this country. Medical care providers must also recognize that population-based health services can be provided more effectively and efficiently by public health agencies.

There seems to be universal agreement that our current health care system is not working very well. In fact, many health policy experts believe that the current health care system is in a state of crisis. This system costs too much; many Americans do not have access to it, and even though we are living longer in this country, the quality of life is quite poor for many older Americans.

A large number of our policymakers are focusing on the millions of Americans without access to the health care system and demanding some form of national health insurance for all. However, is the problem in our health care system really one of access, or does it stem from the fact that the system does not concentrate on wellness but rather allows us to become ill? If it is an issue of a desire for good health, then access alone is not the answer. Individuals can generally obtain and preserve good health by practicing good health habits. If one is healthy, the access problem loses some of its importance. The lack of information concerning good health behaviors—and the question of how to direct health care resources toward rectifying this dearth—are the most significant health care problems we face.

Satcher (2006) points out that our health care spending lacks balance in regard to population-based prevention, which represents less than 2 percent of the health care budget. According to Satcher (2006, p. 1010), "The burden of chronic disease is increasingly making the U.S. health system unaffordable and causing much unnecessary pain and suffering." Turnock (2009) argues that public health remains a mystery to the vast majority of the general public. The amazing accomplishments of underfunded public health departments are now being called upon to defeat the current epidemic of chronic diseases and their complications. However, the major portion of the money spent on health care is allocated for the cure of disease rather being directed toward the prevention of disease through health education and health promotion programs primarily found in public health departments. Public health departments must take the lead role in helping health care system providers appreciate that they cannot provide preventive services as efficiently or effectively as can public health departments (Tilson and Berkowitz, 2006). These go on to argue that our health care system is a very important component of the public health system, because the health care system needs to deliver preventive services if public health is to achieve its mission. As McGinnis (2006) has argued, it is mandatory that the health care system form a partnership with the public health system if the crisis in health care in this country is ever to be solved.

The Need for Improved Accountability of Public Health Professionals

Public health professionals require additional training in order to accomplish the public health objectives of the twenty-first century. Public health departments in this country cannot continue to do business as usual; they cannot continue to use antiquated tools, spend dwindling resources, or rely on visions of past successes to deal with the new and emerging threats to the public's health. The IOM (2002) recommends a system for regularly assessing the adequacy, capacity, and competence of the various public health agencies in this country. Tilson and Berkowitz (2006) call for the use of national performance standards and accreditation for our public health departments to ensure they are prepared for their vital role in health care delivery in this new century. Finally, a means of checking accountability for outcomes needs to be built into public health funding.

Tilson and Berkowitz (2006) argue further that because there are public health employees of varying competence levels, there should be standardized training programs to prepare all public health workers for the tasks ahead. Mays, Miller, and Halverson (2000) maintain that there is increased interest in the establishment of public health performance standards and a national system of accreditation for public health departments. Such standardization could yield comparative data, which all public health departments could use to improve their quality and accountability. Employees and volunteers, especially at a local level, need continuous training in all areas of preventive health care. In addition, it is clear that public health professionals need to receive instruction in the advanced use of computers and marketing techniques; they also require leadership training to assume the new role of guiding communities toward better health. Once trained, they need to be held accountable for outcomes.

Local Health Departments

As discussed in Chapter One, the IOM (2002) acknowledges that public health departments perform three core functions: assessment, policy development, and assurance. These functions are usually performed by a unit of government at the federal, state, or local level. At the local level, they are best performed by a local health department (LHD), which receives its authority and responsibilities from the state and local laws that govern it. The National Association of County and City Health Officials (NACCHO) published an *Operational Definition of a Functional Local Health Department* in 2005 that listed the following functions of an LHD (2005b, pp. 6–10):

1. Monitor health status and understand health issues facing the community
2. Protect people from health problems and health hazards
3. Give people information they need to make healthy choices
4. Engage the community to identify and solve health problems
5. Develop public health policies and plans
6. Enforce public health laws and regulations
7. Help people receive health services
8. Maintain a competent public health workforce
9. Evaluate and improve programs and interventions
10. Contribute to and apply the evidence base of public health

Characteristics of Local Health Departments

NACCHO (2005a) recently completed a national profile of local health departments, reporting on the characteristics of the nation's local health department infrastructure. Because public health programs are services, it stands to reason that the largest costs associated with offering them on a local basis are those invested in hiring, training, and employing their staff. The NACCHO survey was sent to 2,834 LHDs; 2,300 participants returned the questionnaire, representing a 77 percent response rate. The following information represents an overview of LHDs in the United States.

Over 70 percent of LHDs serve a county or combined city-county jurisdiction, and 60 percent serve small populations. The medium-size LHD serves a population base between fifty thousand and five hundred thousand individuals. Almost three quarters of the LHDs are under the control of a local board of health. Most boards of health are appointed by elected county officials. Their functions include governing, policymaking, and advising the county health director.

There is great diversity in the budgets of LHDs, with yearly expenditures ranging from as low as $10,000 to as high as $1 billion. Local sources provide the greatest percentage of revenues for LHDs, followed by sources directly from the state and federal funds passed through to LHDs by state agencies.

Approximately 86 percent of the LHDs have a chief operating officer who may have one of the following titles: health officer, director, administrator, health commissioner, nurse manager, or hometown improvement leader. This position is always a full-time responsibility, and the vast majority of chief operating officers hold an advanced graduate degree. The mean time of tenure for this position across the country is eight years.

Approximately 160,000 full-time workers are employed by LHDs. Most LHDs employ administrative or clerical personnel, nurses, managers, and directors. Other personnel found in LHDs include but are not limited to sanitarians, environmental health specialists, health educators, physicians, information management specialists, disease intervention specialists, and epidemiologists. The average complement of full-time employees for LHDs varies in size depending on the size of the population. That population includes 5 managers or directors, 20 nurses, 9 environmental specialists, 23 clerical staff, 3 nutritionists, 2 health educators, 1 physician, 1 epidemiologist, and 1 information management specialist.

The vast majority of LHDs have received federal funds from the CDC for preparing for bioterrorism, and most LHDs have improved their ability to respond to emergencies over the last few years. The funding has been used to hire and train people in preparedness planning, surveillance and epidemiology, and information technology.

The LHD plays a very important part in transforming a community into a healthier place to live. Turnock (2009) points out that the services an LHD most frequently provides in this country include

- Adult immunizations
- Childhood immunizations
- Communicable and infectious disease surveillance
- Tuberculosis screening
- Food service establishment inspection or licensing
- Environmental health surveillance
- Food safety education
- Tuberculosis treatment
- High blood pressure screening
- Tobacco use prevention
- Maternal and child health programs
- Injury prevention programs
- Oral health programs

Planning and Performance Improvement

LHDs are also very involved in community health assessments and community health improvement planning. These agencies spend a great deal of time gathering, analyzing, and disseminating valuable health data to communities. They also concern themselves with constantly improving the quality of the services they offer to their respective communities.

In recent years, LHDs have spent a great deal of time developing partnerships with other community agencies in the attempt to improve community health. This includes partnerships with schools, businesses, emergency responders, the media, and other health care providers. There has also been an increasing effort on the part of LHDs to reach the disparate populations in their community.

Information management has become a critical component of the LHD. Almost all LHDs have access to computers and high-speed Internet, and can rapidly communicate with federal and state health agencies, increasing LHDs' ability to provide valuable health information to communities. Most LHDs have developed their own Web site, which allows easy access to a wealth of public health data that can be shared with other health agencies and the general public.

Epidemic of Chronic Diseases

As we have already argued, the public health problems our nation faces have changed over the years, moving from very noticeable outbreaks of communicable diseases to the very quiet but more dangerous epidemic of chronic diseases, many of which are caused by our own behaviors. In 1900 the leading causes of death were influenza, pneumonia, and tuberculosis. Today the leading killers are all chronic diseases, including cancer, heart disease, and stroke. Because the chronic diseases have long incubation periods, the health care system usually chooses not to deal with them until they manifest themselves in complications. There is also no real incentive in our health care system to prevent illness, because physicians and hospitals receive payment for treating or curing diseases, not preventing them.

This waste of scarce resources must change through the leadership of public health departments. All providers of health care must move toward a prevention model of medical care for their patients. This is a major shift for the vast majority of health care providers, and public health agencies have to provide the guidance necessary to make this change a reality.

Behaviors like using tobacco, maintaining a poor diet, being physically inactive, and misusing alcohol are responsible for over 40 percent of the premature mortality in this country each year. One of the answers to preventing these high-risk health behaviors lies in behavioral interventions, or the practice of **behavioral medicine.** This type of medicine involves preventing or changing high-risk health behaviors so that chronic diseases do not develop, constituting primary health care delivery, which does not return high profits to those dispensing the care. This is a very difficult concept to sell to a medical establishment that has developed and grown under the rules of capitalism, and at which profits determine the actions of the players. If we are ever going to get the costs of health care to a manageable level and deal with the enormous access problem for many Americans, we are going to have to combat the epidemic of chronic diseases in the United States. This is going to be one of the most difficult tasks the public health sector and our health care system have ever undertaken.

One of the best ways of preventing chronic diseases and their complications is through **health education programs** designed to prevent high-risk health behaviors in individuals and communities. These programs are not hard to develop, but they offer tremendous challenges in regard to their implementation and evaluation. There is also a need for a different type of evaluation to measure the success or failure of health education programs whose goal is the reduction of chronic diseases, because these diseases' long incubation period and multiple causal factors complicate the evaluation process. It has therefore been difficult to discover what types of intervention programs will be successful in preventing or delaying the onset of chronic diseases. It has been even harder to obtain adequate funding to slow the development of high-risk health behaviors on the part of younger Americans. It is very challenging to educate these individuals about their health behaviors, because they cannot relate the practice of risky health behaviors when they are young to the possibility of poor health later in life.

The payoff for reducing the incidence of chronic diseases in this country is enormous. The CDC (2009a) maintains that the medical costs for individuals with chronic diseases accounts for almost 80 percent of the total health care costs in the country. More important than the monetary burden of these diseases are the years of potential life lost for people under the age of sixty-five. These human and monetary costs can be avoided if we work to remain healthy.

Public health departments are making progress in their response to the growing epidemic of chronic diseases in this country, but they cannot win the battle on their own. These departments do not have the resources necessary to triumph against the most difficult public health problem that they have ever faced. They have to become the catalysts in the formation of partnerships with the medical establishment, businesses, and other agencies in order to develop an effective strategy for helping individuals develop and maintain healthy behaviors. These needed partnerships are much easier to develop and nurture on a local level. At this level it is much easier to involve the community, which is a required prerequisite for success in the development and implementation of chronic disease prevention and health education programs. The local community is a potential source of resources, human and financial, for the new educational intervention.

Information Management

The science of public health involves using the tools of epidemiology, conducting surveillance, and preventing disease. Information management is a critical component of these activities, because the most important factor in any effort to improve the health of populations is the availability of accurate information. Very few agencies do a better job at managing and interpreting health information than do public health departments. Because of their responsibility to investigate reportable diseases, they are allowed to receive and use confidential medical information. They can then develop and implement sophisticated passive and active surveillance systems to gather a great deal of very accurate data concerning diseases and other health problems.

The IOM (2002) has argued that the use of information technology to improve surveillance systems for disease reporting, which is so necessary in the improvement of the health of communities, presents great opportunities and challenges. This prestigious group went so far as to recommend that government public health agencies should use information technology to collect and disseminate information more efficiently in order to help the public and public officials better understand what health services should be offered. This would include conveying to a large number of people the advantages of using preventive services for circumventing or postponing the development of chronic diseases and their complications. According to Novick et al. (2008), information management has evolved as one of the most important processes available to public health departments because of the sheer volume of health data available and the emergence of technology to swiftly disseminate these data.

Due to the availability of computing technology, public health departments are now able to rapidly gather health-related data, analyze these data, and share them with those responsible for the improvement of the health of the population (Novick et al., 2008). The future holds great promise for the further development of information technology to be used in delivering public health information to larger audiences. Information delivered by public health departments, especially at the local level, should include notices pertaining to education programs to prevent diseases and their complications, notifications about other preventive services, and data concerning quality of care issues. Also necessary to improve health outcomes is a partnership with medical providers, which should involve sharing medical information with them and helping each patient to understand the relevance of that information to the quality of his or her life and the lives of family members. Information sharing can help patients implement their own prevention strategies in order to avoid chronic diseases and their complications.

Expansion of Health Education Programs

The Healthy People concept, which began in 1979 and continued with the release of *Healthy People 2010* and most recently *Healthy People 2020* (CDC, 1999a, 2009d), has put the concept of good health in front of the American population for their review through media releases to the public. The Healthy People reports have resulted in a change in the attitude of the general public about the value of good health. McKenzie, Neigeral, and Thackeray (2009) note that consumers are now demanding information about their health in order to be part of the medical decision-making process. Today consumers are pressuring health professionals to help them make quality health decisions.

Health education programs have never received the credit they deserve because it is hard to place a value on that which is unable to be seen. However, public health departments are now placing a great value on health education programs because research has been able to demonstrate cost-effective results from many of them. By preventing expensive chronic diseases and their complications, health education programs are becoming an important adjunct to modern medicine. Appreciation for health educators and health promotion programs is only going to increase as we get more serious about keeping Americans healthy.

The success of public health education programs is evident in the reduction of many high-risk health behaviors in this country over the last several decades. The use of tobacco products has dropped dramatically, the incidence of cardiovascular disease has plummeted, much progress has been made in reducing the incidence of cancer, and Americans have become more knowledgeable about the causes of disease. We must now expand on these success stories.

According to McKenzie et al. (2009), many individuals are now motivated to maintain good health, producing a need for accurate health information. Public health agencies can meet this need, especially at the local level. This country has never invested a large amount of resources in health education programs designed to prevent individuals from engaging in high-risk health behaviors. In fact, health education programs are not even a priority in elementary or high schools in the vast majority of U.S. states. This is probably because school districts believe that health education for children is the responsibility of the parents. This lack of health education at an early age is one of the reasons for the epidemic of poor health behaviors among youths, including maintaining an unhealthy diet and getting insufficient physical exercise. This must change if we are ever to solve the problems of our current health care system. It is known that health behaviors develop at an early age, and that once developed these behaviors are very difficult to change. That is why public health departments must play a leadership role in fostering the development and expansion of health education programs for all grade levels in U.S. schools.

Local health departments have the expertise and the ability to provide health education programs to schools and workplaces. They are capable of developing strong educational campaigns with these captive audiences, measuring results and attracting government and foundation resources to accomplish their objectives. The time has come for an expansion of education initiatives that can improve the health of a community and actually be viewed as a community investment. The payoff for this investment will be a reduction in high-risk health behaviors, which in turn should result in a decrease in chronic diseases and their expensive complications. We have to view this investment the way we envision our retirement contributions: we plan for our retirement years by saving money in our working years; and we can plan for our health in our older years by investing in health education programs for ourselves and our children in our younger years.

Therefore, the solution to the vast majority of health problems rests on the use of public health expertise to reduce the expensive chronic diseases that are causing death and disability for so many Americans. This is a challenging but not impossible task, requiring leadership with a vision of reducing the development of chronic diseases through health education programs in schools and workplaces. It also requires a U.S. population that appreciates the value of using health education and health promotion to prevent disease. Public health departments have to lead the effort while the opportunity is present.

Public Health and the Legacy Concept

There is no question that public health departments have had great successes in improving the health of Americans with very limited resources. Unfortunately, it seems that the more success these public health departments achieved, the more their budgets were reduced. Those who fund public health have never looked at the dollars given to public health as an investment that will actually save money if disease is prevented. It is sad that public health departments have done so little to market their successes to those responsible for supplying their funding. It seems that public health has become a victim of the legacy concept, which we will now explain.

Herbold (2007) defines the **legacy concept** as the tendency for successful businesses to believe that they are entitled to continued success. Because of their past successes, they become complacent and stop looking for new opportunities that would serve to further their success in the future. The assumption inherent in this concept is that the past practices that produced success will work in the environment of the future. The legacy concept is responsible for the failure of many businesses that were unprepared to deal with the strategy changes necessitated by shifts in the external environment.

The problem of the legacy concept is not limited to for-profit businesses. It is also at work in the nonprofit sector, and we believe it has become part of public health departments in the United States. The public health sector has collected many success stories over the years, which include winning the war on communicable diseases and increasing the life expectancy of most Americans. Recently, however, public health departments have been content to use the same old set of tools that once helped them succeed—but these tools are not as effective as they used to be, and the successes of the past are not continuing. The chronic disease epidemic requires a new set of tools from public health departments.

Herbold (2007) argues that success often results in the damaging behaviors of entitlement thinking—espousing an attitude that is proud and protective and lacks urgency in responding to problems. This absence of urgency is probably the most serious effect of the legacy concept for those who work in public health. Not only are public health professionals convinced that all of the old tools will eventually work on chronic disease epidemics but also they do not see the urgency of intervention in these severe public health problems. Tobacco, obesity, unsafe sex, and poor diet are major public health issues that require immediate response. The time for simply meeting to discuss these threats is over. Public health departments know what the problems are, and they know what needs to be done. These problems have produced an opportunity for public health agencies to provide leadership in dealing with the health care crisis.

An article in *The Nation's Health* reported in early 2009 that the health of Americans had failed to improve for the fourth consecutive year (Currie, 2009). The reasons listed for poor health included obesity, increasing numbers of uninsured individuals, and the practice of high-risk health behaviors like using tobacco. At least two of these causes of poor health, obesity and tobacco use, are going to result in chronic diseases that cannot be cured and usually result in premature death and disability. This same article reported that the prevalence of obesity has more than doubled in this country in the last nineteen years. This epidemic of obesity has resulted in more than one in four Americans becoming obese, and these numbers are certainly going to rise in the short term. What is more, this tremendous weight gain will most certainly increase the incidence of such chronic illnesses as type 2 diabetes and heart disease.

These public health problems require a different set of tools, which will only be used if the legacy concept in public health is replaced by a new attitude that encourages innovation, risk taking, and the building of new partnerships. This innovation in public health programs will require new ways of thinking about and acting on old and new public health problems. We must expand and rapidly disseminate best practices of health promotion throughout the country for use by all. This cannot be accomplished without the formation of partnerships among strong leaders and empowered followers.

In many cases public health departments are attempting to use the same tools that brought them such great success in dealing with the communicable disease epidemics of the past. Chronic diseases are very different from communicable diseases and, therefore, warrant a different approach by public health departments. This approach requires an emphasis on preventing disease from occurring in the first place rather than allowing disease to occur and then using contact tracing and treatment.

When Ronald Reagan was elected president in 1980, public health departments became the ultimate target for budget cuts and elimination (Sultz and Young, 2009). The subsequent dramatic decline in authority and funding caused these departments to become very quiet because of fear of elimination. Meanwhile, the health care system expanded, spending more and more money on curing disease, and the public health system moved to the sidelines, happy to have any budget at all. The two systems should have been working together to improve the U.S. population's health, but that was not where the money was going.

Sultz and Young (2009) argue that one of the major weaknesses in our current public health system lies in the fact that public health departments are constantly reaching for arbitrary and unobtainable goals that make them look like failed agencies. This is happening despite all of their great successes in the past. In order for public health agencies to move forward, they need to be developing public health leaders with marketing skills who can help them gain political clout to reverse past budget cuts.

The Need for Leadership Development in Public Health

This is a book about how to take the public health system in America to its next great achievement through the development of leadership skills in the administrators and staff of public health programs. Our health care system needs skills of prevention to solve the current health care crisis in America. Public health practitioners have these skills, but must learn how to develop the leadership capabilities necessary to exploit the current opportunities present in our evolving system of health care. Most public health departments already are capable of achieving unbelievable feats if only given the necessary resources for success. The missing ingredient that is needed to improve the health of Americans is public health leadership that is capable of supplying the vision and securing the resources necessary to achieve that vision.

Developing an effective public health system requires bringing together the vast array of public health skills to be found within and outside of government agencies. There are a large number of private agencies, including schools of public health, that have a great deal to offer in the movement of our health care system from an emphasis on curing disease to an emphasis on disease prevention. Public health leadership is needed to achieve collaboration among different entities with varied agendas—to forge community partnerships that involve all stakeholders in the improvement of the health of the population. This is not an easy task; in fact, many would call it impossible to achieve.

Public health leaders have had little to no formal training and development in leadership, mainly because schools of public health have not offered a curriculum that included any business education. The focus in these schools has been on the sciences, including environmental science, epidemiology, health education, and public policy. These are all very important topics, but in order for leaders to accomplish goals in a large agency, they must have had some exposure to topics that help them understand how to lead people from diverse disciplines toward the achievement of a common goal. Any public health leader must also have an understanding of culture, worker empowerment, communication skills, conflict management, and marketing in order to be successful.

The IOM (2002) has been calling for the development of leadership programs for those who work in public health for several years. Whenever large companies in the private sector are in crisis, they usually bring in new leadership to help them change their direction and improve their performance. These businesses are attempting to turn a crisis into an opportunity by looking at new ways of doing business, under the guidance of new leaders. This example also applies to public health agencies in the United States: the health care system in this country is in crisis, and the change that is required entails a new approach of keeping people healthy rather than allowing them to become ill. The obvious choice for leadership assignments in public health would be those with public health expertise; but these people must also have training in leadership that allows them to work with the thick culture found in public health agencies and in the context of our powerful medical care establishments. Such leadership training ought to be available to all public health employees so that they can better use the skills they possess to do their part to make Americans healthier.

Clark and Weist (2000) argue that public health leaders need to spend a great deal of their time organizing communities around embracing the values of disease prevention. This effort requires tremendous leadership skills, and an understanding on the part of leaders that members of the medical community will express little gratitude for their efforts because they fear change and the loss of power.

Public health professionals are being asked to make use of their interpersonal skills as part of a team approach to decision making. This is a real change from the bureaucratic approach of delivering only mandated core public health services. Such interpersonal skills are found in those who have received training in leadership, and there is absolutely no reason that public health employees could not receive ongoing leadership development. They also have to be instructed in marketing principles that they could use to inform the public and political leaders of what they do and how important public health departments can be in solving the health problems in this country.

Public health employees are now being asked to collaborate with other agencies in order to improve the health of the community. These new responsibilities are coming with very little, if any, new funding or even direction. This is why leadership skills are so necessary for those working in public health departments. The old public health departments used power to achieve results by virtue of their being government entities authorized to protect the health of the population. The new public health system has to learn how to empower others to achieve even greater results in preventing disease. Public health professionals must become the leaders of the change in health care that will reduce illness and increase wellness. This new assignment will not be easy, but it can be accomplished if we invest in public health and the programs that public health departments are so good at offering to the population.

Summary

The American health care system is in dire need of change in regard to the delivery of medical care. The medical model of care must be replaced by a primary care model that focuses on healthy behaviors—and on health promotion programs that provide information to individuals on how to avoid high-risk behaviors.

Public health agencies have a long history of dealing with population-based health programs focusing on disease prevention. These agencies have had tremendous success in reducing disease and extending the life expectancy of most Americans. They have skills that need to be employed in the reform of our current health care system.

Public health agencies, health care system providers, and communities need to form partnerships to develop population-based health programs designed to keep people healthy. These programs should focus on the dissemination of health information to communities in order to help reduce the occurrence of disease and prevent complications from diseases already acquired. Public health leaders must be catalysts in this reform effort.

Key Terms

Behavioral medicine

Community health worker

Health education program

Legacy concept

Local health departments

Population-based medicine

Thick culture

Discussion Questions

1. Explain the various functions of a local health department.
2. Discuss some of the major accomplishments of the U.S. public health system. What brought about these successes?
3. Why has it been difficult to expand health education programs in the United States?
4. Explain population-based medicine and its role in the current crisis in health care delivery in this country.

CHAPTER 3

CRITICAL ISSUES FOR THE FUTURE OF HEALTH CARE IN THE UNITED STATES

LEARNING OBJECTIVES

- Understand the major problems found in the U.S. health care system
- Become aware of the ramifications of the epidemic of chronic diseases in this country
- Understand the value of health education in preventing the development of chronic diseases and their complications
- Appreciate the need for reform of the present system of health care delivery in America
- Be able to explain how the problems of cost, access, and health levels in our health care system are interrelated

The American health care system, which was the envy of the world, is not working very well. Even those who manage this enormous system are not happy with the results it has produced. In fact, it is hard to find anyone who supports its continuance in its present state, except for those who profit from the current structure. Those who control the system fear change because they are unwilling to give up their power over system resources. The word *change* is not in their vocabulary. Despite the resistance, however, the system must be overhauled.

Health care costs in this country are increasing at twice the rate of the costs of all other goods and services produced every year. This cost escalation continues to increase as a percentage of gross domestic product (GDP), and is expected to reach 20 percent of GDP in the next seven years. Fuchs (2008) argues that within thirty years the costs of health care could consume 30 percent of everything we produce in this country on a yearly basis. Sultz and Young (2009) point out that every move to control costs over the last several years by government or the health care industry has only escalated the cost increases for health services.

FIGURE 3.1   Personal Health Care Expenditures, 2005

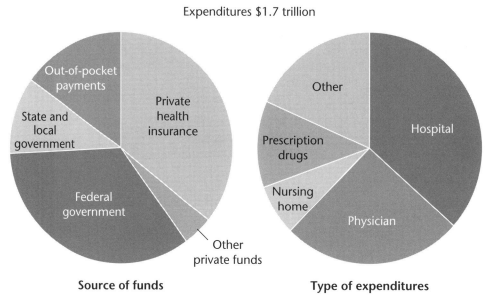

Expenditures $1.7 trillion

Source of funds   **Type of expenditures**

Source: National Center for Health Statistics, 2007, p. 27.

This cost escalation of health care services is perhaps the greatest challenge this country has ever faced. Even though our bill for health care continues to rise, however, our nation is not getting any healthier.

Figure 3.1 shows the various categories of spending on health care from 1960 to 2004. It is interesting to note the very rapid increase in per capita personal spending, per capita national spending, and national spending as a percentage of gross domestic product. Most health economists predict that these increases will become even larger as the costs of chronic diseases and their complications work their way through our health care system.

The aging of Americans, the increasing spending associated with chronic diseases, the treatment of HIV/AIDS, the growing use of expensive technology, and the rising price of drugs are all factors contributing to this escalation in the costs of health care. What is more depressing is that there does not seem to be an answer to the question of how to control the costs of maintaining this most vital system. The outcome associated with a health care system should be good health. According to Emanuel (2008), over $2 trillion, representing $7,000 per person, is spent each year on a system that does not keep people very healthy. Compounding the problem is the fact that the health care system is providing too many services, increasing medical errors that claim thousands of lives every year.

Table 3.1 illustrates the tremendous escalation in the costs of health care services delivery from 1960 through 2006, which are shown as increases in per capita spending and as a percentage of gross domestic product. Our current economic crisis is only going to make matters worse for the cost escalation of

Table 3.1 National Health Care Expenditures by Category (in Billions of Dollars), 1960 to 2006

Category	1960	1970	1980	1990	1995	2000	2003	2004	2005	2006
Hospital Care	$9.2	$27.6	$101.0	$251.6	$340.7	$417.1	$525.4	$564.4	$605.5	$648.2
Physician and Clinical Services	5.4	14.0	47.1	157.5	220.5	288.6	366.7	393.6	422.6	447.6
Dental Services	2.0	4.7	13.3	31.5	44.5	62.0	76.9	81.5	86.6	91.5
Other Professional Services	0.4	0.7	3.6	18.2	28.5	39.1	49.0	52.4	56.2	58.9
Home Health Care	0.1	0.2	2.4	12.6	30.5	30.5	38.0	42.7	47.9	52.7
Nursing Home Care	0.8	4.0	19.0	52.6	74.1	95.3	110.5	115.2	120.7	124.9
Prescription Drugs	2.7	5.5	12.0	40.3	60.9	120.6	174.2	188.8	199.7	216.7
Other Medical Products	2.3	5.0	13.6	33.7	40.9	49.5	54.8	55.9	57.6	59.3
Other Personal Health Care	0.6	1.2	3.3	9.6	23.0	37.0	50.3	53.2	56.8	62.2
Personal Health Care	$23.3	$62.9	$215.3	$607.5	$863.7	$1,139.6	$1,445.9	$1,547.7	$1,653.7	$1,762.0
Government Administration and Net Cost of Private Health Insurance	1.2	2.8	12.2	39.2	58.1	81.8	121.0	129.0	133.6	145.4
Public Health Activities	0.4	1.4	6.4	20.0	31.0	43.4	53.8	53.9	56.3	58.7
Noncommercial Biomedical	0.7	2.0	5.4	12.7	18.3	25.6	35.5	38.8	40.6	41.8
Research New Construction	1.9	5.8	14.5	34.7	45.4	63.2	76.3	83.0	89.1	97.6
National Health Expenditures	$27.5	$74.9	$253.9	$714.0	$1,016.5	$1,353.6	$1,732.4	$1,852.3	$1,973.3	$2,105.5
Per Capita Personal Spending (dollars)	$126	$301	$931	$2,397	$3,214	$4,033	$4,967	$5,264	$5,572	$5,879
Per Capita National Spending (dollars)	$148	$356	$1,102	$2,813	$3,783	$4,790	$5,952	$6,301	$6,649	$7,026
National Spending as a Percent of GDP (%)	5.2	7.2	9.1	12.3	13.7	13.8	15.8	15.9	15.9	16.0

Source: U.S. Department of Health and Human Services, Centers for Medicare and Medicaid Services, n.d., p. 55.

health care, because spending will continue to rise for health services despite a weakened economy. These increased costs are not sustainable.

Cost escalation is found in all parts of the health care system, but it is especially visible in the rising percentage of spending on physician and clinical services. Physicians are paid to do more even if the additional tests and procedures have little if any value and could pose great risks for their patients. We have produced a system that delivers too much health care of marginal value, which might place some patients in danger. The more we do, the more we put the patient at risk by exposing him or her to the many dangers that result from the delivery of modern medical services. According to Brownlee (2007), medical errors kill between forty-four and ninety-eight thousand people every year. It is ironic that thousands of Americans get little or no medical care, while the rest of America receives too much of the wrong kind of medical care.

Table 3.2 shows national health expenditures for 2005, with projections through 2016. National spending will continue to rise per capita and as a percentage of GDP. Despite the escalation of the costs of health care, however, we have been unable to improve the health of the population. This is because the fragmented health care system in our country does not evaluate outcomes. Rather, it concentrates on activities like physician visits, testing, and hospitalizations, which in health care are very expensive and do very little to keep people healthy, but from which many providers profit.

The cost increases for health care are affecting our government, businesses, and consumers, and even our ability to compete with other nations by increasing the prices for our goods and services. These costs have forced millions of individuals either to not have insurance or, if they do have insurance, to contribute a larger percentage of the cost of that insurance, reducing their disposable income. The health care cost crisis has an impact on every aspect of our lives, and many of us are demanding solutions from our political leaders. And it seems that these

Table 3.2   National Health Care Expenditures for 2005, with Projections for 2010, 2015, and 2016

Category	2005	2010	2015	2016
Personal Health Care (billions)	$1,661.4	$2,312.9	$3,227.9	$3,449.4
National Health Expenditures (billions)	$1,987.7	$2,776.4	$3,874.6	$4,136.9
Per Capita Personal Spending	$5,598	$7,485	$10,049	$10,658
Per Capita National Spending	$6,697	$8,985	$12,062	$12,782
National Spending as a Percent of GDP	16.0	17.2	19.2	19.6

Source: U.S. Department of Health and Human Services, Centers for Medicare and Medicaid Services, n.d., p. 56.

leaders keep visiting the past for solutions that have never worked and only make the current problems worse. What is more, those who profit the most from the present system of health care delivery are the ones who are being consulted for ways to improve health services in this country.

Why We Are Failing in Our Health Care Reform Efforts

Our system of health care delivery is failing to solve the main problems with the health of Americans. Fuchs (1998) argues that there are three major problems found in our health care system: **cost, access, and health levels.** He goes on to explain that these are not really problems but symptoms of a much larger dilemma that includes the issue of how to effectively use scarce resources. In order to solve these problems in health care, we have to completely change the way health care is delivered in the United States. This is going to require an emphasis on preventing rather than curing disease, and it will require leadership in the change process.

It seems that most people are concentrating on the problems of cost and access while paying little or no attention to the problem of Americans' poor health levels. This is a very normal response, given that most Americans pay very little attention to their health until they become ill. The medical care system in this country has never been very interested in disease prevention because the payment system for medical care does not usually reimburse efforts that are designed to keep people healthy.

As we have already noted, it is very true that costs have escalated for the purchase of health care services. The main reason for this cost escalation is that individuals are allowed to become ill in the first place. Annual expenditures on personal medical services have increased from over $35 billion in 1965 to over $2 trillion in 2011. This represents an increase from 5 percent of GDP in 1965 to over 16 percent of a much larger GDP in 2008. Despite all of these expenditures on health care services, however, this country still has over forty-five million individuals without health insurance. These are clearly very serious problems, but we must ask whether these problems are more serious than the epidemic of chronic diseases. If we can first eliminate the epidemic of chronic diseases and people remain well, the problems of cost and access will diminish. It is becoming more evident as time passes that prevention efforts may be the answer to the cost and access problems that plague our country. But how do we change the business of health care delivery? How do we change a system that is focused on curing disease into one that concentrates the bulk of its resources on preventing disease? This is where we need answers from public health departments.

According to Williams and Torrens (2008), the costs of Medicare and Medicaid, which already account for 23 percent of all federal spending, will continue to rise well into the future. The increased spending for these mandated health programs can only be controlled if their recipients remain well. It is amazing that there is so little discussion about prevention programs designed to keep people well as a way to control these costs. Even if the recipients have chronic conditions, prevention efforts can reduce the complications from these diseases later in life.

Williams and Torrens (2008) assert that these health programs cannot be allowed to grow at a faster rate than the rest of the economy, and that something drastic has to be done to tame their growth. The question becomes, then, What can be done to lower costs while simultaneously improving the quality of these popular government programs? Making matters worse, the number of Medicare beneficiaries is currently forty-three million and is expected to reach forty-nine million in the next few years, placing further strain on the system. Again, prevention efforts never seem to enter into this debate.

The problem gets worse when we discover that the rising number of aging baby boomers is only part of the predicament. The key trigger in increasing health care costs is not America's aging population, but rather the growing epidemic of obesity and the health problems associated with this weight gain (Centers for Disease Control and Prevention [CDC], 2009a). This country ranks poorly in prevention of health problems when compared with most other industrialized nations. This becomes more difficult to explain when it is revealed that the other countries spend a smaller portion of their wealth on health care, but nevertheless have healthier inhabitants. It seems that the United States is spending its dollars on the wrong types of health care interventions rather than investing in prevention efforts. Why doesn't our country recognize the potential return on the investment in prevention programs? Everyone seems to recognize the value of good health, but that is about as far as the concept of prevention goes. Prevention as a potential solution to the health care crisis never seems to leave the discussion phase.

There is no question that the health care industry in the United States is in trouble, causing tremendous change in the way it delivers services to its customers. Health care costs continue to rise every year, and millions of Americans are losing their health insurance. The practices of unhealthy behaviors are resulting in chronic diseases, and their complications are threatening to bankrupt the health care system in the United States.

The costs associated with delivering health care services to Americans are rising faster than the cost of living every year. This difference in price increases usually indicates a problem with productivity in the sector experiencing the higher costs of production. This nation has tried price controls, managed care, and government management of such programs as Medicare and Medicaid—and has been met with only limited success. The solution to productivity problems is usually better management of scarce resources to improve outcomes. There is also an immediate need for leadership in keeping Americans healthy at an affordable price.

Despite the enormous costs associated with health care, the majority of Americans are not very healthy. They are living longer, but many are developing chronic diseases as they age and suffering the complications associated with chronic illness. Their later years have become plagued by poor quality of life, which is a result of practicing unhealthy behaviors when they were younger.

A large number of our political leaders have determined that this lack of access to health care services is the major problem with our current health care system. These politicians believe that they can solve the problems of health care delivery by instituting a national health insurance program similar to the type of government-sponsored program found in other countries. We do not wish to demean the seriousness of not having insurance for health care services, but this lack of insurance is not the biggest problem in health care that the United States faces. Access alone does not guarantee good health. Having insurance alone does not usually keep people healthy and protect the quality of their health: it only allows them to receive medical care after they have become ill.

Access to health care, usually meaning coverage by health insurance, is a very complicated issue. The access issue has become more important in recent years because most of the newly uninsured are working families who have lost their employment-related health insurance. Recent research indicates that people without health insurance die prematurely, are less productive at work, and usually receive fragmented medical care when they become ill. This fragmentation of care leads to the use of expensive medical tests that may result in increased medical errors. Health care delivery in the United States has become a series of poorly defined problems that lead to other, less clear problems, making solutions seem virtually impossible. Although most people assume that this issue can be solved by issuing some type of universal health coverage plan, there is another choice that involves keeping people healthy throughout their life.

The real problem with our health care system in the United States is that it is not prepared to prevent high-risk health behaviors that are practiced by a large number of Americans. These behaviors usually result in the development of chronic diseases after a long incubation period. These are unlike communicable diseases with shorter incubation periods and available treatment regimens: the health care system cannot offer a cure for a chronic disease once it manifests itself and becomes symptomatic in the patient, and as the individual grows older he or she will usually develop life-threatening complications from that disease.

According to the CDC (2009a), chronic diseases contribute to the greatest morbidity, mortality, and disability in this country. Cardiovascular disease, cancer, and diabetes are the most prevalent and costly—and yet all of these diseases remain preventable. Further, seven out of ten Americans who die each year do so as a result of a chronic disease. Chronic diseases are not contagious, have a long latency period, and are usually incurable. They are usually caused by human behaviors, which, once developed, are very difficult to change. Tobacco use, poor nutrition, being overweight, and physical inactivity are the main causes of chronic diseases. Once these diseases develop, they are nearly impossible to eliminate. They just continue to get worse as the individual ages, and they eventually become the catalysts in producing disability or premature death.

The way to deal with chronic diseases is to prevent them from occurring in the first place, or at the very least to postpone the complications from these diseases. In order to accomplish this, we must emphasize the prevention of high-risk behaviors through health education and health promotion programs. Those responsible for decision making in health care have never had an interest in preventing disease because the money and power are not present in prevention efforts. This is very evident in the way we train physicians, teaching them to cure disease, not to prevent disease from occurring. Population health and preventive programs have been left to poorly staffed and underfunded public health departments.

The question that we need to answer in the near future is, How do we keep people healthy in this country at a price that we can all afford? It seems very clear that a different approach to delivering health services is a prerequisite for saving our health care system from bankruptcy. This solution cannot include more government involvement, because government tinkering with the system has actually caused the severity of the current crisis. The answer must include the development of partnerships among businesses, schools, and public health departments to keep people healthy. We contend in this book that public health departments can provide leadership in prevention efforts if they are freed from bureaucratic government control. This will be discussed later in the text.

Root Causes of the Failures of the Health Care System

There are several contributors to the health care crisis in this country. They include the health insurance industry, providers of health care services, government entities, and individuals practicing unhealthy behaviors. The health care industry and providers of health care services have gained power, prestige, and profits by allowing duplication, errors, disease, and abuse of power to be a large part of the delivery of health care services in our country. Their collective power blocks change to a new model of health care delivery that would encourage wellness instead of illness for a large part of our population.

Health Insurance Industry

The most important determinant of access to health care is health insurance. The majority of Americans cannot afford to pay for expensive tests, hospitalization, surgery, and medical devices. Therefore, they pass on the risk of most costs associated with potential poor health to others through insurance. The financing of health services in the United States is done within a very fragmented system that involves public and private insurers, and it is paid for by employers, taxes, and individuals.

Insurance is protection against financial loss associated with an event. **Health insurance** involves the application of the principles of insurance to protect individuals from the costs associated with medical care. There are two major models for providing insurance to individuals in order to protect them from risks. These models are the casualty model and the social model. The casualty model, used for auto, fire, flood, and life insurance, forces the insured to assume some risks and losses if the insured event occurs. The social model, used in health insurance, does not require the insured to assume any risks or costs if a poor health event occurs. This model allows individuals to practice high-risk health behaviors, like using tobacco, and yet pay no higher premiums for health insurance than someone who does not practice high-risk health behaviors.

The fundamental concept of health insurance is to balance costs and risks across a large number of individuals in order to protect an individual against an unexpected health event. However, health insurance is very different from casualty insurance because of the possibility of adverse selection and moral hazard. Under the concept of **adverse selection,** only those who will benefit from insurance have a tendency to acquire it—unhealthy individuals are more likely to subscribe to health insurance in anticipation of extensive medical claims. Conversely, individuals who consider themselves reasonably healthy may consider health insurance an unnecessary expenditure. Because of adverse selection, insurance companies use a patient's medical history to screen out persons with preexisting medical conditions. Those perceived as high financial risks may be denied coverage or charged higher premiums to compensate; conversely, discounts may be granted to low-financial-risk applicants.

The term **moral hazard** refers to the reduced incentives to mitigate risks that come from having insurance. A person weighs the costs and benefits of an action, and if benefits exceed costs (which sometimes happens when insurance has shifted the risks associated with that action), he or she takes that action. In health insurance, moral hazard means that if you believe that major expenses are covered, you have fewer incentives to take measures to ensure your continued good health. In response, insurance companies attempt to reduce the risk of moral hazard by providing the insured with financial reasons to avoid making a claim, such as by employing deductibles, copayments, and co-insurance. For a society to remain healthy, incentives for both individuals and providers should encourage the provision of preventive services, including those that encourage healthy behaviors. Such incentives are usually not a part of health insurance programs.

The health insurance industry is under tremendous pressure to change the way that it does business. This important component of our health care system can no longer afford to continue to pay for damage done by individuals to their own health by willingly practicing high-risk behaviors. The insurance industry has to include some accountability for outcomes in the insurance process. McGinnis (2006) argues that health care reimbursement should encourage the delivery of preventive care services. This might involve urging third-party payers to pay more attention to preventing illness rather than simply paying bills for health problems that could have been prevented. In other words, structure a payment system that pays for wellness, not illness.

Employer-provided insurance is group insurance under which a single policy covers the medical expenses of many different people, instead of covering just one person. According to Feldstein (2007), this arrangement minimizes adverse selection by spreading the risk of an adverse health event among a large number of individuals, thus lowering the cost of premiums for those participating. For example, if one member of the group has a major health issue and the others stay healthy, the insurance company can use the money paid by the healthy to pay for the treatment of the unhealthy.

Unlike with individual insurance, for which each person's risk potential is evaluated to determine insurability, all eligible people can be covered by a group policy, regardless of age or physical condition. The insurance premium is calculated based upon the aggregate characteristics of the group, such as average age and degree of occupational hazard. This system of social insurance shares the risks, costs, and benefits of the program equally among participants, but has the danger of creating a sense of entitlement to benefits and provides little encouragement for positive health behavior. There are usually no incentives in this type of insurance plan to remain healthy.

Health insurers should be responsible for doing more than just collecting premiums and paying the providers of health care services. Their financial ability allows them to play a major role in the improvement of the health of the population, which could include offering incentives for individuals to practice healthy behaviors, such as a reduction in their insurance premium. The reverse is also true: insurance providers could increase premiums for those who practice high-risk health behaviors like tobacco use, but this is not the case in most health insurance plans.

Insurance companies could also supply public health agencies with the necessary resources to develop and implement population-based health education programs. For nonprofit health care organizations, providing community benefit is the principal standard for maintaining tax-exempt status. However, it is becoming increasingly difficult to differentiate for-profit health care organizations from the nonprofit ones, and as a result, both the Internal Revenue Service (IRS) and Congress have begun to challenge the appropriateness of the community benefit standard. The IRS wants to make tax-exempt entities more accountable for their activities and to quantify the supply of community benefit provided by nonprofits.

Nonprofit health care organizations can benefit the communities they serve by funding local health department programs. This seems like a logical way for a health care organization to maintain its nonprofit status and improve the health of its community. The catalyst in bringing this about would be public health leaders' using the tax code to persuade third-party payers to provide financial resources for community health education programs. This has not happened.

Shi and Singh (2008) argue that changing patterns of morbidity and mortality should cause financers of health care to shift their emphasis from acute care to preventive care. This will require collaboration between the payers for health care and those with knowledge of prevention programs. This is a wonderful opportunity for public health professionals to provide real leadership in acquiring the necessary resources to keep people healthy, reduce illness, and lower health care costs. We must explore this opportunity for public health leadership if we are serious about keeping the U.S. population healthy.

Providers of Health Care Services

The power of the providers of health care services in America has changed dramatically over the years. The key providers of health care in the United States in terms of power and influence over the system are still the physicians and hospitals. Physicians receive less than 25 percent of hospitals' total income, but they influence most of the other 75 percent of expenditures through their decisions (Henderson, 2009). They admit patients to hospitals, recommend treatment, and prescribe medications. If we are serious about dealing with the problems in health care delivery, we must address physicians' current power and their ability to influence health.

The power physicians hold allows them to create their own demand. Sloan and Kasper (2008) argue that because physicians are paid more if they do more, there is probably too much medical treatment in this country. This excessive medical treatment may be good in some cases, but it probably results in a waste of scarce medical resources and danger to many patients. If we are ever to gain control over health care costs, we are going to have to deal with how physicians are paid. This is a very difficult task, however, because the medical market is not a normal economic market.

McLaughlin and McLaughlin (2008) point out that the numbers of physicians in specific areas of medicine usually reflect the perceptions of income potential. When you add prestige, respect, and earning potential for specialists, is there any wonder why we have a surplus of specialists and a shortage of primary care doctors in this country? There is no question that medical care has become big business. In many cases money has replaced caring in one of the most important sectors of our economy. There is too much of the wrong type of medical care, too much duplication, many medical errors, and an excess of greed. There is virtually no interest in preventing disease on the part of physicians, who are paid to do more medicine and less patient education. The profit model that health care providers in this country follow has no time for education to prevent disease. Instead, physicians have been trained to cure disease, and hospitals have expanded to provide the facilities for that process. The whole business model of health care delivery falls apart if people remain well.

The field of medicine and the education of physicians have largely ignored the value of preventive medicine, health education, and health promotion (Sultz and Young, 2009). Physicians are trained to treat and attempt to cure disease, while the disease-prevention aspect is largely ignored. The medical education system in this country has made instruction in health promotion and disease prevention a very low priority. The reasons for this include medical school faculty members' own lack of exposure to prevention education and the clear failure of our payment system to offer incentives for prevention activities to those who provide medical care.

Sultz and Young (2009) argue that recent health care reform efforts have resulted in the reduction of power and prestige of physicians and hospitals. The relationship between physicians and hospitals has also changed in recent years due to restrictions from the government payment mechanism and insurers. The physician still admits patients to the hospital, but his or her power has been restricted. Prospective payment systems require a reason for hospital admission and a diagnosis of the admitting condition, which restricts payment. Therefore, the physician's close relationship with the hospital has diminished.

Millions of dollars have been spent to increase the number of primary care doctors over the last twenty years. This increase in funding has produced more doctors, but they have situated themselves in urban rather than rural areas, and most new physicians have opted for specialization rather than primary care. Starfield, Shi, Grover, and Macinko (2005) point out that adding one primary care physician per ten thousand people produced a 6 percent decrease in all causes of mortality. This is because primary care physicians are more likely to discuss high-risk health behaviors with patients, thus providing the health education that is a prerequisite for avoiding chronic disease.

It seems clear that most physicians are not willing or able to drive prevention efforts within our current health care system. This is especially evident in that the majority of new physicians entering medicine specialize rather than providing primary care. This deficiency must be offset by increasing the number of public health professionals who provide health education programs in communities.

According to Sultz and Young (2009), the U.S. medical care system is ready to move toward an emphasis on prevention, but the finances for such a transition are in disarray. It is very important that medical practitioners begin to assume leadership roles in public education about the benefits of prevention in the delivery of health care services. In order for this to happen, however, public health departments must reach out to physicians in an effort to increase the perceived value of prevention programs as part of the health care system.

Government Entities

The rapid rise in the number of individuals without health insurance in the United States has increased the clamoring for some form of national health insurance system similar to the single-payer plan found in Canada, where taxes pay for health care for the population. The president and Congress are discussing the value of a single-payer plan. These calls for and promise of a national health insurance plan are nothing new—we have heard them before, and nothing has ever happened. Most health policy experts do not believe that more government involvement in our health care system is going to do anything but make matters worse.

Many people are amazed at the government's involvement in health care, given its history of funding health care initiatives and dictating medical decisions without having the money and the expertise to accomplish anything productive in health care delivery. The interest in health care is primarily on the part of politicians getting elected or reelected, and then the serious interest disappears. The government is currently funding almost half of the costs of health care in America, and matters have only gotten worse.

According to Emanuel (2008), 1 out of every 5 dollars of the federal budget ($580 billion) goes to pay for Medicare, Medicaid, and the State's Children's Health Insurance Program (SCHIP). This bill is most certainly going to continue to rise because of the aging of Americans and the complications associated with chronic diseases. These funds are used to pay for health care delivery, with very little of the funding going to prevention activities or health promotion programs.

Medicare has been called a success by most legislators. It has many satisfied customers and has the lowest administrative costs, so it seems to be very efficient in paying health care bills for those covered by the plan. Medicare only devotes 3 to 4 percent of its budget to administrative costs (Emanuel, 2008). However, the unfortunate trade-off for low administrative costs is a 10 percent rate of fraud. This fraud was never more evident than in a recent report from the *New York Times*, which reported that Medicare paid 478,500 claims that contained identification numbers assigned to physicians who were deceased (Pear, 2008). This entitlement program uses price-fixing to keep the enormous health care spending under control. This has not worked, however, as suggested by the fact that Medicare trustees project an unfunded liability of $36 trillion over the next seventy-five years.

A program of national health insurance, although providing access to all Americans, would do little to prevent illness. It would simply transfer payment for health services from employers and consumers to the government, which would then raises taxes to pay the enormous bill. These government-financed plans do not make us healthier so that we can lower costs—they just pay for illness in a different way. But these schemes do get votes that allow politicians to keep their employment.

Individuals Practicing Unhealthy Behaviors

The vast majority of the costs of health care delivery in this country are a direct result of chronic diseases and their complications. Currently, almost 80 percent of health care costs are for treatment of chronic diseases, and these costs are expected to rise rapidly as a result of high-risk health problems, such as obesity, and the increase in diabetes and other diseases with no cure. The incidence of diabetes is expected to double over the next twenty-five years because of the current epidemic of obesity in the United States (Bodenheimer, Chen, and Bennett, 2009). The practice of high-risk health behaviors over a long period of time causes and aggravates these chronic diseases. One of the only ways to stop these behaviors from developing is through well-developed health education programs for children that begin with the parents, continue during school years, and are reinforced in the workplace. Our current health care system ignores health education as a form of medical care. Health education programs have never become a priority for schools and workplaces, and the result has been an epidemic of chronic diseases.

Shi and Singh (2008) maintain that the epidemic of chronic diseases will eventually force the incorporation of wellness and disease prevention into the health care system. This change will not come easy to a system that makes money on illness. Further, it will shift cost increases over to individual patients, requiring them to make changes in order to comply with recommendations for health behaviors. In order for this to be successful, the patient must become educated in regard to how chronic diseases develop and, more important, how to prevent their occurrence. This is a wonderful opportunity for the expansion of public health prevention programs that have been shown to be effective when properly implemented.

The major causes of most chronic diseases in this country are a few high-risk health behaviors that are addictive to the individual, are encouraged by society, and are beginning earlier and earlier in life. A very good example is found in the increasing rate of obesity, resulting from poor diet and lack of physical activity, which is causing an epidemic of type 2 diabetes that is rapidly moving to the adolescents in this country.

Table 3.3 shows the major causes of mortality in the United States in 2004. It is interesting to note that for the most part these diseases are preventable.

Table 3.3   Ten Leading Causes of Death in the United States, 2004

Rank	Causes of death	All persons	Causes of death	Male	Causes of death	Female
	All causes	2,397,615	All causes	1,181,668	All causes	1,215,947
1.	Diseases of heart	652,486	Diseases of heart	321,973	Diseases of heart	330,513
2.	Malignant neoplasms (cancer)	553,888	Malignant neoplasms (cancer)	286,830	Malignant neoplasms (cancer)	267,058
3.	Cerebrovascular diseases	150,074	Unintentional injuries	72,050	Cerebrovascular diseases	91,274
4.	Chronic lower respiratory diseases	121,987	Cerebrovascular diseases	58,800	Chronic lower respiratory diseases	63,341
5.	Unintentional injuries	112,012	Chronic lower respiratory diseases	58,646	Alzheimer's disease	46,991
6.	Diabetes mellitus	73,138	Diabetes mellitus	35,267	Unintentional injuries	39,962
7.	Alzheimer's disease	65,965	Influenza and pneumonia	26,861	Diabetes mellitus	37,871
8.	Influenza and pneumonia	59,664	Suicide	25,566	Influenza and pneumonia	32,803
9.	Nephritis, nephrotic syndrome, and nephrosis	42,480	Nephritis, nephrotic syndrome, and nephrosis	20,370	Nephritis, nephrotic syndrome, and nephrosis	22,110
10.	Septicemia	33,373	Alzheimer's disease	18,974	Septicemia	18,362

Source: National Center for Health Statistics, 2007, p. 9.

In recent years, for example, there has been a very noticeable decline in heart disease: between 1970 and 2002, the mortality from heart disease declined from 362 deaths per 100,000 to 241 per 100,000 (Feldstein, 2005). The cause of this decline was most likely lifestyle changes associated with reduced cigarette smoking, reduced serum cholesterol levels, and increased physical activity. Interventions to encourage lifestyle changes that promote health behaviors do very well in a cost-benefit analysis.

According to The Commonwealth Fund Commission on a High Performance Health System (2009), a focus on prevention and improving the outcomes that result from chronic diseases could be the solution to our health care cost crisis in America. This goal could be met with the movement of scarce health care resources away from curing diseases and toward preventing them in the first place. This prevention effort will require the expansion of health education programs in schools, workplaces, and communities. These education programs can help prevent the practice of high-risk health behaviors.

Changing health behaviors is going to require a combination of broad public health incentives and health education to become part of every aspect of health care delivery (McGinnis, 2006). In order to accomplish this objective, public health professionals will need advanced training and increased funding. This will not happen until they are able to take risks and grasp the opportunities that are presenting themselves as the reform of the health care system gets into high gear during the next few years. They will also need to receive the leadership training they greatly need to bring all of the necessary prevention partners together.

Other Problem Areas

There are many other less obvious causes of the failures of our current health care system. They include:

Increase in Lobbyist activity

Whenever the government has large amounts of money to spend in a given area, there is an increase in interest groups' involvement in how that money gets distributed. These interest groups include many of the associations that represent health care providers, such as the American Medical Association, the American Hospital Association, and third-party payers like Blue Cross. This phenomenon is very evident when interest groups use their economic resources to shape opinions on ways to improve the health care system in this country. Their recommendations also increase the power, influence, and, ultimately, income of their members. It must be noted that lobbyists and special interest groups do absolutely nothing to improve the health of Americans. This interest group involvement will virtually eliminate healthy competition that can bring the consumer higher-quality and lower-cost health care services. "But who cares," we might say, "it is the government paying the bills"... until we realize that we *are* the government, and all of us are paying those bills.

The End of the Primary Care Physician

The primary care physician should be the health educator for the patient. This type of doctor is concerned with keeping his or her patient healthy, which requires a major emphasis on prevention. As previously noted, preventing disease does not benefit the medical care sector in this country. Physicians and hospitals in the United States get paid for doing more, not for doing less. This is the major reason why primary care doctors do not command a high salary; this is also why new doctors avoid primary care. There is currently no monetary incentive at work in health care delivery to keep individuals healthy. Physicians have found that they can have a higher salary and live a more comfortable lifestyle by becoming specialists rather than general practitioners. The specialist does not have the time or the motivation to educate his or her patients about the dangers of practicing high-risk health behaviors.

According to Starfield et al. (2005), there is lower mortality from disease in geographical areas with more primary care physicians. Therefore, increasing the supply of primary care physicians has a positive effect on communities' health. Sadly, the number of physicians choosing primary care has diminished.

Epidemic of Medical Errors

Medical errors, especially in hospitals, represent a well-known problem that has received very little attention from those in power (Sultz and Young, 2009). In many instances physicians and hospitals are reimbursed for making the error, and then reimbursed again for rectifying the error if the patient lives. Types of errors include diagnostic and treatment errors, surgical errors, drug errors, and delays in treatment, to name a few. It is frightening to know that one of the major causes of medical errors was miscommunication among health care professionals. Brownlee (2007) points out that a lack of cooperation among the players in the current health care system is one of the major reasons for the epidemic of medical errors. Up to ninety-eight thousand patients die each year from preventable medical errors (Institute of Medicine, 1999). This is another opportunity for public health leaders to intervene.

Minimal Political Appreciation of Public Health Activities

Public health leaders have never done a very good job of marketing their many success stories to the legislators funding their departments. They are frightened by the media, unless they are given the green light to speak freely when asked questions about sensitive topics. The result is that many people think of public health as part of the welfare department, and don't really care if the sector's funding is increased or even reduced. One of the missing skills of public health leaders has been the ability to work with the public and legislators through the media in an effort to convey how important public health departments' contributions are to the improvement of the U.S. population's health.

To be successful in helping people change their high-risk health behaviors requires time and resources. Many of these behaviors are addictive and will take intensive, time-consuming interventions to change. People want to know how much it is going to cost to correct these behaviors. The other question that is frequently asked is why more resources are not dedicated to preventing high-risk behaviors from developing in the first place.

Solution to the Problems in Our Health Care System

The solution to our array of health problems must begin with an honest attempt to stop diseases before they begin. This will require the development of partnerships and the leadership of public health agencies in the improvement of the health status of the vast majority of Americans.

Businesses and Employers

Businesses across the country are realizing that they can increase worker productivity and reduce their health insurance costs by keeping their employees healthy. Productivity diminishes when an employee is unable to come to work because of illness or disability. The environment of the workplace can have a major—and often negative—influence on the overall health of the workers, and requires much greater study in order to protect the worker from injury, disease, quality of life issues, and premature death. The average worker spends the most productive years of his or her life in the workplace, and if that worker's health is affected in a negative way, he or she has an overall negative payoff for all that hard work. There is nothing more important than personal health. Although some economists attempt to place a monetary value on life, there does not seem to be much interest in putting a price on the quality of life, especially when this quality begins to diminish because of injury or disease.

There are still too many Americans becoming disabled, developing chronic diseases, and reducing their quality of life in later years as a direct result of their work environment. There is a real need for the expansion of time-tested public health programs, including those that provide information about chronic diseases and their prevention in the workplace. The starting point will be improving the methods of gathering data concerning workers' health. These should encompass all health data, including statistics on such chronic diseases as heart disease, cancer, diabetes, and other incurable conditions with high medical costs that affect both employer and employee.

Although the workplace has been shown to be very dangerous for many workers in many occupations, over the last several years the nation has made significant improvements in the health of working people. There is much more work to be accomplished, however, as employers are asked to assume a greater responsibility for the future quality of life of their employees.

The quality of health care services is becoming a very serious component in controlling both the outcomes and the costs of health care delivery. Those with the responsibility of paying for health care in the United States are starting to demand that providers reduce errors in the delivery of medical services. Further, businesses are capable of playing a key role in reducing these costs while simultaneously improving the health of their employees through the development of workplace wellness programs.

Rather than seeking one big fix for our ailing health care industry, we believe that success can be achieved through small, continuous, well-thought-out, and incremental changes that keep the focus on the customer or the patient. The workplace is an ideal location to provide health information to a very large segment of the U.S. population. This can be accomplished by dedicated individuals who already possess the requisite public health expertise to improve the health of all workers.

Innovation in Health Care Services Delivery

Innovation entails a new way of doing something, and may be incremental or radical. When business models fail, leaders usually innovate and come back with new ways of achieving their goals. Our health care system has failed in keeping us healthy at an affordable cost. This fact is very hard to sell to those in power in health care because they are so very impressed by the strengths of the current system that they are blind to its very obvious shortcomings.

Our current health care system is ineffective in that it cannot provide evidence that what it is doing is actually working. The system breeds inefficiency through overuse and unbelievable duplication of services, thereby wasting valuable resources. Hospitals and doctors are paid to do more rather than to keep people healthy. Christensen, Bohmer, and Kenagy (2000) argue that it is time for the application of disruptive innovation to health care delivery in the United States, which entails using unexpected new programs that shake up the current way business is conducted. Disruptive innovation is actually a new model of doing business that capitalizes on the opportunities presented by a changing environment.

It seems that applying this concept to health care is not all that difficult if we start with the belief that the health care system should be keeping people healthy, not using scarce resources to cure those who become ill. The catalysts for this disruptive innovation are information technology and patients' involvement in their own health. This changing model of the way we deal with our health will disrupt one of the largest industries in our economy, providing a once-in-a-lifetime opportunity for public health departments to provide leadership in designing wellness programs for the nation. The only missing link in this process is the leadership development within and empowerment of our public health departments.

New Model of Health Care Delivery

There are those who believe that somehow health care is different from other businesses in the United States. This is true because of the nature of the health care business, but this is no excuse for not trying to improve the delivery of health care services. This delivery process needs to be evaluated by those implementing the new approach and developed through the use of business analysis. There needs to be accountability for the enormous quantity of resources that are inefficiently used to create less-than-stellar outcomes.

As discussed in Chapter Two, Herbold (2007) argues that most businesses that are failing to produce results have been seduced by their own past success—a phenomenon he refers to as the legacy concept. He has noticed three very negative factors present in failing organizations that follow the legacy concept: a lack of urgency, protective and proud attitudes, and an entitlement mentality among employees and business leaders. These elements are evident in most of our large health care organizations in the United States. They not only revel in their past successes but also believe that they are entitled to provide medical care in America even if their services cost more than they are worth. They have become convinced that they can even cure death if given enough resources.

Notice the key word in the last sentence: *cure*. You do not hear the word *prevention*, because there are very few if any economic returns associated with prevention. Therefore, the health care system dedicates very few resources to preventing anything. Herbold (2007) asserts that there is a need to change the focus from an emphasis on curing disease, which has been continued for years with little impact on good health outcomes, to an emphasis on preventing disease. The American health care system is the best in the world, but it is not keeping people healthy. It allows individuals to become ill even though there are enormous resources available that could have prevented their illness at a much lower cost. It is a wonderful collection of health resources that have been focused on the wrong outcomes. This needs to change.

The lack of focus on prevention does not seem to be deliberate or the result of any medical conspiracy. The fact that the American health care system has been so successful has made its leaders incapable of even considering a change in focus. The system was born and grew up dealing with communicable diseases that could be cured. These diseases have been replaced by chronic diseases that cannot be cured and are responsible for major health complications as time passes. Although the diseases have changed, the system has refused to change with them because of its past successes. This is truly an example of the legacy concept at work.

Herbold (2007) also argues that businesses that achieve success begin to believe that if they continue doing business in the same way they are entitled to future success. This sense of entitlement leads companies to block change, even when their current business processes are failing. The legacy concept will usually cause businesses in the for-profit sector to go under. This does not happen to entities in the nonprofit sector as long as they have access to some continued source of funding. This is especially true for the health care system in the United States.

Members of the health care sector claim that business is done in a certain way because that is the way that they have always done business. If health care delivery were not subsidized by the U.S. government and employers, however, this type of attitude would result in health care providers going out of business. It makes little sense to support a system of health care delivery that waits for individuals to become ill before the system responds. The system should be preparing individuals to remain well and thus avoid illness. Instead, this system has successfully managed to avoid pressures to change the way health care is delivered—it is broken and refuses to allow any type of plan for repair.

The old system has failed to deliver cost-effective care for a number of years, and there is a real need to change the way we deliver health care services to Americans. Unfortunately, there are many who demand a shift to universal coverage, which would be funded, for the most part, by the government. But the government is already funding one-half of the health care bill with Medicare and Medicaid, and both of these programs are in financial trouble. It seems obvious that more government involvement in health care delivery is the last type of change needed.

Many health policy experts touted managed health care as a new model of health care delivery over twenty years ago, expecting that this new model would eliminate waste and reduce the costs associated with delivering health care to most Americans. In retrospect, this new model increased costs and in many instances reduced the quality of care. We cannot afford more incremental tinkering with the largest sector of our economy, especially by individuals who profit from the change whether it is successful or a complete failure. There is a need for both real discussion about how best to restructure the health care system and time to evaluate new models of health care delivery that could work.

The medical establishment in this country has always feared and resisted the words *innovation, change,* and *new ways of delivering health care.* Physicians developed the current model of health care delivery, and these same professionals are reluctant to give up their power to others—including other doctors and medical personnel—with respect to creating their own demand. Almost all businesses in this country have had to make changes in the way they do operate in order to survive. Health care has been the exception to the business model and impervious to business cycles because it is considered a necessity that we must have no matter what the cost.

It is not that those responsible for delivering health care do not know how to be innovative. Instead, they do not want to change the way they do business, and there are currently no incentives to change. Christensen et al. (2000) argue that the phenomenon of disruptive innovation would require health care organizations to look for ways to reduce the cost of care by making it easier for customers to access that care. But this type of change will also upset the way business is done, hence the resistance to innovation in health care delivery.

Those responsible for keeping the population healthy need to employ the new and inexpensive technology that has been shown to improve health in order to facilitate the delivery of health care to all parts of the country. This type of technology uses the Internet to share health education programs with large segments of the population at little or no cost. The old business model in health care was designed to help people return to wellness after they suffered illness. Once reimbursement for disease management and preventive care becomes widespread, the problem of access to health care will be lessened, because wellness will become the new business model for health care. Once we pay for wellness, those paying for health insurance will embrace and expand the new model.

There are many people working in health care who actually view technology as an enemy that is driving up health care costs. To these individuals, technology is a cost of doing business rather than a solution to the problems in our health care system. This is because of the way they define technology as an expense rather than an investment and their inability to see the secondary effects that usually result from the adoption of such new technology. For businesses in America, for example, new technology has the secondary effect of empowering consumers, once this technology becomes widespread and customers better understand it and become more comfortable in its use.

Another modification of the business model of health care delivery must be a change in the reimbursement process to a pay-for-performance model. The current system of reimbursement pays for input but does not even remotely correspond to health care outcomes. A large number of outcomes are very poor, including medical errors, wrong diagnoses, inappropriate testing and hospitalizations, and focusing scarce resources on curing diseases that cannot be cured. And, as discussed earlier, providers quite often get reimbursed for poor work, and then get reimbursed again for correcting their own mistakes.

Business models in most industries recognize the need for a company to regularly improve its product and delivery of services. Intense competition pressures businesses to innovate and pursue quality in order to survive and grow. These competitive incentives have never really been present in the health care industry, in which government regulations concerning the payment for health care delivery (for example, the implementation of prevention programs) usually prevent innovation and competition under the rationale that the health care system is somehow different from other business ventures. These regulations serve to protect the inefficient and discourage new ways of delivering health care.

Health care organizations need to look at continually making small changes rather than always considering the big changes, all while keeping a constant eye on the patient, or customer. Physicians' relationships with their patients are also a critical component in the new world of health care delivery. The doctor is still one of the most important players in delivering of quality health care in this country and must, therefore, assume a leadership role that will require better knowledge of all parts of the delivery process. New physicians also need to receive more training in preventive medicine while in medical school, along with continuing education in ways to keep individuals well.

Public Health as a Potential Solution to the Health Care Crisis in America

In his book *Hot, Flat, and Crowded,* Friedman (2008) discusses how a green revolution can renew America. He points out that when dealing with the new "energy-climate era" we need new tools, a new infrastructure, and new ways of collaborating to solve our environmental problems. We can apply Friedman's arguments to the case of the health care crisis our country faces. If public health departments choose to take the leadership role in helping America become healthy, they will need new tools, a new infrastructure, and, most important, a new way of collaborating with the various power players in the evolving health care system.

A primary goal of public health departments is to enhance the health in human communities and assure the conditions in which those communities can remain healthy (Holmes, 2009). Achievement of this goal would solve the bulk of the major problems found in our current health care system. However, although public health professionals have the expertise necessary to resolve these problems, the American health care system overall was never designed to prevent illness and promote wellness. Further, the patient—the consumer of health care services—has been given a passive role in maintaining his or her health status. The physician, who is more knowledgeable about the value of health services, has been assigned the responsibility of deciding what is needed to keep the patient healthy. The problem with this approach is that the patient has to know when to see the physician, which requires that patient to be educated about disease and how it can be prevented. Unfortunately, the patient has not been prepared to assume this role.

Public health departments are usually government-funded agencies that deal with the health of community populations rather than the health of the individual. Shi and Singh (2008) argue that public health has always been separated from medicine due to fear that the government will interfere with the delivery of health care. This is very unfortunate because collaboration between the public health and medical care systems could improve the health of the population. Both medicine and public health suffer from the legacy concept of thinking that their way of improving health is superior, and both have become very comfortable in how they go about their work. Both block change and continue to live on past accomplishments, with minimal success in solving our country's new health problems.

Our health care system has always undervalued prevention activities (Satcher, 2006). This point is supported by the fact that less than 3 percent of the money spent on health care in this country goes to population-based programs. It is interesting to note that many of the greatest gains in better health over the years have had very little to do with treating illness, resulting instead from health promotion programs that attempted to change the high-risk health behaviors of community populations. Such community-based health programs are usually developed and delivered to communities by public health agencies.

McGinnis (2006) argues that one of the most important issues in health care today is getting public health and medicine to form a real partnership. Physicians have struggled to consider anything other than treatment of disease as a logical way to deal with patients. Also, as these medical professionals have tended increasingly toward specialization, they have become further removed from the teachings of public health. At the same time, public health departments have been reluctant to engage with those delivering medical care, except for brief legal encounters over specific disease problems. These interactions have usually been power displays rather than collaborative efforts. Both the medical care system and the public health system share equal blame in this lack of unity to improve the health of the U.S. population. The disconnect between these two powerful forces must be replaced by cooperation in working toward goals that are larger than either one.

Chronic diseases are responsible for one-third of Americans' being disabled or experiencing severe limitations on daily living activities (Siegel and Lotenberg, 2006). Yet the vast majority of Americans do not even recognize these enormous health problems, and most individuals blame the aging process for disabilities and limitations in daily living rather than behavior-induced chronic diseases. Siegel and Lotenberg point out that even those working in public health are not well-equipped to deal with the challenges of addressing the multiple causes of chronic diseases, improving social and economic conditions, and reforming social policy. Nevertheless, they are the ones who are able to provide the leadership necessary to bring other community agencies together in a united effort to reduce the incidence of and complications from chronic diseases.

It is very difficult to see what public health departments do on a daily basis. If these agencies prevent disease from happening through their efforts, there is often nothing tangible that can support a claim to their effectiveness. And even if the accomplishment were to become visible, how would agencies be able to prove that their efforts were responsible for that success? It could have been caused by any number of random occurrences.

Satcher (2006) argues that the increasing epidemic of chronic diseases has triggered the escalation of health care costs and decreased the quality of life for many aging Americans. This former surgeon general offers a prescription for good health that requires no medication. Instead, he recommends moderate physical activity, a diet that includes fruits and vegetables, avoidance of toxins like tobacco and alcohol, and responsible sexual behavior.

There is a need for leaders in public health to take advantage of the opportunities present in the current health care crisis. The future of health care delivery in this country is being shaped, and if the public health sector wants a seat at the table, it is time to embrace these opportunities and assume a leadership role in the change process.

The solution to the chronic disease epidemic is not to be found in the medical care system or in public health departments (Bodenheimer et al., 2009).

This epidemic will require collaboration among health educators, schools, the media, and health care organizations to promote a culture that encourages the practice of healthy behaviors. This epidemic has provided the opportunity for public health departments to fill a leadership vacuum in order to contend with the culture of high-risk health behaviors that has grown in this country.

Public health departments are facing both opportunities and a threat as a result of the health care crisis. The opportunities are found in their ability to improve the health of the public. The threat lies in the demand for public health departments to provide more services with the same or fewer resources. This book is about how public health departments can respond to this need for public health leadership as our new health care system evolves over the next few years.

Summary

The American health care system costs too much, is not available to a very large number of citizens, and is failing to keep many Americans healthy. What is more, all of these problems are getting worse each year. Clearly there is a need for immediate change, or the best health care system in the world is going to self-destruct.

Because costs and access are dependent on population health, it would seem that the answers to these problems are found in preventing illness and reducing the complications from our current epidemic of chronic diseases. In order for this to happen, our health care system has to change, and begin to espouse more widely the public health approaches designed to keep the population healthy. This is not an easy task, but it can be done.

Practitioners from the medical care and public health systems must begin to form partnerships. This will require leadership from both sectors in order to move beyond distrust to collaboration in order to develop programs to keep people healthy rather than attempting to cure them after they have become ill.

New incentives are necessary to get the major contributors to the health care crisis—insurance companies, employers, the government, health care organizations, and consumers—working together. Once again, this is going to require leadership rather than management of scarce health resources. Further, the leadership effort must begin with those organizations that have successfully used public health skills in the past to prevent high-risk health behaviors. It is time to change from a curative model to a prevention model of health care delivery in this country.

There are two major problems in moving prevention programs to the forefront. The first is that of how to market the prevention success stories to those making health care expenditure decisions in this country. The second involves determining how to eradicate the legacy concept in public health departments. The elimination of these problems requires the emergence and subsequent development of leadership in the U.S. public health system.

Key Terms

Access

Adverse selection

Cost

Health insurance

Health levels

Moral hazard

Discussion Questions

1. Discuss the many causes of the fragmentation of the health care system in the United States.
2. Explain the difficulty associated with the epidemic of chronic diseases and their complications.
3. How can the members of the public and their legislative representatives be made to appreciate the value of prevention in dealing with the health care crisis in the United States?
4. Why is this country failing in its efforts to reform the health care system?

CHAPTER 4

APPLICATION OF EPIDEMIOLOGICAL CONCEPTS TO HEALTH CARE DELIVERY

LEARNING OBJECTIVES

- Comprehend the major uses of epidemiology in the restructuring of the health care delivery system
- Become aware of the value of epidemiology as an adjunct to making medical decisions
- Understand the value of information management in the improvement of health outcomes
- Recognize the use of epidemiology in determining best practices in health care delivery

Epidemiology has been part of both medicine and public health since the first recorded outbreak of disease. Epidemiologists examine the health of the population, not the health of the individual—a practice often referred to as population-based medicine. Epidemiology has served public health departments well over the years by helping solve many of the mysteries surrounding the causation of morbidity and mortality associated with communicable and noncommunicable diseases. The principles of epidemiology are now being applied more widely for use in medical decision making, and should be particularly helpful as we reorganize the health care system. A very important piece of the new world of public health is going to be the expanded use of epidemiological tools to investigate the problems inherent in combating complicated chronic diseases and implementing evidence-based prevention programs.

Hippocrates, who lived between 460 and 377 BCE, probably made the first use of epidemiology when he recorded outbreaks of such communicable diseases as plague, cholera, and dysentery. As the science and art of epidemiology grew in stature and understanding, its many possibilities in the scientific field also expanded. In recent years those working in health care management positions have used epidemiology to solve many managerial and marketing problems. Its important place in medical decision making is evident in that it has become a vital component of the graduate curriculum in health care administration programs around the world.

Epidemiology is a sound method of data gathering and investigation that employs statistical techniques to evaluate hypotheses concerning the causation of any given disease or health problem (Merrill and Timmreck, 2006). Investigators, or medical researchers, frequently use the epidemiology of chronic diseases, injuries, environmental and occupational exposures, and personal behaviors. There is no reason why the science of epidemiology cannot be expanded for use in offering solutions to many of the major problems found in our current health care system. Merrill and Timmreck (2006) further define epidemiology as the study of the determinants, distribution, and frequency of disease.

Like a detective methodically solving a crime, the epidemiologist attempts to understand a disease by determining the various causative factors. Detectives work with motives, circumstances, and profiling of the victim and the criminal; epidemiologists analyze the disease, injury, or other health problem, and profile the victims and circumstances—the environments, habits, and motivations for healthy or unhealthy lifestyles. Epidemiologists evaluate ill and well individuals in an attempt to find the reasons some people become ill and others do not. They usually begin this type of investigation by gathering data from ill and well individuals through surveys. They then attempt to uncover the determinants of the disease, and document locations and numbers of old and new cases. The data investigators gather from potentially exposed sick and well individuals allows them to develop a rough hypothesis to explain the causes of the problem.

The epidemiologist now begins building a **case definition,** which includes standardized criteria for determining whether a person has a disease or other health-related condition (Turnock, 2007). This case definition also incorporates clinical and personal qualities of the health event under investigation, eventually becoming the problem statement applied to that health event. Health care managers can also use this tool when gathering other types of health data that will help improve our health care system.

An epidemiological study can also be the starting point for a plan to control and prevent occupational injuries and disease. The first thing epidemiologists would need would be a well-defined case definition for each of the possible health hazards found in the various businesses throughout the United States. This would allow them to label health events according to location, time, and person, lending a degree of standardization to the process of investigation.

A good understanding of the principles of epidemiology can be beneficial to managers in all facets of health care management. It is really a science of decision making that is very useful for anyone faced with clinical or managerial responsibilities in health care.

Descriptive Epidemiology

The field of **descriptive epidemiology** involves the characterization of events such that investigators can explore common traits exhibited by those who are ill. By describing health problems according to time, place, and person, the epidemiologist is better able to communicate those problems in terms that can be understood by all (Merrill and Timmreck, 2006). Therefore, descriptive epidemiology allows public health departments to determine who is at risk of developing a particular health issue, enabling agencies to evaluate the proposed method of preventing that adverse health outcome. It is the most basic form of epidemiology, but it has great value when beginning to investigate a health event. The individual using descriptive epidemiology simply describes what happened in a way that makes sense of the available data, helping to offer a possible explanation of phenomena. This form of epidemiology is useful for evaluating any problem, not just an outbreak of disease.

Exhibit 4.1 is a list of diseases whose appearance must be reported to the Pennsylvania Department of Health. According to state law, medical facilities and physicians who examine and treat patients have to report these diseases whenever they encounter them. Efforts by this and other public health departments to deal with communicable diseases have as their goal the treatment of infected individuals and the discovery of new cases of disease in order to reduce the incidence of disease and protect communities from an epidemic. Through thorough investigation, epidemiologists and public health professionals are able to trace the step-by-step process of a disease's development.

The epidemiologist operates using a concept called the **chain of infection** to explain how disease is transmitted from an infected individual to someone who is not infected. It is a time-tested method used to solve medical problems with no known cause. Figure 4.1 shows the chain of infection for disease. A disease usually

FIGURE 4.1   Chain of Infection for Disease

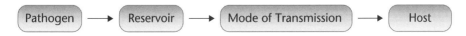

Source: Healey and Walker, 2009, p. 29.

EXHIBIT 4.1
LIST OF REPORTABLE DISEASES

1. **AIDS** (Acquired Immune Deficiency Syndrome) **$**

2. **Amebiasis**

3. **Animal bite #**

4. **Anthrax #**

5. **An unusual cluster of isolates**

6. **Arboviruses** (includes Colorado tick fever, Crimean-Congo hemorrhagic fever, dengue, Eastern equine encephalitis, St. Louis encephalitis, West Nile virus infection, Yellow fever, et al.) **#**

7. **Botulism** (All forms) **#**

8. **Brucellosis**

9. **Campylobacteriosis**

10. **Cancer** ^

11. **CD4 T-lymphocyte test result with a count <200 cells/microliter, or a CD4 T-lymphocyte % of <14% of total lymphocytes $**

12. **Chancroid**

13. **Chickenpox** (*Varicella*) (Effective 1/26/05)

14. ***Chlamydia trachomatis*** infections

15. **Cholera #**

16. **Congenital adrenal hyperplasia** (CAH) (<5y/old)

17. **Creutzfeldt-Jakob Disease**

18. **Cryptosporidiosis**

19. **Diphtheria #**

20. **Encephalitis** (all types)

21. **Enterohemorrhagic *E. coli* # ***

22. **Food poisoning outbreak #**

23. **Giardiasis**

24. **Gonococcal infections**

25. **Granuloma inguinale**

26. **Guillain-Barre syndrome**

27. *Haemophilus influenzae* **invasive disease # ***

28. **Hantavirus pulmonary syndrome #**

29. **Hemorrhagic fever #**

30. **Hepatitis, viral, acute and chronic cases**

31. **Histoplasmosis**

32. **HIV $**

33. **Influenza** (laboratory-confirmed only)

34. **Lead poisoning #**

35. **Legionellosis #**

36. **Leprosy** (Hansen's Disease)

37. **Leptospirosis**

38. **Listeriosis**

39. **Lyme disease**

40. *Lymphogranuloma venereum*

41. **Malaria**

42. **Maple syrup urine disease** (MSUD) (<5y/old)

43. **Measles** (Rubeola) #

44. **Meningitis** (all types—not limited to invasive *Haemophilus influenzae* or *Neisseria meningitidis*)

45. **Meningococcal invasive disease # ***

46. **Mumps**

47. **Perinatal exposure of a newborn to HIV**

48. **Pertussis** (whooping cough)

49. **Phenylketonuria** (PKU) (<5y/old)

50. **Plague #**

51. **Poliomyelitis #**

52. **Primary congenital hypothyroidism** (<5y/old)

53. **Psittacosis** (ornithosis)

54. **Rabies #**

55. **Respiratory syncytial virus**

56. **Rickettsial diseases/infections** (includes Rocky Mountain Spotted Fever, Q fever, rickettsialpox, typhus, Ehrlichiosis)

57. **Rubella** (German measles) and congenital rubella syndrome

58. **Salmonellosis ***

59. **Severe Acute Respiratory Syndrome (SARS) #**

60. **Shigellosis ***

61. **Sickle cell hemoglobinopathies** (<5y/old)

62. **Smallpox #**

63. *Staphylococcal aureus*, **Vancomycin Resistant** (VRSA) or Intermediate (VISA) invasive disease

64. **Streptococcal invasive disease** (Group A)

65. *Streptococcus pneumoniae*, drug resistant invasive disease

66. **Syphilis** (all stages)

67. **Tetanus**

68. **Toxic shock syndrome**

69. **Toxoplasmosis**

70. **Trichinosis**

71. **Tuberculosis**, suspected or confirmed active disease (all sites) including the results of drug susceptibility testing

72. **Tularemia**

73. **Typhoid fever #**

For health care practitioners and health care facilities, all diseases are reportable within 5 workdays, unless otherwise noted.

\#   Health care practitioners and health care facilities must report within 24 hours.

> For clinical laboratories, all diseases are reportable by next workday, unless otherwise noted.
>
> $ Clinical laboratories must report within 5 days of obtaining the test result.
>
> * In addition to reporting, clinical laboratories must also submit isolates to the state laboratory within 5 workdays of isolation.
>
> ˆ Hospitals, clinical laboratories, and health care facilities must report within 180 days.
>
> *Source:* Pennsylvania Department of Health. (PA Code, Title 28, Chapter 27 | Updates 1 & 2 requiring electronic reporting.)

follows a step-by-step process, from infection to the manifestation of the signs and symptoms that become present with communicable and most chronic diseases. Documenting this process helps public health departments better understand how a disease develops and spreads from person to person.

The investigation of a disease also enhances our understanding of its major components, better known as the **triad of disease:** agent, host, and environment (see Figure 4.2). It is the intersection of these three factors that usually leads to the occurrence of disease. The agent is the cause of the disease, the host is where the agent lives, and the environment surrounds the host.

The starting point in the investigation of any problem is an observational study (Webb, Bain, and Pirozzo, 2005). In this type of study the investigator does not intervene in the problem being explored, but merely observes and records what is happening. Such observational studies can further be classified as either descriptive or analytical. Those using descriptive epidemiology are looking for common patterns of disease or other health problems.

One of the most famous uses of descriptive epidemiology occurred in 1854 during a London cholera epidemic. John Snow, a physician, used epidemiological techniques to observe the spread of cholera through the water supply coming from a water pump located on Broad Street. Prompted by knowledge acquired during his prior years of observing and describing the transmission of cholera through contaminated water, Snow surveyed households of cholera victims and traced their water supply to one of the town's three wells. Once the suspect well was closed at his urging, the illness in the town ended. This is one of many instances of the successful use of epidemiology to suppress an outbreak of a communicable disease.

FIGURE 4.2   Triad of Disease

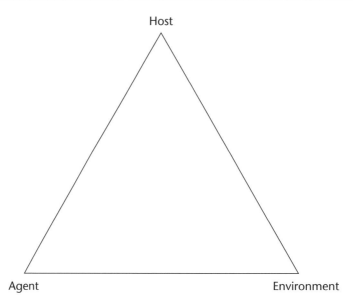

Source: U.S. Department of Health and Human Services, CDC (2010).

Once descriptive epidemiology is completed there are several types of studies that can help prove causation in epidemiological investigations, many of which are conducted in order to follow up on associations that are suspected during the practice of descriptive epidemiology. Merrill and Timmreck (2006) maintain that randomized controlled trials are the most scientifically rigorous. These are experimental studies and usually fall at the end of a sequence of less-demanding and less-costly studies, which have already helped investigators develop a hypothesis about causation that will usually require more work to prove. These studies are very complex and expensive in their development, implementation, and evaluation. Therefore, descriptive epidemiology is usually the best starting point for investigating any health problem.

A case control study involves looking at retrospective data on both cases and controls in an attempt to determine the cause of the event under observation. According to Christoffel and Gallagher (2006), the case control study allows investigators to perform an odds ratio—a representation of the odds in favor of individuals' incurring a disease or injury when an associated factor is present.

An outbreak of a communicable disease has always been a serious concern for communities in this country. A communicable disease, also called a contagious or infectious disease, is capable of being transmitted rapidly from one person to another as well as from contaminated foods or water. Communicable diseases have been around since the beginning of time, and although their incidence has declined, they still are capable of causing panic in communities, schools, or workplaces.

Using descriptive epidemiology is a very rapid way to determine the criteria for cases and then select experimental controls from the pool of individuals who remained well after exposure, and discover the cause responsible for the outbreak of illness. Once the cause of the health problem is determined using epidemiological principles, control measures can be implemented to stop the problem. For example, frightening outbreaks of typhoid fever, cholera, and influenza have become more infrequent thanks to clean water, better personal hygiene, and the united efforts of environmental and public health specialists dedicated to controlling these past killers.

The success in controlling most communicable disease outbreaks has resulted in a relaxed attitude concerning the possibility that these diseases could ever return. One the one hand, we must remember that although most of these pathogens are under control, they have not been destroyed. In fact, only one communicable disease, smallpox, has actually been eliminated, despite the best efforts of public health professionals. On the other hand, descriptive epidemiology allows us to better evaluate any problem—new or old—and look for clues as to why the problem exists and what its solution might be.

Epidemiology of Communicable Diseases

As we have already noted, the epidemiology of communicable diseases has been studied since ancient times. Hippocrates, in an essay titled "On Airs, Waters and Places," actually suggested that environmental and host factors were at the root of many diseases. Scientists have always been interested in how disease agents are spread from one person to another. McKenzie, Pinger, and Kotecki (2005) define communicable diseases as those caused by biological agents and spread to others, usually in a short period of time.

It bears mention that a number of diseases that are spread from person to person can also be classified as chronic diseases if they remain for a long period of time, as does tuberculosis. They can be acquired from another person, but can last for a long period of time. The best examples of such chronic and communicable diseases are acquired immune deficiency syndrome (AIDS) and tuberculosis (TB). AIDS is caused by the human immunodeficiency virus (HIV), which is spread from person to person by certain high-risk behaviors. It is considered a chronic disease, because once infected there is no cure, and the infected person will probably live for many years with the disease before he or she dies. Similarly, TB is caused by a bacterium that is spread from person to person; it becomes a chronic disease as time passes, and remains with the infected for an extended period.

The acute diseases that are easily transmitted from one person to another represent a serious threat to individuals in the workplace. The threat may include the dangers of illness and perhaps death, not only for the worker but also for family members, should that worker bring the disease home. The threat also manifests itself in a fear of the unknown, because communicable disease occurrence is a very rare happening, and nonmedical people often do not know the full extent of what exposure to a communicable disease means.

An agent is the catalyst that must be present for a disease to occur. If the agent can be eliminated, the disease usually caused by the agent will not appear. For example, poultry products quite often are contaminated by salmonella, a bacterium. If the contaminated poultry is cooked at the right temperature for the appropriate amount of time, then the agent is destroyed and no one consuming the product will also consume salmonella. This agent must be present for a disease to appear. Many such agents are well-known and occur on a frequent basis among individuals. Most people have heard of bacteria, viruses, and even protozoan parasites. Unfortunately, most people are unaware that these agents can be deadly, and also that they can be spread to others very easily under the right circumstances.

Public health departments are responsible for controlling outbreaks of disease caused by these agents. In fact, communicable disease control programs have always been a mandated public health function in all health departments throughout the country. The word *control* has been used in association with these agents because they have never been eliminated. They may be transmitted in different ways, their incidence may remain low, but they are always present and capable of causing large outbreaks of illness that can terrorize a community.

Communicable diseases are spread in a very specific way that epidemiologists and other medical personnel have studied for hundreds of years (McKenzie, Pinger, and Kotecki, 2005). Research into the chain of infection for various illnesses has been useful in developing an information base concerning the majority of infectious diseases that occur frequently throughout the world. Public health epidemiologists who investigate outbreaks of infectious diseases complete reports of their investigations and share them with other health agencies and the medical community. The *Morbidity and Mortality Weekly Report* (*MMWR*) offers up-to-date information on outbreaks of communicable diseases in reports written by disease investigators, helping medical personnel and public health professionals better understand how infectious diseases are spread from one person to another.

If any piece of the chain of infection is broken, the disease in question is stopped from spreading to a new host. This has been the case with vaccine-preventable diseases. If an individual is properly immunized and then exposed to the disease, there is no infection because the exposed individual is no longer susceptible to that particular disease.

The mode of transmission is the way an infectious agent travels from an infected person to a new person who is currently not ill. The route of transmission can be either direct or indirect. **Direct transmission** involves immediate transmission of an infectious agent to a new host, whereas indirect transmission may involve the air, a vehicle, or a vector (McKenzie, Pinger, and Kotecki, 2005). **Indirect transmission** usually involves an inanimate object, or fomite, is not immediate, and causes a panic situation among individuals who believe they may have been exposed.

Epidemiology of Emerging Infections

The resistance of some pathogens to antibiotics and the importation of diseases into this country from around the world have produced new and emerging communicable disease threats. Satcher (2006) argues that infectious diseases maintain a large reservoir of agents that are always available to create epidemics under the right conditions. Recent large outbreaks of infectious diseases like tuberculosis in this country underscore how easy it is to have an epidemic if public health professionals do not remain vigilant about the threat of disease. As discussed in the previous section, many infectious diseases, although they are currently under control, remain capable of reemerging as major health threats to the United States and the world.

One example illustrating the serious nature of these infectious diseases occurred in Milwaukee, Wisconsin, in 1993. Contamination of the water supply in this city resulted in an outbreak of cryptosporidiosis that affected an estimated four hundred thousand people, resulting in over four thousand requiring hospitalization. On a broader scale, TB reemerged in the United States in the 1980s as a formidable disease threat, especially in cases of drug-resistant strains. E. coli has also become a major threat to the public in recent years. Finally, pneumonia and influenza cause tremendous morbidity and mortality every year, and mutations of the influenza virus—like avian flu and swine flu (H1N1)—pose the threat of worldwide pandemics of disease capable of reaching this country and killing thousands.

The epidemiological approach has over time been employed to investigate chronic diseases that are noncommunicable; have long incubation periods; and have no cure once developed, usually resulting in serious and costly complications. Many of the chronic diseases are the result of practicing poor health behaviors like using tobacco, maintaining a sedentary lifestyle, and having a poor diet. The major reason for our escalating costs in health care in this country involves an epidemic of chronic diseases that require prevention, not a cure.

Analytical Epidemiology

Moving beyond descriptive epidemiology, investigators use the techniques of **analytical epidemiology** in an attempt to prove the cause of a given health event (Webb, Bain, and Pirozzo, 2005). Proving causation is the major objective of analytical epidemiological studies. Rothman and Greenland (2005) argue that the ability to make causal inferences is self-taught, and that we learn about causation at a very early age through our own life experiences. For example, when we are young we learn that certain behaviors are praised whereas others are not. These authors then define the differences between sufficient and component causes of an occurrence. A cause, in general, is a condition that was necessary for a certain outcome, in this case a health problem. A sufficient cause is an event that by itself can cause an outcome. A component cause is one of several events that must occur in some order to lead to an outcome. The strength of the causal relationship, if high, usually offers an incentive for more researchers to study the cause or causes. The result repeated through several well-run studies offers stronger support to their final determination of the root of the health problem.

Analytical epidemiology involves using data to test hypotheses (Merrill and Timmreck, 2006). Analytical epidemiologists, for example, make comparisons between those with a disease or condition and those without the disease or condition, who had previously been identified through the use of descriptive epidemiology, quantifying associations of variables being observed and determining the cause or causes of the given problem. An analytical epidemiologist uses a comparison group to test the strength of the association between exposure and a disease variable.

Figure 4.3 shows an example of a matrix that displays study outcomes and is very useful in analytical epidemiological studies. (This matrix compares using tobacco and not using tobacco.) This table incorporates cases and controls who were either exposed or not exposed to the variable under study. A very good example of the use of analytical epidemiology is seen in a study conducted by Doll and Hill (1950) that implicated the use of tobacco in the development of a rare form of cancer at that time, lung cancer. This landmark study paved the way for additional chronic disease studies that linked secondhand smoke to the same deadly form of cancer. Tobacco became identified as the leading cause of death

FIGURE 4.3   Sample Matrix Displaying Study Outcomes

	Cases	Controls
Exposed	A (90)	B (40)
Unexposed	C (10)	D (60)

A = Number of persons with disease and exposure of interest.
B = Number of persons without disease but with exposure of interest.
C = Number of persons with disease but without exposure of interest.
D = Number of persons without disease and without exposure of interest.

Source: U.S. Department of Health and Human Services, CDC (2010).

for 430,000 Americans every year (Centers for Disease Control and Prevention [CDC], 2008d). Secondhand smoke was also found to be a cause of over 80,000 additional deaths from lung cancer. This association has been very visible for a number of years, and epidemiologists have described it thoroughly in the medical literature. The maturing principles of epidemiology can now be applied in the investigation of other chronic diseases in this country, with the goal of preventing of these chronic diseases and their complications.

After Doll and Hill's study (1950), it seemed like a natural follow-up to start using epidemiology to evaluate high-risk health behaviors as potential causes of other chronic diseases. The Framingham Heart Study, beginning in 1948 in the town of Framingham, Massachusetts, did just that. This cohort study involved 5,209 men and women between the ages of thirty and sixty-two who were initially free of coronary heart disease (CHD). The study followed residents of this town for over fifty years in order to discover how people develop heart disease.

Turnock (2007) refers to the twenty-eight thousand residents of Framingham who volunteered for this first longitudinal study of heart disease as having given a gift to this country. This study evaluated the effects of blood pressure, blood triglyceride and cholesterol levels, age, gender, and psychosocial issues on the development of CHD. The Framingham study was instrumental in helping to define the term *risk factor* as it relates to heart health.

This study revealed that by changing a few health behaviors—for example, by quitting smoking, maintaining a better diet, losing weight, and being physically active—one can reduce the chance of developing heart disease. The success of this study signaled that epidemiology was moving rapidly into the important and complex area of chronic disease causation. Epidemiology was now ready to deal with diseases with very long incubation periods and no visible starting point. As a consequence, the epidemiology of chronic diseases was now becoming a crucial part of public health departments in the United States.

One of the most feared words in the epidemiologist's dictionary is *epidemic*. This much-abused term simply indicates more cases of a certain disease than one would normally expect. The word *epidemic* can be used in the context of communicable and chronic diseases, injuries, and environmental and occupational health problems. Rowitz (2006) classifies an epidemic according to "the level of contagiousness, small facts or events that have large and long-lasting consequences, and how to prevent additional cases which can occur suddenly or at a dramatic moment." Examples of epidemics are all around us on a daily basis. The city of New York is suffering from an epidemic of diabetes, the nation has prepared for an H1N1 pandemic, women are experiencing an epidemic of heart disease, and some occupations are undergoing an epidemic of homicides. All four of these epidemics can be prevented with the help of public health expertise.

The epidemiologist has many tools that are helpful in determining the cause of an outbreak of disease. One of the most important tools an epidemiologist uses in an investigation is a rate. In fact, it is noted by those in public health that what separates epidemiologists from other scientists is their comparison of rates in order to develop and test a hypothesis. A rate is a measure of some event, condition, disease, injury, or illness in relation to a unit of population during some specific time period.

It makes it much easier to compare health events if the population exposed and infected is taken into consideration. The rate of illness, disease, or injury is easier to comprehend if evaluated in terms of some type of morbidity rate. A morbidity rate is the rate of a given illness in a certain location during a certain period of time. A comparison of the causes of death makes more sense if the health event is evaluated in terms of mortality rate. Many of these rates are used when describing health events in the workplace.

Epidemiologists use many other rates in making comparisons within communities. The incidence rate, for example, is useful in a short-term evaluation of a developing epidemic of some type of illness. This rate is a calculation of the number of new cases of some illness over a short period of time. Further, the prevalence rate is a measurement of disease over a longer period of time, such as a year. The rates most important to an epidemiologist when investigating a disease or other illness are the incidence rate, prevalence rate, and attack rate.

Epidemiology and the Centers for Disease Control and Prevention

The Centers for Disease Control and Prevention (CDC), headquartered in Atlanta, Georgia, employs over eight thousand health professionals, who are involved in health surveillance designed to monitor and prevent disease. The CDC is also responsible for the preparation and distribution of health statistics for the nation. This federal agency develops sophisticated epidemiology systems and provides training and certification programs for those employed as epidemiologists in the United States and several other countries throughout the world.

The founder of the use of epidemiology at the CDC was Alexander Langmuir in 1949. He was the main epidemiologist for the CDC for over twenty years, and helped to develop the *Morbidity and Mortality Weekly Report* (*MMWR*), which is responsible for reporting regularly on disease prevalence and current outbreaks (CDC, 2009b). This agency was a descendant of the wartime agency Malaria Control in War Areas, and its original focus was on the effort to fight malaria by killing mosquitoes. The initial budget was under $10 million, but over the next fifty-plus years the CDC developed into the nation's premier health promotion, prevention, and preparedness agency and a global leader in public health. It is the world leader in health data management and expertise in epidemiology.

Data Management

Data management is the collection and analysis of information and the sharing of data with multiple audiences. Aschengrau and Seage (2003) point out that a great deal of information is available concerning diseases, injuries, disabilities, and mortality, much of which it is the responsibility of public health departments to manage and disseminate in order to the improve the health of various populations—such as those of cities, counties, and states—rather than individual patients. According to Webb et al. (2005), a very large part of public health practice is acquiring and disseminating information about a community in order to better understand the overall health of the group being studied or evaluated. Many of the health data are gathered and analyzed using the principles of epidemiology. Such data management has always been a required function of public health departments at the federal, state, and local levels.

Morbidity represents the incidence or prevalence of disease in a given population during a specified period of time. As discussed earlier in the context of rates, the incidence of disease is the number of new reports of disease, whereas prevalence usually refers to the number of reports of disease over a longer period of time. These data are available from physicians and laboratories, and federal and state law supports the right and obligation of public health departments to receive reports of certain diseases when they occur. Local or state public health departments then report these diseases to the CDC. The sheer volume of these data is enormous, but the information needs to be gathered and analyzed in a systematic way. These morbidity data were made reportable in 1878 when the U.S. Marine Hospital Service was ordered to collect reports on certain diseases that could easily be spread from person to person.

The term *mortality* refers to the deaths that occur during a given period of time. A pioneer in the gathering and reporting of mortality data was the seventeenth-century English epidemiologist John Graunt. He published the *Bills of Mortality* in 1662, which was a weekly count of deaths in London. The reporting of these data allowed him to categorize deaths according to their cause.

Public health data can be invaluable in completing a community health assessment, which usually includes the health data for a given population (Novick, Morrow, and Mays, 2008). The CDC is a major source of all types of data, many of which can help in the evaluation of preventive measures. These include health outcome data, risk factor data, and resource data.

Health Outcome Data

Outcome data are used to measure the presence or absence of health events (CDC, 1995). These data can be indicators of health status, and include death certificates and birth certificates that local health departments have issued. Such data can be used to evaluate the health of a local population, and they enable epidemiologists to look for clues as to the sources of particular health problems.

Risk Factor Data

According to Turnock (2009), risk factors include biological, environmental, lifestyle, and psychosocial elements, as well as the failure to use health-related services. These risk factors have been associated with diseases and certain adverse health outcomes. There is an enormous amount of secondary data available on the many factors that can predispose one to poor health. There are also ongoing epidemiological studies that provide new primary data on the extent of dangerous health practices.

Resource Data

Resource data inform communities of the health resources that are available to them for the prevention or treatment of disease. These include hospitals, physicians, clinics, and various other health care resources. Such data are very useful for public health planning purposes, including emergency preparedness.

Surveillance Systems

Public health surveillance encompasses data collection for infectious and chronic diseases, injuries, environmental and occupational exposures, and personal behaviors that may contribute to the development of illness (CDC, 2009b). The techniques used in public health surveillance are not disease-specific, but can instead be applied to surveillance data concerning a variety of health conditions, exposures, and behaviors within a community. Public health surveillance is based on a very simple premise: understanding the problem is essential to solving it. Surveillance is the ongoing, systematic collection, analysis, and interpretation of health data integral to the planning, implementation, and evaluation of public health practice; it is closely integrated with the timely dissemination of these data to those who need to know.

Analysis of surveillance data often begins by summarizing them according to event or problem, person, place, and time. That is, it is a process of looking for patterns of disease or health outcomes among different groups, in different places, at different times. Identifying who got sick, where they went prior to and during illness, and when and for what duration they were sick yields valuable information about the types of disease control and prevention efforts that are needed and who should be targeted in order to most efficiently limit or prevent the spread of disease.

Looking for trends in surveillance data focused on health promotion and disease prevention behaviors is as important as focusing on the occurrences themselves. For example, knowing about patterns of vaccination coverage helps us understand why cases of vaccine-preventable diseases are declining, and patterns of caloric intake and physical inactivity help explain changing trends in the incidence of obesity and the subsequent increase in cases of type 2 diabetes.

The epidemiological concept of the triad of disease—agent, host, and environment—is extremely useful in explaining how diseases and injuries happen. It provides a starting point to begin viewing any health problem or issue. Researchers are now able to consider the reasons why a health problem might occur, and can move to a strategy focused on prevention rather than on finding a cure.

The process of surveillance starts with a statement of the health problem for which data are being gathered. The problem in question can relate to disease, injury, environmental contamination, or anything that researchers want to investigate. Problem statements have even been used successfully in solving marketing and management dilemmas. It is crucial to define the real problem, and not symptoms of a larger problem.

The second step in surveillance involves risk factor identification, or finding out the cause of the problem. The risk factor might be bacteria, a virus, secondhand cigarette smoke, obesity, or faulty machinery in the workplace. The techniques of epidemiology have given our country significant success in determining the cause or causes of many health problems.

The third step in the surveillance process is to find out what works to solve the problem under consideration. The best way to do this is to look at a number of potential solutions and conduct a cost-benefit analysis to find the one with the greatest chance of success at the lowest cost in terms of resource use. This step forces researchers to make a value judgment about various options for solving health problems while also considering the costs associated with their decision.

The final step in surveillance is the implementation of the system. Should it be an active or a passive surveillance system? A passive system would require researchers to alert the sources of their data, such as physicians and hospital laboratories, that they are interested in monitoring their data and are requesting their cooperation in the process. The assumption is that if these data sources see the data the researchers have requested, those researchers will be informed. Alternately, an active system would require researchers to alert the sources of data that they will be in contact at a prescribed time each week to ensure a timely reporting process. The active system works best when researchers are expecting the possibility of an epidemic, and this type of surveillance system is used every year during flu season.

Consider that in 1900 the leading killer was a communicable disease (tuberculosis), compared to 2010, when the leading killer was a disease often caused by avoidable health behaviors (heart disease). McGinnis and Foege (1993) took these data one step further and determined that the real causes of the disease are tobacco use, a poor diet, weight gain, and physical inactivity. With this revelation, the country was ready to use epidemiology to develop health promotion programs to educate people to prevent chronic diseases. It is interesting to note that life expectancy in 1900 was only forty-nine years of age, which has now increased by almost thirty years. This increase in life expectancy is not due to better medical care; it is the result of a better understanding of how disease occurs and how to prevent it. Thanks to this information concerning the real causes of disease, many in health care have started to look toward the idea of primary care that focuses on the prevention of illness and disease.

Epidemic Intelligence Service

The Epidemic Intelligence Service (EIS) is headquartered at the national Centers for Disease Control and Prevention. It is a two-year postgraduate program of service and instruction for physicians and other health professionals who are interested in receiving on-the-job training in epidemiology. After being trained in epidemiology, these medical officers are then assigned locations throughout the country for conducting epidemiological investigations, research, and public health surveillance. They are typically assigned to state health departments for a two-year assignment.

Epi-X

Epi-X is the CDC's Web-based communication system, which is available to most public health professionals. The system is used by CDC officials, state and local health departments, poison control centers, and other public health workers in order to communicate preliminary surveillance health information on a daily basis. Recipients of this information have been approved by the federal government, and have installed a secure certificate for their computer.

Managerial Epidemiology

The Affordable Care Act passed by Congress and signed into law by President Obama in 2010 is in part an attempt to reduce health care costs by billions of dollars over the next several years. In order to attain these cost reductions, there is going to be a greater demand for efficiency from health care facilities and their managers. This will be accomplished through the use of comparative effectiveness research (CER), the findings from which will require better decision making by those in charge of health care delivery decisions. CER will subject many clinical procedures to rigorous evaluation to determine whether or not they are worth the cost, and if these procedures place the patient at unnecessary risk.

CER is one of the most promising parts of the new health care reform law, but it is going to change the way health care is delivered in this country. Nussbaum, Tirrell, Wechsler, and Randall (2010) point out that part of the new health care reform legislation includes an appropriation of $500 million more a year for the evaluation of medical services. This should reduce the costs of wasteful medical tests and procedures, producing $700 billion in annual savings every year. This process represents an attempt to control runaway health care costs through the elimination of waste, without reducing the quality of care.

CER represents an intense evaluation of different treatment options for a given medical condition. Weinstein and Skinner (2010) argue that CER offers a potential solution to the escalation in the costs of delivering health care in this country. What is more, the vast majority of countries that have reformed their health care system have included some form of CER in their final product

(Mushlin and Ghomrawi, 2010). They have done so to protect patients from harm while attempting to simultaneously improve the quality of care and reduce health care costs. This law will produce an even greater demand for a new type of health care management.

This new emphasis an accountability in health care is an attempt to eliminate what has long been called "flat of the curve" medicine. This concept, made popular by economist Alain Enthoven (1978), suggests that as we continue to increase medical inputs in an episode of medical care, there will be successively smaller increases in medical output or value from the input. This does not imply that there is no benefit in completing additional medical tests and procedures, but that these additional inputs probably cost more than they are worth. They also may be dangerous for the individual, despite adding little if any value. Therefore, the concept of "flat of the curve" medicine underscores the need for vigorous evaluation of all inputs in the delivery of health care services. Public health program managers will bear this concept in mind when deciding how to eliminate the ever-growing list of threats to the public's health.

Looking to the science of epidemiology can offer managers of public health programs a better chance of success when making medical decisions and seeking to implement these effectively. **Managerial epidemiology** is a science to be practiced in the decision-making process concerning how best to make use of scarce health resources (Fleming, 2008). Managerial epidemiology can be highly useful, not only in gathering the requisite data to manage the outcomes associated with particular health care interventions but also in improving the functions of management that are most important for public health leaders and their program managers, including planning, finance, assessment of quality issues, and evidence-based public health practice.

Fleming (2008) argues that the planning function has a critical bearing on all of the management functions, and is by far one of the most important components of the changing health care system. Planning establishes the action steps that should be followed in order to achieve a successful outcome. Using the tools of managerial epidemiology should help those responsible for planning do a much better job at gathering the data necessary for making thoughtful decisions about how to distribute scarce resources. Managers could, for example, explore the descriptive epidemiological data in order to better frame the problems their agency encounters. They could then use the tools of analytical epidemiology to look for statistical relationships among the various data sets. This will allow more accurate predictions of outcomes resulting from medical interventions. A very good example of the use of managerial epidemiology is found in the development, implementation, and evaluation of community health planning found in the series of Healthy People reports, completed by the Department of Health and Human Services, each of which was developed and used for a ten-year time period.

It is obvious that managerial epidemiology can help leaders and managers work with the guidelines and procedures of evidence-based public health practice. This will enable public health departments to use epidemiological techniques in evaluating their interventions and sharing the success stories with other community health facilities. In fact, managerial epidemiology will allow these departments to continually develop and share best practices in disease prevention efforts with the entire health care system. This allows the application of evidence derived from observational and experimental studies to medical decision making.

Fleming (2008) argues that preventive medicine is not practiced as often as necessary in order to improve population health, probably because of the lack of appropriate information systems. Managerial epidemiology may very well be the missing component required to bring evidence-based preventive medicine into widespread use among the majority of individuals who work in health care and who have responsibility for the use of scarce health care resources. Health reform efforts that include the expansion of proven preventive programs may have the ability to reduce health care costs while maintaining the quality of health care delivery.

Application of Epidemiological Concepts to Health Care

The health care system is well on its way to developing best practices that will be part of an overall shift toward evidence-based approaches in medicine and public health. The tools of epidemiology can be extremely powerful in helping reform the way health care is delivered in the United States. Sophisticated surveillance systems, community assessment techniques, descriptive epidemiology, analytical epidemiology, and managerial epidemiology are scientific concepts that public health departments must share with the rest of the health care system.

There is very little disagreement that there is tremendous waste in our current health care system. So the question has become, How do we determine what should and should not be done in health care? This is where the science of epidemiology comes into play, by helping decision makers gather and evaluate all of the available outcome data that are so necessary when making decisions that involve population health. This is a movement away from operating on hunches about causation of disease toward seeking more precise definitions of causation.

According to Lee and Mongan (2009), in order to bring health care costs under control, the diffusion of the development of new health technology must be slowed. We must be able to determine the costs and benefits of new technology tools, which has always been a serious challenge for providers of health care services. This is where epidemiologists can help decision makers understand costly changes before they are incorporated into medical practice. This is of particular importance because once these technology tools become part of health care delivery, they are very difficult, if not impossible, to control.

Christensen, Grossman, and Hwang (2009) argue that it takes disruptive innovation to change the way we deliver goods or services. Disruptive innovation entails a process through which complicated and very expensive products or services become simplified and less expensive. This happens when innovation and creativity become incentivized in the business model; and this concept would certainly apply to the delivery of health care in this country.

Now let's apply the concept of disruptive innovation to improving the health of the population at a cost that we can afford. In order to be successful in this venture, we need to develop and apply a model of health care that is different from the one we have been using. We must apply the idea of disruptive innovation to the delivery of good health to the U.S. population, not just to individuals.

In their new book titled *The Innovator's Prescription: A Disruptive Solution for Health Care,* Christensen, Grossman, and Hwang (2009) assert that health care is attempting to move from an intuitive to a precision approach. They define intuitive medicine as a craft that deals only with symptoms and a treatment for the symptoms that is uncertain. Precision medicine, however, focuses on precise diagnosis of a disease, which is then treated with proven therapy. This is where the science of epidemiology can serve us well by providing statistical data that show the real causes of many medical conditions.

The way that the health care system in our country is structured, especially in regard to how we reimburse providers, means that it is incapable of sustaining innovation. Therefore, we need the same type of disruptive innovation found in the business world to move the health care system away from a preoccupation with curing disease and toward disease prevention. At the same time, public health departments must shift their focus from the control of disease to the prevention of disease.

In order for disruptive innovation in health care to prosper and grow, we have to change the way we pay providers for the delivery of medical services. The current payment system offers incentives for more care, which allows illness to occur and discourages providers of care from spending time on prevention efforts.

What is more, this same type of disruptive innovation has to become the norm in the delivery of public health programs. Just as the science of epidemiology can be a necessary adjunct to the development of precision medicine, a better understanding of epidemiology allows public health departments to change their emphasis on communicable diseases to a stronger focus on the causes and prevention of chronic diseases. Epidemiology can become the catalyst of disruptive innovation to help reduce the costs associated with the development of chronic diseases and their complications.

Summary

Epidemiology is one of the great assets of public health, and should be essential in dealing with the health care crisis. Decision makers who are responsible for the distribution of resources in health care delivery have to understand and use epidemiological principles. Several of the tools that are available to the epidemiologist can also be helpful to medical care professionals who must decide how to bring costs down and improve the outcomes associated with various medical procedures.

The increase in life expectancy since 1900 is not because of better medical care, but rather due in large part to a better understanding of how disease occurs and how to prevent it. By learning the real causes of disease, physicians have started to shift away from the concept of curing disease and toward the idea of primary care that focuses on disease and illness prevention. Epidemiology is a science that can assist health care professionals in making informed decisions about how to use scarce resources; it can also facilitate the gathering of the requisite data to help better manage the outcomes associated with particular health care interventions. What is more, epidemiology is also useful in the improvement of the major functions of public health management, including planning, finance, assessing quality issues, and evidence-based public health practice.

Key Terms

Analytical epidemiology

Case definition

Chain of infection

Descriptive epidemiology

Direct transmission

Epidemiology

Indirect transmission

Managerial epidemiology

Triad of disease

Discussion Questions

1. Explain the use of epidemiology in many of the successes public health departments have achieved over the last one hundred years.
2. What are some of the major differences between descriptive and analytical epidemiology?
3. Offer a thorough explanation of managerial epidemiology. How can this concept be used in making better decisions concerning the allocation of scarce health resources?
4. How can the principles of epidemiology be applied to the process of innovation to solve the problems of cost and quality in our current health care system?

CHAPTER 5

SHIFTING THE FOCUS FROM COMMUNICABLE TO CHRONIC DISEASES

LEARNING OBJECTIVES

- Comprehend the widespread problems that will result from the increasing incidence of chronic diseases in the United States
- Become aware of the fact that chronic diseases cannot be cured
- Recognize that if chronic diseases cannot be cured, they must be prevented
- Acknowledge the need for partnerships in dealing with the health problems associated with chronic diseases
- Understand the necessity of increased funding for chronic disease prevention programs

The United States spends over $2 trillion on a health care system that is not producing great value for the recipients of its medical care. Despite spending all of this money every year on health care, millions of individuals become ill from communicable and chronic diseases that are entirely preventable. Shouldn't the goal of the health care system include preventing diseases in the first place rather than waiting for them to develop? If so, our health care system is failing to meet this goal while wasting precious resources that could be better spent in other areas. This has to change. The current health care system should be renamed the "disease cure system" to better reflect an emphasis on curing rather than preventing disease. The system does not adequately attempt to prevent disease, especially chronic illness. The emphasis of the health care system remains on curing disease—but once acquired, chronic diseases cannot be cured.

Brownlee (2007) argues that over one-third of the money spent on health care is wasted on treatment and testing that have very little if any effect on health outcomes for most Americans. In fact, much of this additional care may actually be very dangerous for its recipients. Making matters worse, over 50 percent of Americans do not receive the treatment they require in a timely fashion. In other words, the health of the U.S. population is not in very good shape, despite the enormous amount of resources expended. We need to begin making better decisions in regard to how we use of our scarce resources, seeking to keep people healthy rather than allowing them to become ill. It is regrettable that in the present health care system there is no reward for preventing diseases, because almost all of the money is used to treat and attempt to cure illnesses after they occur.

Where do public health departments fit into this disease-oriented system of health care? Why aren't public health departments more openly critical of the way medicine is currently practiced in this country? Holmes (2009) argues that the field of public health in the United States arose from the government's attempt to reduce the morbidity and mortality resulting from infectious diseases. Public health departments have had many successes and failures in responding to communicable disease threats. However, public health's victory over most communicable disease epidemics has fostered a feeling of complacency leading to frequent, isolated outbreaks of communicable diseases and the current epidemic of chronic diseases throughout every segment of our population. Public health departments in the United States have long focused on the prevention of disease through a system of care that treats illness as a failure of the health care system. For this reason, public health departments have used immunizations and health promotion activities to prevent rather than cure communicable diseases.

Over time the diseases have changed, and devoted servants of public health departments have seen their budgets and manpower decline as more serious public health threats have contributed to increased morbidity and mortality in the United States. The new epidemic of chronic diseases calls for public health departments to develop new strategies in order to achieve even a modest victory over these new public health challenges. However, public health departments are not prepared to consider different strategies because of their past success with communicable disease epidemics. A great deal of change has occurred since the victories over smallpox, polio, and measles some forty years earlier, beginning in the early 1970s. It seems that public health departments have been seduced by their own success; and today they still believe that their old strategies will continue to work with the current chronic disease epidemic. They are very wrong.

Herbold (2007) argues that when individuals and businesses achieve extraordinary success over time, they begin to believe that they are entitled to this success in the future—a phenomenon he calls the legacy concept. Further, they become convinced that their past success will ensure future success, as long as they employ the original practices. This is what has happened to public health departments over time: they will not even consider new ways of looking at public health problems because the ways of the past have worked so very well. We must at least think about other ways of dealing with very different types of diseases, whose costs and prevalence continue to grow. When failure continues to occur, we need to begin looking for alternate ways of approaching the problem.

Public health departments should be building on their past successes and developing the new skills that are necessary to continue preventing disease in the future. These departments need to recognize that the current epidemic of chronic diseases does not lend itself to control or curative measures. We need to develop new strategies in order to reduce chronic diseases' threat to the quality of life of our population and, perhaps, to the very survival of our health care system. The U.S. health care system and its public health departments must learn how to deal with illness before it occurs, a strategy that must be driven by disease prevention programs and a greater focus on population health.

The mission of public health departments in the United States has always been the prevention of disease. Public health departments moved away from this mission, however, when dealing with sexually transmitted diseases, including human immunodeficiency virus (HIV). Public health departments have used a strategy with this category of disease that involved counseling and testing of infected individuals. They see this approach as the only way to deal with the epidemic, and have not considered prevention, which can only be accomplished by education at an early age. Health education efforts in this country, especially in schools and workplaces, have never received a great deal of attention from public health departments. There may have been a health promotion program offered from time to time, but never a sustained, measurable effort to educate children and employees in the prevention of disease. In the case of sexually transmitted diseases, it seemed like a better answer to locate infected individuals, get them to treatment, and then find their contacts and also treat them. This type of strategy does not prevent anything except the spread of the current infection—and there is no question that the strategy has failed, given the increasing incidence of sexually transmitted diseases. The approach will certainly not work with chronic diseases, because finding individuals with these diseases does nothing to prevent others from becoming ill.

As we have argued throughout this book, the United States is now faced with an epidemic of chronic diseases that do not lend themselves to curative or counseling and testing approaches. These diseases are unlike communicable diseases in their etiology, incubation period, prevalence, and burden to society. They are also very different in regard to the strategy required to deal with them. Although this country has had great success in controlling communicable diseases, such ailments remain a threat, and some communicable diseases like chlamydia and HIV are still increasing in incidence. This is a direct result of not using resources to prevent these diseases. Further, chronic disease rates in the United States show no signs of leveling off in the near future because of Americans' lifestyle choices. Chronic diseases are extremely expensive in terms of morbidity, mortality, and the cost of care. We must address these illnesses through education programs designed to prevent the development of such poor health behaviors as using tobacco, maintaining a poor diet, being physically inactive, and abusing alcohol.

These diseases are affecting American families; government programs at all levels, especially Medicare; businesses; insurers; and the entire health care system. This increase in chronic diseases is not a silent epidemic, but the medical community is ignoring its potential consequences. Doctors are trained to care for those with diseases, but they receive very little if any education concerning disease prevention. They then earn their living by diagnosing and attempting to cure diseases, not by preventing them—and that remains a societal problem. What is more, physicians' focus is on their patients, and not on the population. There needs to be a system of payment that focuses on outcomes not only for individual patients but also for the entire community. This is why public health departments have to work with physicians in an attempt to improve the health of the population. Halvorson (2009) points out that there is not even a payment code for insurance plans that accounts for curative measures or medical outcome. He also argues that almost 80 percent of health care costs come from chronic diseases and their comorbidities. These comorbidities involve more than one disease and also more than one doctor, making the process of treating the chronic diseases even more difficult.

Communicable Disease Threat

It is useful to classify diseases as either communicable or noncommunicable. Communicable or infectious diseases are caused by agents that can be transmitted from one individual to another and also from contaminated foods or water, including pathogens as bacteria, viruses, and parasites, and they usually have a very short incubation period from exposure to illness. These diseases have been a major contributor to morbidity and mortality since the beginning of time. Although these diseases are still a major threat to our population, many communicable diseases—for example, smallpox, measles, polio, and malaria—have been largely eliminated. It must also be mentioned that even though we have had great success in controlling communicable diseases, we have only been successful in the eradication of one communicable disease, smallpox. In fact, many communicable diseases are actually increasing in incidence in this country because of global travel and reduced funding for public health programs.

In 1900 the leading causes of mortality in the United States were communicable diseases, including pneumonia and tuberculosis. These diseases have been replaced by such chronic illnesses as heart disease, cancer, and diabetes. Although the chronic diseases are increasing in their numbers and are capable of breaking our health care budget, we cannot let down our guard on the old and new versions of infectious diseases. Communicable diseases, like influenza, are still capable of causing enormous morbidity and mortality for our population in a very short period of time. A comparison of Tables 5.1 and 5.2 shows this very real change in the diseases the U.S. population experienced between the years 1900 and 2000. Even though there has been a shift from communicable to chronic diseases as the major threat to the health of the population, however, communicable diseases still require our attention and funding.

According to a 2008 report (Trust for America's Health, Prevention Institute, The Urban Institute, and New York Academy of Medicine), the threat of communicable diseases is shaped by three factors that the U.S. health care system need to take very seriously:

1. *The dynamic nature of infectious diseases.* Infectious or communicable diseases are constantly changing, producing more virulent pathogens or entirely new

Table 5.1   Number of Deaths and Crude Mortality Rate for Leading Causes of Death in the United States in 1900

Cause of Death	Number of Deaths	Crude Mortality Rate per 100,000
Pneumonia and influenza	40,362	202.2
Tuberculosis	38,820	194.4
Diarrhea, enteritis, and other gastrointestinal problems	28,491	142.7
Heart disease	27,427	137.4
Stroke	21,353	106.9
Kidney diseases	17,699	88.6
Unintentional injuries (accidents)	14,429	72.3
Cancer	12,769	64.0
Senility	10,015	50.2
Diphtheria	8,056	40.3

Source: National Center for Health Statistics, n.d.

Table 5.2   Number of Deaths and Crude Mortality Rate for Leading
Causes of Death in the United States in 2000

Cause of Death	Number of Deaths	Crude Mortality Rate per 100,000
Heart disease	710,760	258.1
Cancer	553,091	200.9
Stroke	167,661	60.9
Chronic lower respiratory diseases	122,009	44.3
Unintentional injuries (accidents)	97,900	35.6
Diabetes mellitus	69,301	25.2
Influenza and pneumonia	65,313	23.7
Alzheimer's disease	49,558	18.0
Kidney diseases	37,251	13.5
Septicemia	31,224	11.3

Source: Miniño et al., 2002, p. 8.

strains of communicable diseases. Because these new infectious diseases are quite often found in developing countries, they usually become epidemics before serious investigations uncover the source, spread, and incubation period. Therefore, communicable disease epidemics remain a constant threat to this country, requiring constant surveillance using the most advanced technology that is available.

2. *Globalization.* The globalization resulting from international trade has expanded our wealth, but it also has increased the opportunities for infectious diseases to cross international boundaries, making us all susceptible to communicable disease epidemics. This threat from globalization is only going to escalate as world trade expands along with immigration from countries that have not gained control over infectious diseases. Further, this escalation in infectious diseases imported to our country is happening at a time when we are losing many of our senior public health employees to retirement, and insufficient funding makes it difficult to attract and train suitable replacements.

3. *The effects of poverty.* Poverty can be the catalyst that spreads communicable diseases throughout a population at a very rapid rate. Poor personal hygiene and sanitation in many third world countries make the possibility of new epidemics of infectious diseases a very real threat that will be carried into the future.

The proper management and eventual eradication of communicable diseases could exhaust the funds currently allocated for public health departments in this country. If we add to this burden the costs associated with dealing with the epidemic of chronic diseases, it becomes clear that public health departments are going to fail in their effort to win the war against disease in this country.

We need to change how we look at resources used to combat diseases, especially those diseases that can be easily passed from person to person. We must also consider monies used to prevent or eradicate infectious diseases as an investment in preventing future infections that would cost more than the amount initially spent. In realty, many prevention efforts to combat both communicable and chronic diseases result in increased spending in the short term (Russell, 2009). If disease is prevented or postponed, however, long-term savings replace the initial costs, making the investment in prevention an exceptionally good use of scarce resources.

Public health programs that deal with the prevention of all diseases need to develop sophisticated surveillance systems, rapid detection and communication mechanisms, and new education initiatives. Those responsible for communicable disease prevention programs must have the resources required to deal with communicable diseases as early as possible in order to prevent epidemics. There is no acceptable excuse for outbreaks of communicable diseases in the twenty-first century. Unfortunately, communicable diseases have not been eradicated in our country, only controlled, because when an outbreak occurs very little attention is paid to preventing the next outbreak through health education. The CDC reports that there are still over four thousand food-borne outbreaks every year; tuberculosis has remained a stubborn problem; rates of infection for sexually transmitted diseases, including HIV, are on the rise; and outbreaks of other vaccine-preventable illnesses still occur on a regular basis (Mead et al., 2010). In the case of food safety, the Food and Drug Administration (FDA) has to do more to protect our foods from harmful bacteria. Foods that are infected with bacteria and toxic substances must be stopped from ever reaching production for final human consumption. This mandate must include foods produced both nationally and internationally. Again, there can be no excuse for failure in the protection of our food supply and the protection of the population from epidemics of communicable diseases in general. This is another example of investing more resources in prevention that will result in a reduction in costs over the long term.

The Challenge of Chronic Diseases

Chronic diseases pose an even greater challenge to public health departments than do communicable diseases. There is no question that chronic diseases have surpassed communicable diseases as the major threat to the health of most

Americans. According to the CDC (2009a), over 50 percent of Americans are living with one or more chronic diseases, and 70 percent of the mortality in this country is attributable to chronic diseases. The CDC is very concerned about the increase in high-risk health behaviors, such as using tobacco, maintaining a poor diet, abusing alcohol, and being physically inactive, that is not only fueling the development of new cases of chronic diseases but also leading to more of the complications that result from chronic diseases over time. This is evident in the growing numbers of Healthy People 2010 objectives that have been put forth at the national and state levels of public health departments (U.S. Department of Health and Human Services, 2010a). This interest in chronic disease control is very important because much of the death and disability attributable to chronic diseases can be prevented through a broad array of lifestyle changes. This epidemic of chronic diseases is producing an enormous burden and challenge for our entire medical care system. Because these diseases cannot be cured, our current medical care system is not capable of doing very much about this epidemic—in fact, the medical care system is at a loss as to how to handle patients with these diseases, other than to treat the resulting complications. The system makes patients comfortable through prescriptions that do very little to improve their quality of life as they age and become disabled from the complications of diseases that could have been prevented in the first place. The solution to the raging epidemic of chronic diseases in our country remains a mystery to the medical community.

One in three Americans ages nineteen to thirty-four, two in three of those ages forty-five to sixty-four, and nine out of ten of the elderly have at least one chronic disease (Christensen, Grossman, and Hwang, 2009). According to Paez, Zhao, and Hwang (2009), chronic diseases increase with age, with the greatest increase occurring from early adulthood (ages twenty through forty-four) and middle age (ages forty-five through sixty-four). These figures indicate that over ninety million Americans currently have at least one chronic disease. We are currently directing very few resources toward preventing these diseases from occurring in the first place. The key to averting chronic diseases rests with primary prevention, which usually involves health education and health promotion programs.

The costs associated with these chronic diseases are capable of bankrupting our health care system as affected individuals age and develop the complications associated with most chronic diseases. These diseases usually do most of their damage to individuals as they age, causing the costs of health care to escalate over time. This is a very significant because it demonstrates the need for prevention activities that begin very early in life and continue as individuals age, which in turn highlights the value of health promotion activities beginning in school and continuing in the workplace. This revelation supports the argument for early implementation of chronic disease prevention programs. It also calls for health care professionals to develop and implement education programs to help those with chronic diseases avoid expensive complications.

The American Medical Association (2010) reports that the insurance provider Humana is bolstering its chronic disease management service in response to the increased costs associated with treating individuals with chronic diseases. Humana plans to hire 270 employees to work at its home office in Florida to coordinate care for its chronically ill Medicare and commercial plan members. These new employees will work with a multidisciplinary team that coordinates each member's care in cooperation with his or her primary care physician, pharmacies, relatives, and community. A registered nurse will be the team leader, guaranteeing regular contact with the patient. This program is designed to reduce the costs associated with chronic disease complications. This is a very good idea, but it would be a much better option to develop community-based programs to prevent chronic diseases in the first place.

The epidemiology of chronic diseases is much different from that of communicable diseases. Chronic diseases are not caused by exposure to one agent, and they are for the most part self-inflicted through the practice of unhealthy behaviors. This is a category of diseases that do not lend themselves to the development of vaccines and that cannot be cured by medication. These diseases are capable of causing tremendous disability and pain, a reduction in one's quality of life, and premature death. Because of their long incubation period it is difficult to determine the true catalyst of chronic diseases' onset. Epidemiological studies have confirmed that risky behaviors begun early in life and practiced for many years usually are found to be the major cause of chronic diseases. There are tools available for use in primary prevention and screening processes that can help either prevent or detect a disease in an early stage, when the treatment can postpone disease complications and improve one's quality of life. Chronic diseases are also preventable if individuals are educated to never begin practicing the unhealthy behaviors that are at their root. It is therefore unfortunate that the majority of providers working in the medical care system have been trained to treat and cure diseases, not to keep people healthy in the first place.

The epidemic of chronic diseases in the United States is going to have a profound effect on the financing of health care services. The increase in life expectancy of Americans is in turn increasing the duration of chronic diseases and their complications. The physical and monetary costs are going to be staggering unless this nation can devise a plan to prevent chronic diseases and their complications from developing. The tools of prevention are available through public health departments, which house the expertise in preventing disease, and public health professionals are now being called upon to provide leadership in stopping the epidemic of chronic diseases. Public health leaders will require tremendous communication skills to convince those who control resources to work with communities in preventing chronic diseases or at least avoiding their complications.

Morewitz (2006) argues that chronic diseases are a result of complex interactions among environmental, social, and genetic factors that can be prevented through lifestyle changes. Chronic diseases are also considered a much greater threat for the disparate population, which represents those with low income, minimal education and family resources, and poor living conditions. The health care system is currently investing less than 3 percent of its resources in chronic disease prevention activities. If this same type of epidemic were being caused by infectious diseases, unlimited resources would be made available to prevent the illnesses. The chronic disease epidemic has been an ignored epidemic because its victims are usually older, and the combination of aging and disease has become an accepted norm for many older Americans. There is no reason, however, why illness should simply be accepted without even an attempt at prevention.

The most distressing part of the current epidemic of chronic diseases in this country is that they can be prevented, just like communicable diseases. Both communicable and chronic diseases are not receiving the prioritization or funding necessary for successful intervention. The current model of the delivery of health care services must change, focusing resources on preventing disease rather than on curing disease—a tremendous challenge given that those who control resources in health care profit from illness. This is where the need for community partnerships as a national priority in the United States becomes evident. This is also where the need for strong leadership in public health prevention programs becomes a requirement for saving our health care system from financial destruction.

The Need for Investment in Preventing Chronic Diseases

The most important difference between communicable and chronic diseases is the role of the individual: eliminating high-risk health behaviors can prevent the development of chronic diseases, and can also circumvent the complications from these diseases if they are already present. According to Sultz and Young (2009), many individuals do not believe that they are responsible for their illnesses. This assumption may be true with many communicable diseases, but it is not the case with the majority of chronic diseases and their complications. This "no responsibility" attitude may explain individuals' lack of interest in practicing healthy behaviors and avoiding high-risk ones. Look, for example, at the change in public attitudes toward and concern about AIDS ever since the effectiveness of treatment of this disease has improved. AIDS has become a chronic disease, allowing an individual to live longer by using an array of drugs on a daily basis. Once this disease became chronic and treatment seemed to work, the fear of infection seemed to disappear, along with the attention of the media. We are a country that does a much better job of responding to an emergency than preventing one.

The costs associated with allowing chronic diseases to develop and present complications for an individual are much higher than the costs associated with communicable diseases. These differences in costs are in part explained by the fact that chronic diseases have no cure—only ongoing and costly treatment. The CDC (2009a) reports that chronic diseases account for almost 80 percent of the 2.7 trillion dollars spent on health care services this year. These diseases are taking a larger proportion of the health care budget while also entailing lost productivity in the workplace and increasing the years of potential life lost (YPLL). Chronic diseases and their complications are robbing Americans of the quality of life years, defined as years free of disease, that they could have enjoyed had they been able to avoid becoming ill.

Chronic diseases are preventable with only a small investment in programs designed to change the health behaviors of a large portion of the population. There are many proven best practices in health promotion, a number of which are available as case studies at the end of this book, that are designed to prevent or modify the high-risk health behaviors responsible for the development of many chronic diseases. There is mounting evidence that investing resources in the prevention of chronic diseases is the only way to deal with the present cost crisis in health care. TFAH (2008) argues that investing only ten dollars per person per year in programs designed to increase physical activity, improve nutrition, and prevent tobacco use could save the payers of health insurance in the United States more than $16 billion annually within five years. This represents a return on investment of $5.60 for every dollar invested. These very positive projected results need to be communicated to all communities so that they can begin to take charge of their residents' health through community-based prevention programs.

TFAH (2008) also asserts that out of the $16 billion in savings that could be realized from healthy lifestyles, Medicare would save $5 billion and Medicaid could save more than $1.9 billion. These savings are far too high for the government to ignore. It is interesting to note that these proposed prevention programs do not require medical care—only a dramatic shift toward lifestyles that encourage healthy behaviors for all Americans.

The federal government and private businesses have the most to gain by reducing the incidence of disease through the expansion of wellness programs. The federal government, through the CDC, needs to do more in the way of disseminating research and analysis supporting the return on investment available to businesses and communities. Simon and Fielding (2006) argue that public health agencies have to provide public health information of value, including cost-effective intervention strategies, to chambers of commerce, trade associations, and businesses. What is more, in each region there needs to be a public health practitioner assigned the responsibility of liaising with the business community.

Neumann, Jacobson, and Palmer (2008) maintain that there ought to be a way to measure and share the value of government public health agencies. The fact that public health programs continue to be underfunded every year is a clear indication that the public is unaware of the tremendous benefit these programs offer. Chronic disease prevention efforts represent a way for public health leaders to prove the value of their efforts by actually reducing the costs of medical care in the United States. Many individuals require incentives to develop and maintain lifestyle practices that reduce the risk of chronic diseases (Paez et al., 2009). Such incentives should be part of all health insurance programs in our country. This is an opportunity for everyone who pays for health insurance—including the government, employers, and individuals—to improve the health of the population while reducing the cost of health care. Public health departments need to take a leadership role in helping everyone understand the positive economic effects associated with wellness programs.

Health Education

Our current medical care system allows individuals to become ill, and then attempts to cure that illness. Medical care developed as a system devoted to curing communicable diseases, which are usually transmitted from person to person and cured through a short course of antibiotic treatment. The providers of care in this system waited for illness to happen and then rapidly responded with medications designed to cure the acute infection. Family doctors spent little time and energy preventing the communicable diseases. The prevention of outbreaks of illness was left to underfunded government public health departments. Medical care professionals gave little thought to changing the system of health care delivery because it seemed to work so well, especially when a communicable disease was involved.

As we argued earlier, our health care system is bankrupting the country while still leaving forty-five million Americans without health insurance. Primary prevention requires the reduction in risk factors that cause disease (Turnock, 2009). If individuals do not become ill, then there will be an immediate reduction in health care costs as well as a reduced need for health insurance. In order to keep individuals well, our health care system must educate the population about how to prevent the bad health behaviors that cause disease.

Although implementing health education programs is considered one of the basic functions of local health departments, these programs have never been given a high priority or received adequate funding. Public health departments have always used their limited resources to control rather than prevent disease, in large part because of the rigidity of communicable disease programs and their funding guidelines that advocate contact tracing if no vaccine is available. This fact is evident in the lack of attention paid to implementing health education programs in school districts and workplaces. This is also evident in public health departments' strategy for dealing with sexually transmitted diseases. Proponents of the Sexually Transmitted Disease Control Program, previously called the Venereal Disease Control Program, uses all of their resources to interview and treat infected individuals and then find their sexual partners and get them treated. Personnel hired for this program are told that their only priority is contact tracing and treatment, not education to prevent infection. This has obviously been the wrong strategy, given that we never stopped the escalation of the sexually transmitted disease epidemic—it has only been controlled on a temporary basis, and most of the sexually transmitted disease rates continue to increase every year.

Frieden (2004) argues that the local public health infrastructure has not been able to transition from dealing with communicable diseases to the more dangerous chronic diseases. This is primarily a result of many public health officials' attitude that public health strategies cannot be successful in dealing with this type of epidemic.

Because chronic diseases cannot be cured, the only intervention available is the development and implementation of prevention programs. This will require an expansion in the demand for health educators, who are far less expensive than physicians and take fewer years to train. Health education programs and the health educators that direct these programs have never received the attention that they deserve. The compensation for these positions is low, and there are not that many positions available at the present time. This lack of attention to primary prevention programs is about to change. The shift will occur because we as a nation cannot continue to waste precious resources on a failed system of health care that allows individuals first to develop chronic diseases, and then to develop deadly complications from these diseases.

The sheer desperation of our health care system is forcing it to shift to an emphasis on disease prevention, which requires community populations to reduce their high-risk health behaviors and replace them with healthy ones. This change will require more health education programs in schools and workplaces as our country attempts to expand prevention efforts and reduce the need for the cure of chronic diseases.

The prevention of disease in our health care system seems to begin and end with the use of vaccines to prevent illnesses. Health education programs are almost nonexistent in our school systems, and we are allowing our young to develop unhealthy behaviors that lead to the onset of chronic diseases later in life. It would seem that investment in the prevention of illness would be the number one priority of a modern health care system. It would also seem that businesses would have seen the value of healthy workers long ago and would be doing everything possible to keep members of their workforce free of disease and productive throughout their working years. Yet this has not been the case because the reimbursement system compensates for illness rather than wellness. Physicians and hospitals are paid for activities aimed at curing illness rather than preventing illness from ever occurring.

Prevention includes interventions designed to reduce or slow the advancement of illness and disability (Goetzel, 2009). The problem is that there are no incentives in place for prevention efforts to flourish. The health care system does not make money if people remain well. It is only when individuals become ill that the system prospers. This has to change if we are ever going to solve the major problems of health care delivery in this country—problems produced by chronic diseases, which cannot be cured, only prevented.

The 2010 **Affordable Care Act** has responded to growing recognition of the need for increased prevention programs in the United States. This act was the result of an attempt by the federal government to reform the current health care system in our country. Koh and Sebelius (2010) argue that this new law draws attention to the value of preventive health in the following ways:

- The Act provides individuals with improved access to clinical preventive services.
- The law promotes wellness in the workplace, providing new health promotion opportunities for employers and employees.
- The Act strengthens the vital role of communities in promoting prevention.
- The Act elevates prevention as a national priority, providing unprecedented opportunities for promoting health through all policies.

The Need for Partnerships to Combat Chronic Diseases

Public health departments have had great success in dealing with many of the chronic diseases that plague our health care system. Their prevention efforts have reduced the incidence of heart disease, cancer, and stroke over the last twenty years by focusing on reducing tobacco use, improving diet, and increasing physical activity. Their progress with reducing chronic diseases has slowed in recent years, however, because of the reduced funding that resulted from public health leaders' inability to prove the value of primary prevention to those in control of distributing resources.

The only way to deal with the epidemic of chronic diseases is through population-based medicine. This strategy requires a movement from concentrating on individual health concerns toward devoting attention to the health of communities. Public health departments have always practiced population-based medicine because of their previous work with community-wide outbreaks of communicable diseases.

Chronic diseases are such a large public health problem that they require **community partnerships** to deal with the epidemic. These partnerships involve most health care providers and other health-related agencies in a given community. The escalation in the numbers of individuals developing chronic diseases and their complications is best handled at the local or community level. Because the problem of chronic diseases is too large for public health departments alone to solve, partnerships need to form among local health departments and several other community agencies in order to make a real difference in the epidemic.

Partnerships allow partner agencies to move forward when an individual agency does not have the required expertise, authority, or resources to bring about change (Bailey, 2010). This is the case with the challenge of chronic diseases that faces both public health departments and communities. As Tennyson stated in *The Partnering Toolbook* (2003, p. 3), "The hypothesis underpinning a partnership approach is that only with comprehensive and widespread cross-sector collaboration can we ensure that sustainable development initiatives are imaginative coherent and integrated enough to tackle the most intractable problems." Partnerships would allow public health professionals to maximize resources by pooling talent from various organizations. Despite the different mission statements found among potential partners, there is common ground in the desire to combat the greatest public health threat to ever face our nation: every community as a whole is paying for the chronic disease epidemic in terms of lost wages, increased disability claims, higher health care costs, and a lower quality of life for large sections of the community.

Some of the community partners that are vital to any population-based community prevention program are local, state, and territorial health departments; federal agencies; health care providers and facilities; and public and private organizations, industrial entities, and academic institutions. Public health departments have not heretofore been particularly interested in working with businesses for a variety of reasons (Simon and Fielding, 2006). The public health sector and the business community have generally only encountered each other in a regulatory capacity during outbreaks of communicable disease. It is very difficult to become partners in this type of relationship. Partnerships offer great opportunities for public health departments to assume a leadership role, uniting communities in defeating the awesome challenge of the epidemic of chronic diseases. This is a starting point for the development of community partnerships in the delivery of population-based health services. Exhibit 5.1 shows many of the advantages and potential disadvantages of community partnerships.

EXHIBIT 5.1

ADVANTAGES AND DISADVANTAGES OF COMMUNITY PARTNERSHIPS

Advantages of Partnerships

- Maximizing community resources

- Reducing duplication of health care services

- Gaining the support and respect of the entire community

- Increasing the chances of obtaining government and foundation support

Disadvantages of Partnerships

- Reducing the autonomy of member agencies

- Losing independence

- Experiencing potential conflicts of interest

According to Shortell (2010), there should be further discussion about partnerships developed:

1. Partnerships need to be both internally and externally aligned. Partners should achieve domain consensus among themselves with sufficient overlap of goals and should understand what is expected of the partnership by external groups.
2. The partnership should gain legitimacy and credibility within the community. Drawing on the developing literature on social capital would improve this process.
3. Partnerships can gain legitimacy by understanding their centrality in the political economy of the community. Social network concepts involving direct and indirect ties, the strength of ties, network density, and structural holes are relevant.

4. Every partner has a core competence and comparative advantage. Partnerships can fail because individual members either overestimate or underestimate their comparative advantage and misdiagnose their core competence.

5. Leadership should be explored more fully: the kind of leadership needed, the kind of partnership that can deliver it, and the stage of the partnership's life cycle that is best suited for it. The role of individual leadership versus organizational leadership should be discussed.

6. Forming a partnership has a transaction cost. The literature on transaction cost economics originally developed by Williamson may be relevant.

7. The process of selecting partners, including tradeoffs and timing, should be more fully explored.

8. Population health improvement can be perceived as simply a resource for organizations to advance their own agenda and cause.

The development and expansion of partnerships to improve the health of our community populations is our only choice if we are ever to gain ground in meeting the challenge chronic diseases pose. There are certainly risks associated with this bold strategy, and that is why a neutral participant like public health must take on the leadership role and become the catalyst required to develop partnerships for improving the health of every community population in the United States.

Opportunity to Improve the Way Health Care Is Delivered

The emerging communicable disease threat and the escalation of the epidemic of chronic diseases is making it necessary to change the way health care is delivered. Not only is the current medical care system too expensive but also, and more important, it was never designed to deal with epidemics of both emerging communicable infections and chronic diseases. These two categories of diseases require a health care system with providers who get paid to keep individuals healthy and to not allow them to suffer from illness. This system will treat illness as a failure on the part of medical professionals, resulting in lower rates of reimbursement.

Gladwell (2000) argues that change happens because of the convergence of three factors: contagiousness; the ability of small causes to precipitate a large effect; and the coming together of the first two factors at one dramatic moment, or **tipping point.** In public health the example of an outbreak of disease caused by bioterrorism can easily explain this concept. A terrorist group introduces a contagious agent into a susceptible population. If this agent is introduced to a large group of susceptible hosts at the same time, the tipping point will most likely be reached. A similar scenario may also be present in our health care crisis in this country: the explosion in health care costs and the resulting increase in the costs of health insurance are causing those paying the bills to demand change in how we deliver health care and to come together to cause a tipping point that is capable of shifting health care delivery in this country. This tipping point is also producing a tremendous opportunity for public health departments to take a leadership role in the transitioning health care system.

This opportunity is also presenting significant challenges for public health departments—particularly in regard to the need for improved data collection and better cost-utility analysis (Neumann et al., 2008). Public health investigators must develop core data sets that are acceptable to those involved in output measurement. How do we know when public health interventions are successful? A cost-utility analysis incorporates and measures some of the intangible benefits. Without a sustained effort to define and measure the value of public health services, the public health system will have an increasingly difficult time competing for scarce resources—especially now, with a reduced federal budget.

Figure 5.1 illustrates how risk factors precede disease, which is the cause of the escalating costs of health care. It stands to reason that in order to prevent increasing costs we need to invest resources in the prevention or reduction of the high-risk health behaviors that are the risk factors for chronic diseases.

Table 5.3 shows four different methods the CDC has used for evaluating health interventions. The CDC proposes **cost-utility analysis** as the method of choice to make public health resource decisions. This type of analysis is used to compare interventions that have morbidity and mortality outcomes, measuring the health effects in terms of years of life adjusted for quality of life.

The number of quality of life years a program intervention adds is a very important measure when dealing with chronic diseases and their complications. Because there is no cure for chronic diseases, the prevention of the complications from these diseases is of paramount importance in attempts to improve the health of communities and at the same time reduce the costs of health care in this country.

TFAH (2008) points out that only four cents of every dollar spent on health care delivery in this country are used to prevent the occurrence of disease, even though the research clearly demonstrates the value of investing in prevention. The rest of the money, spent on medical care, represents an enormous amount of

FIGURE 5.1   Cause of Cost Escalation in Health Care Delivery

Risk Factor → Disease → Cost

waste. Brownlee (2007) argues that over $700 billion was spent on medical care in 2006 that offered no medical value and was capable of causing unnecessary harm to individuals. The public health system could better use this money to develop sophisticated programs designed to deal with chronic diseases. Traditional public health strategies hold tremendous potential for dealing with the chronic disease epidemic we face. The most important public health strategy involves the development of education programs that use available technology to disseminate information to large segments of the U.S. population.

Bernstein (2008) argues that our current model of health care delivery was not developed to deal with chronic diseases. He therefore proposes the use of a **Chronic Care Model** of evidence-based health care practices that allow practitioners to measure the outcomes of care. This model requires active participation by an informed patient who has become empowered to self-manage his or her particular chronic disease. This management is geared toward the prevention of the complications of chronic diseases, which are the real issue for those with chronic conditions. The current model of medical care focuses on curing a disease after it has occurred, with the patient acting as a passive recipient of a physician's information concerning the disease that affects him or her.

Table 5.3   Economic Evaluation Methods

Economic Evaluation Method	Comparison	Measurement of Health Effects	Economic Summary Measure
Cost analysis	Used to compare net costs of different programs for planning and assessment	Dollars	Net cost Cost of illness
Cost-effectiveness analysis	Used to compare interventions that produce a common health effect	Health effects, measured in natural units	Cost-effectiveness ratio Cost per case averted Cost per life-year saved
Cost-utility analysis	Used to compare interventions that have morbidity and mortality outcomes	Health effects, measured as years of life, adjusted for quality of life	Cost per quality-adjusted life year (QALY)
Cost-benefit analysis	Used to compare different programs with different units of outcomes (health and nonhealth)	Dollars	Net benefit or cost Benefit-to-cost ratio

Source: Centers for Disease Control and Prevention, 1995, p. 11.

This model of an ignorant patient who lacks empowerment in his or her own health care decisions is designed to fail. In order to prevent chronic diseases, individuals have to be empowered, must avoid high-risk health behaviors, and need to recognize the possibility of acquiring an incurable chronic disease. The investment in providing the prerequisite health information to individuals has the potential for an enormous payoff—a reduction in the incidence of chronic diseases and their very expensive complications.

Summary

There are significant differences between communicable and chronic diseases that all Americans need to understand. These types of diseases vary in regard to incubation period, mortality, quality of life implications, and root cause. Our success with curing communicable diseases has led us to believe that we can cure all diseases, including chronic ones. This has become a very costly error—we are unable to cure chronic diseases, and we continue to allow some patients to experience their complications. We must correct this error if we are ever to gain control over the escalating costs of health care in this country.

Public health departments need to develop partnerships with businesses and community leaders in order to funnel valuable information to every community concerning the importance of preventing chronic diseases. Each department must appoint a staff member as a liaison between the department and businesses in order to obtain resources for the expansion of prevention programs for a given community.

The chronic disease epidemic is providing public health departments with an opportunity to lead the reform efforts necessary to make our health care system work. It is time for the emergence of public health leadership similar to that present in the early years of our successful battle against communicable diseases. The tools public health professionals use will have to change, but that shift can occur as part of retraining efforts and strong leadership development. Public health departments must exploit this opportunity through assuming leadership roles and forming community partnerships.

Key Terms

Affordable Care Act

Chronic Care Model

Community partnerships

Cost-utility analysis

Tipping point

Discussion Questions

1. Name and explain the major differences between communicable and chronic diseases.
2. What special competencies does the health educator require in order to work effectively with community partners?
3. What are the advantages and disadvantages of community partnerships in dealing with the epidemic of chronic diseases?
4. Explain the use of the Chronic Care Model in dealing with the epidemic of chronic diseases.

PART TWO

ISSUES AND METHODS OF PUBLIC HEALTH LEADERSHIP AND MANAGEMENT

CHAPTER 6

LEADERSHIP AND POLITICS IN PUBLIC HEALTH

LEARNING OBJECTIVES
- Understand how power develops in organizations
- Become aware of the need for leadership skills in public health
- Recognize the role of leadership and politics in the changing health care environment
- Acknowledge the need for new roles and responsibilities for those who work in the field of public health
- Be able to explain the various styles of leadership and relate them to worker empowerment and innovation

The world of business, which includes health care services, is changing every day, catching many companies unprepared to deal with the new customer. The new customer wants quality in both the products and the services he or she purchases, and often does some research before buying anything. The world of business is in a revolution, changing very rapidly to better serve the customer. This is also true in the realm of health care services.

It is a proven fact that bureaucratic organizations do not work well in times of rapid change. A bureaucratic structure often exhibits redundant layers of management that prevent a business from responding rapidly to competition and the needs of its customers. They can only respond rapidly to consumer demands by talking to their customers and empowering their employees to rapidly respond to consumer needs. Health care is no exception to the rapidly changing consumer. Because of the changing nature of the health care system, health care managers relying on rules and regulations need to be replaced by strong leaders who can empower workers to deliver services that meet the needs of the consumers of health care—the patients. This will require a movement from a bureaucratic organizational structure and decentralization of decisions to lower-level employees. This change is also affecting public health departments as they attempt to do their job and retain their funding.

This is not to say that management does not have a role to play in the health care industry, including public health departments. We will always need to have elements of management and control in any business. Managers will assume responsibility for using nonhuman factors of production like technology and equipment in delivering health care services in order to provide for planning for future activities. In fact, managers do very well when they are responsible for things rather than people.

The health care industry is a part of the service sector of our economy, using human beings to provide extremely important services to other humans. This is where management principles do not work very well. Health care workers require leadership and empowerment to rapidly respond to the patient's ever-changing needs. Therefore, there needs to be a separation of the human and nonhuman components of the delivery of all health care services in order for *things* to be managed and *people* to be led.

Most leaders in health care delivery have the unique ability to separate the real problems from the symptoms that resonate from those real problems. They are usually very capable of developing and sharing a vision of what the future could be if we work together and concentrate on the real problems of health care delivery in this country. Leaders are also skilled in productively using their power to make change happen. In other words, they can define the real problems such that people understand why change is necessary in any serious effort to improve health care delivery.

Effective leadership is not about personal success. It is about uniting people in the business around a vision or common purpose. **Leadership** involves the ability of an individual to influence others to accomplish a predetermined goal. Further, Yukl (2010) argues that leadership involves having influence over individuals to guide or facilitate group activities. It is that special something that separates successful organizations from those that fail. It seems to be one of the most important components in determining the effectiveness of organizations. It is the glue that holds a thick, positive culture together, allowing the achievement of greater success.

Development of Power in Health Care Delivery

The use and abuse of power remain the major reasons for many of the failures in our current system of health care delivery. The power needs to shift to the consumers of health care and away from the providers of care. There are a number of people who believe that the majority of the income the various players in health care delivery receive is a direct result of health laws and regulations.

Legislation determines who can and cannot practice medicine, dispense drugs, and admit and discharge patients from hospitals. The rules and regulations actually determine all income in health care. They are responsible for the development of power in health care, which in turn has shaped the way we deliver health care to our citizens. It will be virtually impossible to make positive change in health care without first dealing with the power of those who currently control this very large and vitally important sector of the American economy.

Power is nothing more than the ability to influence the way things are done or how goals are accomplished. There are several types of power, including legitimate power, coercive power, reward power, expert power, and referent power. Legitimate, coercive, and reward power originate from the position one holds in an organization. Expert and referent power are found in the individual and are considered personal power. Legitimate power comes from the top administrators of an organization and usually produces a bureaucratic organization run by a manager who follows the rules and regulations put forth by those top administrators. This is the way health care operates and the major reason why change is usually blocked. Those in power fear the loss of control if things are done differently. Personal power, however, is found in many individuals and is owned by each person, not the organization.

Figure 6.1 shows the sources of both position power and personal power. It is interesting to note that power is necessary to make change happen but that it can also block change from ever occurring. Both types of power take time to develop and are very important to getting anything done in any organization or relationship. You lose position power when you leave your position in an

FIGURE 6.1 Sources of Power

Power of the POSITION: *Based on things managers can offer to others*	Power of the PERSON: *Based on the ways managers are viewed by others*
Rewards: "If you do what I ask, I'll give you a reward."	**Expertise:** As a source of special knowledge and information
Coercion: "If you *don't* do what I ask, I'll punish you."	**Reference:** As a person with whom others like to identify
Legitimacy: "Because I am the boss, you *must* do as I ask."	

Source: Lombardi, 2007, p. 248.

organization, whereas you take personal power with you. Leaders usually have personal power, but they may or may not have position power.

I (Bernard) experienced the abuse of power very early in my career. My first position in public health involved investigating venereal diseases, now called sexually transmitted diseases. My duties included interviewing those infected with syphilis and gonorrhea, and finding their sexual contacts and bringing these individuals to treatment. In this position I was not allowed to educate young people to prevent infections, but rather was required to spend all of my time finding infected people. In fact, it negatively affected my annual evaluations if I used my time educating children in school districts. When I questioned my supervisors about the value of prevention rather than control, I was told that I was not paid to educate.

This is a very good example of the power of program directors forcing a system not to change even though it is obvious that the wrong approach to solving a problem is being used. Many more types of sexually transmitted diseases have become epidemic among younger and younger children in this country over the years. The misuse of power is at the root of this failure, and even today the majority of money allocated for coping with sexually transmitted diseases goes to contact tracing and not education.

This is the same type of arrogant abuse of power that is keeping our health care system focused on treating expensive illnesses rather than on supporting wellness, which would lower costs, reduce access to health services, and diminish monopoly profits for those in control. Those in control resist change because they cannot envision a new health care system that preserves their power and wealth. They are probably right—if we had a health care system that kept people well, the large monopoly profits of many providers would disappear. This change-resistant mentality must shift if the greatest health care system is going to survive. Effective leadership has been difficult to find in health care because of the development of power in the various groups that control how the system functions. In order for leaders who want to change the system to emerge in health care, they must have the courage to face the tremendous power of those who control the resources of, and therefore rule, the health care industry. In order to begin to deal with the problems of health care delivery, the workers in health care must become empowered to offer quality and cost-effective services to their customers. Further, the leader must first be empowered before he or she can empower others.

The normal response by a business when a given strategy is not producing the desired results is to change the strategy. Systems of health care delivery do not seem to follow this business practice, even though health care outcomes are less successful than desired. There has always been a very strong resistance by those who are rewarded and have power, especially those who control payment and those who receive the payments, to changing the way health care is delivered in this country. This is because there is no incentive to change. In fact, it seems that all of the financing in the payment for health services helps to make problems in health care worse. It is probably the only industry that is paid more for failed services. The system attempts to do too much of the wrong things, including treatment measures that have very little if any value in their contribution to good health.

Even though everyone understands the need for wellness efforts in order to improve the health of our nation, the financial incentives still favor illness rather than wellness. This is because the American system of health care has been built around illness and does very little to encourage individuals to stay healthy. In fact, the only time when you get anything back from your health insurance is when you become ill and start receiving bills for treatment of your poor health that you can pass on to your insurance company. There is very little incentive for you to practice healthy behaviors that would help you remain free of disease as you grow older.

This paradigm of health care must be shifted. It makes absolutely no sense to allow individuals to become ill when it is well known that a large majority of illnesses could have been prevented if the delivery system were changed. This required change should also include modified incentives and reimbursement structures, and will most certainly affect the incomes and power of those who currently control the system.

The right change in our health care system could solve simultaneously the problems associated with cost escalation, uneven access to health care, and diminishing quality of life as we age. This change would require action rather than discussion about the value of wellness programs. It is possible to produce financial incentives that can slowly transform an illness-based health care system to one that incentivizes keeping people well. This change will not occur while all monetary incentives encourage treatment of illness and ignorance toward the value of preserving the population's health.

There is enough blame to go around for our failures in producing better health for our population. Everyone in health care, especially public health departments, have to get involved with the change process, empowering their followers to recognize and respond to the need for change in health care delivery. Extraordinary achievements require active support of others. This requires trust, and trust can only grow when the leader and the followers work together according to their common vision.

In a recent report titled *The Future of the Public's Health in the 21st Century* (Institute of Medicine [IOM], 2002, p. 4), a very prestigious group of health experts made the following recommendations to public health departments for improving population health:

1. Adopting a population health approach that considers the multiple determinants of health;
2. Strengthening the governmental public health infrastructure, which forms the backbone of the public health system;
3. Building a new generation of intersectoral partnerships that also draw on the perspectives and resources of diverse communities and actively engage them in health action;
4. Develop systems of accountability to assure the quality and availability of public health services;
5. Making evidence the foundation of decision making and the measure of success; and
6. Enhancing and facilitating communication within the public health system (e.g., among all levels of the governmental public health infrastructure and between public health professionals and community members).

In order for these recommendations to become reality, leaders must emerge from among those who work in public health in the United States.

Maciariello (2006) offers a systems view of executive leadership and effectiveness put forth by Peter Drucker a number of years ago. Figure 6.2 provides a systems view of the internal and external components of leadership that are prerequisites for accomplishing the actions and changes the Institute of Medicine proposed in 2002. Drucker points out that this figure shows the three interconnected areas of leadership and effectiveness—personal attributes and practices, special skills, and particular tasks that a leader must perform in order to improve his or her effectiveness (cited in Maciariello, 2006). Individuals can develop these attributes through leadership training programs. We will discuss the skills public health administrators require in Chapter Nine.

Leadership and Politics in Health Care Delivery

There are many who believe that we have a crisis in our health care system in regard to the leadership of health care institutions—a crisis that involves the politicians who develop and ultimately fund policy decisions related to health care. The government is the largest payer of health care services and concentrates on paying for medical procedures rather than reimbursing for the outcomes associated with medical interventions in the overall health of the patient. The

FIGURE 6.2   Systems View: Executive Leadership and Effectiveness

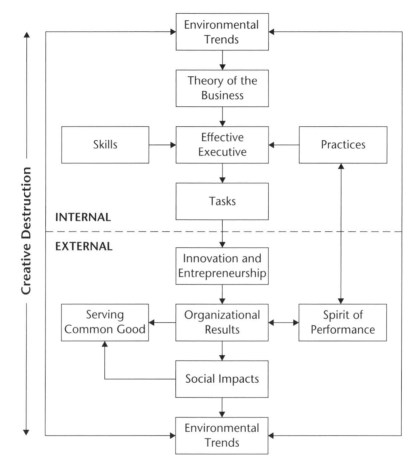

Source: Maciariello, 2006, p. 4.

U.S. health care system is in desperate need of strong leadership in order to solve the problems that poor management and a lack of attention to the patient have caused. Other sectors of our economy, such as automobiles, computers, and software development, have been restructured in response to a crisis, and actually began to perform better after leaders came forth and made appropriate changes in the way they were managed. In its own state of crisis, the health care sector needs the wisdom of leaders who can diagnose the real problems and respond with the necessary solutions. These health care leaders must be able to bring together followers in a united vision of better health for all at a price that we can afford.

The health care sector has not seemed to require leadership in the past, primarily because of the way health facilities and physicians were reimbursed for care. The old retrospective reimbursement system actually rewarded inefficiency by paying for care regardless of its outcome. The result was tremendous waste of scarce resources, inappropriate tests and hospitalizations, and the expansion of poor managerial decisions. The health care industry became a hopeless bureaucracy that received rewards for poor choices. Many powerful coalitions such as medical and hospital associations still exist, hold tremendous power, and are blocking the needed change to a system that advocates preventive care as the model for delivering health services.

Bureaucratic management techniques have not worked very well in most organizations in recent years. Decisions need to be made rapidly and usually require an empowered workforce capable of immediately responding to consumer demands. **Bureaucracies,** which are organizations run according to rigid rules and regulations and directed under centralized authority, are not designed for rapid response to consumer needs because of the rules and regulations the management imposes. Leaders rather than managers have a much better chance of inducing a rapid response to shifting consumer demands, especially in the delivery of services. The health care delivery system is a business that provides very special services for its customers. It is no secret that these services have been poorly managed in the past, and the system is seeking leadership, just as are other sectors of our economy that are also facing troubled times and having difficulty responding to rapid change.

Never have the problems facing our health care system been so numerous and so very difficult to solve. These challenges can only be resolved by strong leadership. Although there are problems in health care delivery, there are also numerous opportunities present to actually improve health care outcomes as the health care sector reorganizes. The industry needs to carefully reevaluate how its practitioners deliver health care and to try to improve the entire process. This is clearly a time of profound change in the paradigm of how medicine works. There is no reason why they cannot shift the health care system's focus to prevention and away from waiting for people to become ill and then attempting to cure them. The old system may have worked well with communicable diseases, but it has failed utterly in regard to chronic diseases that cannot be cured.

It is interesting to note that the public health sector is also changing the way it seeks to improve the health of all Americans. Public health departments are focusing more attention on the need for leadership development in order to accomplish their goals, and are also attempting to increase their responsibilities and learn how to better evaluate the success of their own health interventions. Although the challenges are enormous, the opportunities to improve the health of all Americans have never been more abundant. In order to exploit these opportunities, public health departments must learn how to lead communities in the improvement of their health.

A landmark report concerning the state of public health, *The Future of Public Health* (IOM, 1988), demanded leadership development for those charged with delivering public health services in this country. The report argued that "the need for leaders is too great to leave their emergence to chance" (p. 6). The report went on to recommend that public health leaders develop greater leadership effectiveness, and that schools of public health add leadership to their curriculum. This report has influenced the increased provision of leadership education to individuals pursuing a career in public health.

The Institute of Medicine's report (1988) also called for the emergence of a special type of leader for public health departments in the new century. This new leader will perform traditional management functions, but will also work with stakeholders, community groups, and other government agencies in order to push public health goals to acceptance and achievement. This new leader will require special talents, including a firm understanding of public health problems to be overcome and the leadership skills needed to unite followers in the accomplishment of the new mission of public health. Assuming such a leadership role would be a challenging task for those placed in leadership positions in public health departments, but it could be accomplished if those in charge possess the appropriate leadership skills.

The public health leader needs to continue to build a thick departmental culture that empowers dedicated public health workers to become the key sources for motivating new tasks, and encourages them to accept changes as opportunities for growth. We must understand public health leadership to be a never-ending process. The vision has to include the protection of all Americans from the many dangers of their environments and from their own high-risk health behaviors. Strong, consistent, visible leadership is essential for sending a message of support to all Americans. Public health leaders must also work to bring together the medical establishment and public health departments in an attempt to improve health, and ultimately to reduce health costs and increase the quality of care.

Public Health Leadership Styles

Some of the older theories of leadership assert that leadership qualities are inherited. In other words, leaders have **leadership traits** built into the genes their parents gave them. According to Lussier and Achua (2004), leadership traits are distinctive characteristics (like physical appearance or self-reliance) that account for the effectiveness of a leader. From these theories there emerged the belief that several traits are responsible for one's ability to lead. Pierce and Newstrom (2006) define traits as general characteristics that could include individual motives, capacities, or patterns of behaviors. There are many who believe that these and other general traits may contribute to what makes someone a good leader. Traits do matter in leadership, but they are not enough to define a good leader. Because traits cannot be taught, it makes very little sense to include trait theory when considering the development of public health leaders. If an individual requires certain traits to be a leader, then the old adage "he or she is a born leader" would seem to be true. There is no question that being gifted in speech or exuding self-confidence does not hurt your leadership capabilities, but having these traits does not guarantee that you will become a leader.

Novick, Morrow, and Mays (2008) argue that having a certain trait, like being tall, does not in itself guarantee success as a leader. It is true, however, that certain traits help the leader communicate his or her vision to followers in a more believable format. If the followers agree with the vision, the voyage to successful goal attainment becomes much easier. These are communication skills, and it is likely they are learned rather than inherited.

There is no question that leaders are different from nonleaders, whether in regard to their traits, the situations they have to face, their exposure to leadership training programs, or a combination of all of these conditions. It is important for public health leaders to come in contact with all of the various leadership theories in order to understand the importance of leadership and learn how to grow as leaders to face the near-impossible tasks that will continue to confront public health departments in the future.

The way a leader behaves influences his or her followers. From the moment a new leader is introduced in an organization, the followers begin to watch and evaluate his or her behaviors. Northouse (2007) argues that leaders generally exhibit two kinds of behaviors: task behaviors and relationship behaviors. Task behaviors focus on the job, whereas relationship behaviors concentrate on interpersonal abilities. Both kinds of behaviors work very well in some situations but fail in others. There seems to be solid agreement among most researchers that the situation is the controlling variable that determines which leadership style works best. Leaders of public health programs may require a combination of these behaviors to accomplish public health goals. Therefore, possessing people skills may not be enough to be a successful leader of a public health department, especially in the twenty-first century. In order to attract more resources from tight government budgets, public health departments must continue to solve public health problems. This may require the leader to revert to task behaviors when goals are not being accomplished.

A leader's style—the way he or she behaves—is of great importance when he or she interacts with those purchasing a service from his or her organization. Public health is a service industry that for the most part shares information with individuals regarding their health. This type of business usually requires an administrator with a people-oriented leadership style. Public health departments have a small staff and limited resources available to accomplish very large goals. They are forced to rely on community support to achieve these goals, and in order to gain such support their leaders need strong people skills—including the ability to communicate with community stakeholders.

There are times when a leader must exhibit task behaviors in order to be successful at a given mission. The public health team is responsible for accomplishing the goals, whereas the leader is responsible for giving the team the resources they require in this process. Quite often a leader's task behaviors may facilitate the goal accomplishment. Relationship behaviors come into play when a leader helps team members feel good about and supported in whatever they are trying to achieve. It seems obvious that in order to lead public health departments in this new century, leaders require both people- and task-based skills . . . yet many current administrators in these departments are devoid of either type.

In order to better understand leadership, it is helpful to understand the motives an individual might have for seeking and accepting a leadership role. Manning and Curtis (2007) argue that there are three motives to lead—the desire for achievement, the desire for power or the ability to influence others, and the desire for affiliation interpreted as an interest in helping others. There is no question that the majority of people who seek a career in public health do so because of a desire to help other people. The problem is that most top positions in public health departments are given to political appointees, who usually have a short tenure. These appointees have usually helped the governor or county administrator win the election, and are then rewarded with a position in a government agency. Many of these political appointees have a motive to survive and keep their job rather than to take the risky road of leadership. If a potential improvement poses a risk to the political appointee, you can be certain that the improvement will not occur. This is why public health departments are so very conservative in their approach to change.

According to Kouzes and Posner (1995), every leader seeks challenge, exploits change, and understands the great risk that is present in all of his or her actions. By definition, managers are not expected to go beyond the planned outcome that has been determined by their superior. Leaders, however, allow the larger vision and not the planned outcome to determine the results of their activities. It is very difficult to push for a vision that is controversial and may cost you to lose power and even your employment. This is why public health administrators have been reluctant to criticize our current health care system—being critical of this system is risky because those responsible are afraid to take on the medical elite for fear of losing their political appointment.

The style of the leader is contingent on the way he or she behaves. This style is especially visible in the leader's interaction with the employees of the organization or group of which he or she is in charge. It seems obvious that the way a leader behaves affects employees' response to him or her as well as their performance. Lussier and Achua (2004) argue that several studies of leadership theory conducted over the last thirty years have continued to focus on two major types of leader behaviors: task- or work-centered behaviors and employee-centered behaviors. Again, the type of behavior that works best for the leader depends on the situation he or she faces.

The motivation of both the leader and the followers is also important in determining followers' behavior and their response to that leader. A bureaucratic leader who is afraid of risk will not be able to achieve public health goals in the twenty-first century. It won't take long for bureaucratic leader behaviors to destroy the thick culture of public health workers, and once this culture is ruined it will take years to repair the damage.

Leadership is a small component of the entire process of public health management, but also one of the most important—especially to organizations that supply services. Novick et al. (2008) point out that those responsible for the management of public health programs may not offer leadership to practitioners because of their own lack of training or experience. This must be changed in order for those in charge of public health departments to understand the value of leadership.

Transformational Leadership and Public Health

There are many styles of leadership, but the gold standard in service organizations seems to be the **transformational style of leadership.** According to Trompenaars and Voerman (2010), transformational leadership involves the leader's ability to change the consciousness of his or her followers through identification of desires that were previously unconscious. This type of leader represents the ultimate change agent.

This is certainly the case when dealing with a volatile environment that is ripe for change and in need of innovation in the delivery of services. The health care industry has been attempting to change the way it delivers care for the last twenty years. The new health reform law passed in 2010 has become a catalyst for improving the health of the population by including a number of provisions that focus on disease prevention. Because of this new law, public health departments have a once-in-a-lifetime opportunity to be catalysts for reforming the way health services are delivered in our country. Exploiting this opportunity will require strong leadership that supports empowered workers.

Northouse (2007) points out that the transformational style of leadership does not include assumptions about how a leader should act; rather, this style encompasses a way to think about leading. This style's emphasis is clearly on inspiration and innovation in the way the organization does business. The transformational leader works to inspire followers to look for change on a daily basis and exploit that change to improve the business. The transformational leader is very interested in both developing a vision and achieving this vision through his or her followers. This leader wants not only to achieve personal and organizational goals but also to see his or her followers achieve their personal goals and grow in the process. In order to accomplish this, the leader has to share power.

Tichy (1997) argues that the transformational leader seeks to transform his or her follower into leaders themselves. This implies that the major role of a transformational leader is to positively motivate those around him or her, directing followers' energy toward goal accomplishment. This synergy allows the impossible not only to become possible but also to become the norm for the organization. This is exactly the leadership style that is needed to provide direction through the ambiguity confronting public health departments in the United States today. These departments need to better define how they plan to accomplish their long-term goals in accordance with Healthy People 2020. The U.S. public health system is faced with increasing demands, limited or declining budgets, and politicians who want no part of public health until there is an emergency. Then the politicians throw money at the emergency and try to make it go away, when it could have been prevented in the first place.

Novick et al. (2008) believe that transformational leadership in public health requires true empowerment of all team members to accomplish predetermined goals for their program. Such empowerment may create serious problems for the department head due to the political nature of public health departments. These problems might include offending individuals or groups of people who disagree with a particular public health program, such as one that dispenses condoms to younger children. This is one of the reasons for the short tenure of many leaders in public health departments: doing the right thing for the health of the people entails risk to employment, even from the very people leaders are attempting to help.

Northouse (2007) points out that a transformational leader has the unique ability to get all team members interested more in the current project or organizational goal to be achieved than in their own personal interests. This type of leader should be communicating the goals of public health to all of the various constituencies, including community leaders, that have the resources and support to make these aspirations achievable. People are attracted to the transformational leader because he or she is able to explain his or her cause in such a way that supporters understand and want to be part of the movement toward better health for all.

According to Beltsch, Brooks, Menachemi, and Libbey (2007), public health departments have to manage old programs that have never finished accomplishing their goals as well as new programs that add to their responsibilities—all with a dwindling resource base. Public health has never been funded very well in this country because it has never been truly understood by those who control funding. There are many reasons why public health is not fully understood, but the answer to this dilemma may very well be found in the dearth of leadership skills among the top executives of public health agencies. Beltsch and colleagues argue for a change in this country's investment in public health activities. This investment has to command accountability for resource use and the development of a well-trained cadre of public health program leaders. These goals are large, but they can be accomplished through the development of public health leadership and through partnerships with other community health agencies, businesses, and school districts.

According to Novick et al. (2008), one of the major problems the transformational leader faces is the tendency for followers to change back to their old ways of doing things if the leader is not always present. Once the transformational leader is not available to support followers, the old ways of delivering services tend to reemerge and become dominant. Followers are often dependent on the charisma that is always present with the transformational leader. This makes the short tenure of a public health leader a very real liability in the transformation of a public health department. The followers who are left when the transformational public health leader departs are unable to function with the same energy because they feel that part of their team is no longer available. In these instances, the former leader usually has not had the time to fully develop his or her replacement. Further, because most public health departments are funded by government and, therefore, political, there is no guarantee that another leader with transformational leadership skills will be appointed.

Public Health as a Change Agent

A profound change in operations is needed to save the U.S. health care system. Kotter (1995) argues that managers are usually engrossed with complexity, whereas leaders devote their time to change. The pace of change has quickened in recent years, and nowhere is the change process happening at a faster pace than in the service sector of our economy. Public health departments offer services, and they too are caught up in the accelerated process of change. Public health leaders must be capable of responding to change in the form of new crises and new responsibilities that present themselves on a daily basis.

Strong leadership is never in greater demand than when there are dramatic shifts in the way business is done. Pierce and Newstrom (2006) discuss how leaders require the ability to frame reality for their followers. This framing or structuring of the future must be done in a meaningful way for members of the organization to accept and work to achieve the goals associated with that future. Leaders today must learn to manage change rather than simply react to it (Lussier and Achua, 2004). In fact, leaders must be able to exploit change for the opportunities that it can open up for their organization. Change can also bring threats of which the organization needs to be aware, and to which the organization must develop a proactive response in order to continue growth. Finally, those in leadership positions in public health have frequently seen change as the enemy because they fear loss of position power.

The leader and followers need to develop a concept of change as more of a process than a product (Lussier and Achua, 2004). This entails acceptance by the entire organization that environmental change is the catalyst that will transform the organization to meet the vision espoused by the leader and accepted by his or her followers. Change can then become a continuous process of quality improvement and growth for the public health agency. Stadler (2007) points out that one of the prerequisites for leading on a long-term basis is to be conservative about change. This author advocates the exploitation of change, but does not advocate for radical change without appropriate planning. In other words, the leader needs to prepare the organization for opportunities that present themselves through change, but he or she must do so with caution. This is very good advice for public health departments that are always in the media spotlight when public health problems develop.

Public Health Leaders and Power

An individual requires a power base in order to lead any group or organization. Northouse (2007) argues that in order for a leader to influence individuals, a power relationship must exist between the leader and the followers. Because goal achievement requires change, the use of some form of power is required to make change happen.

Northouse (2007) also points out that there are usually two major types of power found in individuals, which are derived from the position or are found in the individual. They are position power and personal power. Lussier and Achua (2004) argue that perceived power may be the key ingredient in developing the ability to influence others. In other words, to influence others, leaders may only need followers to think that they have either position or personal power. These are interesting concepts to keep in mind when evaluating public health leaders' ability to influence followers toward the achievement of public health goals.

Because the vast majority of public health agencies are government sponsored, their structure is usually bureaucratic. A bureaucratic organization relies heavily on position power to achieve its goals. This type of power is derived from the top management or the chief executive of the government entity and flows from the top of the organization downward. Position power involves legitimate, coercive, and reward power, which are owned by the organization and not the leader (Lussier and Achua, 2004). This type of power can be taken away from the individual if he or she makes mistakes. Therefore, bureaucratic leaders are always at risk of losing their position power if they anger those above them in the organizational chart. This makes these leaders very cautious about making decisions, especially if they involve risk.

Risk is part of making change happen, and if the bureaucratic leader's career is in jeopardy every time change is required, he or she will be less inclined to take part in the change process. This has always been a recognized impediment to making rapid change happen in government. Public health leaders are well aware of the implied risk in any actions they undertake to deal with public health issues. There is always the chance that being part of change that affects large numbers of people may anger some politically powerful individuals. The end result of this type of confrontation can be a public health leader's having to relinquish position power.

Lussier and Achua (2004) also discuss the personal power that some leaders possess. Personal power comes forth from the leader and is owned by the leader. When an individual leaves an organization, he or she takes along personal power. Personal power confers on a leader the ability to influence individuals because they like him or her and respect his or her expertise (Northouse, 2007). The two types of personal power usually found in leadership research are charisma and expertise. Charisma, or referent power, consists of certain traits found in an individual that are appealing to followers (Lussier and Achua). This type of power results from relationships with others and usually involves friendship or loyalty between the leader and the follower. This type of power can be developed through education and training programs. It is interesting to note that personal power can also be found among followers who are not in any type of leadership position.

The transformational style of leadership relies more on the personal power of the leader than it does on position power, and the transformational process requires the leader to be considered a competent role model by his or her followers. Such a leader has a vision of the future, and everything that leader does is part of the road map to the attainment of that vision. Getting followers to espouse the vision through the use of personal power is one way to speed up progress in making the vision a reality. Healthy People 2010 is a vision for population health that requires transformational leadership to achieve all of its objectives. Novick et al. (2008) argue that in order to accomplish large goals that have an impact on the American public—like those put forth in Healthy People 2010—public health leaders must collaborate with others in the political landscape. This is where the transformational style of leadership can serve the public health leader. By collaborating with others on the achievement of community goals, the leader can avoid the political dangers of trying to accomplish broad public health goals.

Public Health Leaders and Conflict Management

In order to attain the goals of public health in the twenty-first century, public health leaders will have to experience and learn how to manage conflict. Bureaucratic organizations usually see conflict as bad and attempt to suppress conflict with a heavy reliance on rules and regulations that prevent it from arising. In the new world of public health, we should view conflict as normal and even energizing, and top management should actually support it. Manning and Curtis (2007) argue that conflicting goals and personalities are expected among people in a healthy, vibrant organization. The leader needs to be aware that change is the breeding ground for conflict and that part of the leader's role as change agent is dealing with this conflict. The leader must also be aware that while he or she is attempting to improve the health of the community there will be conflict among some segments of the community population.

Leaders need to realize that the success of a public health agency may depend on how well it handles conflict. Lussier and Achua (2004) argue that conflict management may take up to 20 percent of leaders' time and a great deal of their energy. The ability to handle that conflict may be one of the public health leader's most important skills; the leader cannot and should not try to avoid conflict. Conflict resolution can build collaboration throughout the organization and sometimes the community—and collaboration is needed to make public health departments stronger and able to achieve greater goals as they address twenty-first-century health problems (Lussier and Achua).

Can Political Appointees Lead Public Health Departments?

The predominant form of public health department in the United States is a local health department (LHD). The LHD is most often the responsibility of the city or county government, and its powers and duties are granted by the state. There are approximately three thousand LHDs functioning in the United States, all of which provide mandated public health services and many of which are responsible for the development of new and innovative public health programs.

The major power (control of resources) is usually found at the state level. The leadership positions in public health at the state level are almost always politically appointed by the governor or his or her designee. The IOM (2002) reports that a state public health official's term in office is tied to the governor's term, making the average tenure for these appointments 3.9 years, with a median of 2.9 years. This is certainly too short of a time frame for an appointee to use any leadership skills that he or she may have, given the learning curve necessary to fully understand the role of public health in the community. Tenure, or time in the job, is a critical component in the development of leadership skills. The politics of public health leadership needs to be studied at length if we are ever going to be able to develop strong public health leaders and empowered followers as we work to keep our nation healthy, free of disease, and protected from the many threats to the public's health.

Public health leaders need to learn how to develop their staff and share the power of the agency with all of the workers involved in serving the public, even though this is very difficult to accomplish within a short tenure. The public health system in this country is most dependent on its greatest resource—its workforce. These dedicated individuals come from a wide range of professions, educational backgrounds, and motivations for pursuing a career in public health. These are individuals whom the public health leader needs to energize toward accomplishment of public health goals. It is these people who can develop and implement the prevention programs to deal with the epidemic of chronic diseases.

These followers, because of their diverse training experiences and their thick professional culture, cannot be managed for very long in a bureaucratic organization. They are different—because of the nature of their duties—in that they need to be empowered both for personal growth and for the accomplishment of organizational goals. It takes political appointees in management positions in public health agencies a long time to understand how very different these followers are. They cannot be managed; they must be led and truly empowered or they lose their motivation to perform—at which point they get frustrated and move on to the private sector, where their skills are better appreciated.

According to Pierce and Newstrom (2006) it is very important to understand the role of the follower if one is ever to understand the process of leadership. In other words, we must understand the traits that make up the followers if we are to gauge their receptivity to certain leadership styles. If the leader is ever going to be successful at gaining the support of followers, he or she must pay a great deal of attention to followers' needs, perceptions, and expectations. The vast majority of followers in public health have longer tenure in their positions than the leader. They also have been through changes in management in the past. They are conditioned by what happened and did not happen with the previous leaders.

Empowerment then becomes a process in which the leader shares power with followers so as to develop their own personal power. Position power is absent from this definition of empowerment by choice. One never really owns position power, because the risk of losing this type of power is always present. Every time position power is used to influence or lead, there is always the risk of loss associated with that action. The tendency for individuals with only position power is to not take chances for fear of losing power and damaging their career. To those who only have position power, change becomes the enemy and is, therefore, resisted. Leaders who fear change tend to avoid empowering their followers because this empowerment increases the leaders' chance of losing position power. Public health departments have been the victim of many administrators who did not seek to empower their followers. Fortunately for the American public, some leaders with personal power and the ability to empower followers also have been part of the history of public health. Even with short tenure they have been able to produce admirable public health accomplishments. It is unfortunate that this is such a rare occurrence in public health leadership, however, it being very difficult to respond to public health challenges when you are in constant fear of losing your appointment because of angering politically powerful groups.

Communication Skills of the Leader

Novick et al. (2008) argue that the most important skills required of a leader in the twenty-first century are communication skills. A leader needs communication skills to present the mission statement and goals of the organization, which is essential in getting all stakeholders to become supportive of the leader's vision (Lussier and Achua, 2004).

Northouse (2007) discusses the concept of emergent leadership in which followers believe that the leader has gained influence over the group through his or her communication skills. By being able to communicate with employees the leader can gain the trust and support of the individuals that are so important in the achievement of short-term and long-term goals of public health departments. Communication is actually a major part of the leadership strategy (Lussier and Achua, 2004). There is a very strong relationship between communication skills and the effective performance of a leader. Communication tools are essential to leadership development and goal attainment in public health. The IOM (2002) argues that leaders in public health must be able to communicate internally and externally in order to distribute vital health information to their staff, other agencies, the media, and the community. They must also be able to gather information from the public about disease occurrence and rapidly distribute to the public information concerning emerging public health problems.

Communication skills along with an understanding of the value of technology for health promotion can become very effective tools in responding to the epidemic of chronic diseases in this country (IOM, 2002). The IOM recommends that all partners within the public health system make communication skills a critical core competency of public health departments. The IOM further advocates for the expansion of vital information systems that can help leaders rapidly disseminate public health information to those who need to know. The public health leader must understand and embrace the value of communication skills in the world of public health in the twenty-first century.

Leadership Development in Public Health

Mays, Miller, and Halverson (2000) argue that the demand for professional development, especially leadership training, has grown in response to a multitude of external forces. One of these forces is the need for collaboration among many community agencies trying to make their constituents healthier while also dealing with emerging infections and the threat of bioterrorism. The IOM recognized the need for leadership training in the executive summary of their 2002 report, in which they recommend that Congress increase funding for public health training, especially leadership training, for state and local health department directors. The Centers for Disease Control and Prevention (CDC) also has responded with programs like the Public Health Leadership Institute and the National Public Health Leadership Development Network, which offer leadership development and training to public health professionals throughout the country.

As noted earlier, leadership skills are usually not part of the curriculum in schools of public health. "Getting an MPH [master's degree in public health] does not necessarily confer on you the realities of practicing public health, just as medical schools do not necessarily train doctors to handle money or management issues," said Stephanie Coursey Bailey, chief at the CDC's Office of Public Health

Practice (quoted in Gale Reference Team, 2007, p. 25). The IOM (2002) points out that the MPH is the degree that many public health workers earn, especially those who remain in public health long enough to become program managers. However, a large number of individuals found in leadership positions in public health have academic preparation in areas other than public health and usually have not received any leadership training. This is because they are political appointees, especially at the state level. Despite the academic certification of the public health leader, it is very rare to find individuals with strong leadership training credentials. This means that the individuals appointed to these positions may require training in public health along with leadership training in a very short period of time.

A very small part of the current workforce in public health departments receive training in public health before they begin their career. The average public health worker usually receives on-the-job training in a specific area of public health, such as epidemiology, public health nursing, laboratory science, or health education. Further, even if a worker has a degree or certification in the specific discipline of public health in which he or she is employed, there is almost no chance that the worker received training in leadership or communication skills as part of his or her formal education.

The Nation's Health offered an excellent article titled "Leadership Institutes Help Public Health Workers Advance Careers" (Gale Reference Team, 2007). This article highlights the value of public health workers' attending one of the many public health institutes that offer professional development opportunities to public health practitioners across the United States.

Geoffrey Downie, program manager of the Mid-American Regional Public Health Institute, said that all institutes "share the belief that system thinking is a key component to effective leadership and that community health will improve if the public health infrastructure is sustained and supported" (quoted in Gale Reference Team, 2007, p. 25). Joyce R. Gaufin, executive director of the Great Basin Public Health Leadership Institute in Salt Lake City, commenting about those who complete leadership training, said, "One of the most important individual benefits of participation is an increased sense of confidence about their own abilities and the actions they take as a leader" (quoted in Gale Reference Team, p. 25) These leadership training programs usually entail a one-year commitment, and the training is provided by expert faculty from leading schools of public health, business programs, and the private sector. Funding for these programs comes from a variety of sources, including the CDC, state and local public health agencies, and public health foundations.

We must continue and expand these efforts at providing leadership training opportunities to the public health workforce if we are serious about improving the health of our nation. "The need for leadership in public health is well documented, and many would agree that at no time in the nation's history has the need been greater," said Kate Wright, director of the National Public Health Leadership Development Network. There is a great deal of discussion about standardization by the various organizations that are providing leadership training programs to members of the public health workforce, suggesting the need for schools of public health to develop best practices in public health leadership and to share them with leaders and followers in all public health departments throughout the country.

Culture of Public Health Workers

A culture is a combination of learned beliefs, values, rules, and symbols that are common to a group of people. Kotter and Heskett (1992) argue that developing a strong culture can have powerful consequences, because this culture can enable a group to become proactive in the way its members deal with the problems that confront them. In public health, the creation of a strong culture also results in most managers sharing a set of relatively consistent values and methods of completing work (Kotter and Heskett).

Hickman (1998) argues that a company with a corporate culture that pushes positive change understands the value of the individuals and the processes that create change. Such a company truly believes in its workers and respects its customers, and it shows every day in the way top management acts in the workplace. This company demonstrates a performance-enhancing culture that takes pride in its workers and customers and would never do anything to intentionally hurt either group.

The culture of an organization forms through a process of successful interaction that causes it to be assimilated throughout the workplace (Keyton, 2005). This interaction is a learning and teaching experience for workers in regard to how the process of work is accomplished. The leader needs to obtain from the workers a commitment to a shared set of values. This attempt at culture formation will only work if all workplace members are part of the process. Participation must be voluntary, and it must be a result of the workers' buying into the leader's vision. It is a continuous process that will never end because there will always be room for improvement in the work process.

The successful leader must work very hard at empowering workers to sustain a thick culture, spending a great deal of time and energy encouraging employees to embrace the goals of the organization and to actively work with him or her to accomplish the organization's stated goals. Empowerment is the complete sharing of power with lower-level employees who are critical to successful goal attainment. The leader is most effective when he or she has the ability to make a task for a follower meaningful. This task of building a culture of continuous quality improvement in the workplace is probably the most important responsibility of a leader in today's work environment. We will further discuss the culture of public health workers in the next chapter.

Expertise concerning the work process is a form of power that is usually already present among the workers and just needs to be activated by the leader. There are several ways that the workplace leader can empower the employees. The leader needs to consistently search for people who want to win and who can be empowered to translate short-term wins into long-term successes. Leaders have to create a culture in an organization in which workers are really the key sources for motivating new tasks, and in which employees accept changes as opportunities for growth. Smircich and Morgan (2006) argue that leadership situations consist of an obligation and right of the leader to structure the real world, which includes the leader's vision for others. In other words, the leader has the ability to control the behavior of followers to allow them to see and believe in his or her vision. The leader must recognize that followers need to agree to the vision he or she proposes and the work process that flows from this vision. Leaders should not make changes in the way work is done unless they rethink the process of work through discussions with those who actually do the work. This process should produce a culture that becomes adaptive to continuous change in the improvement of the process of work.

There are so many descriptions and definitions of leadership that it becomes virtually impossible to discover one definition that is accepted by everyone. As we have seen in previous sections, leadership is quite often described in terms of some type of power relationship between the leader and followers. The concepts of power development and power sharing can provide us with a better understanding of what the leader can and cannot do for the organization. The leader's potential for success diminishes if the followers in the workplace do not validate his or her power.

Leadership involves the ability to acquire the respect and support from members of an organization that are necessary to accomplish organizational goals (Dubrin, 2007). Leaders are responsible for developing the culture of the company to emphasize accountability and help managers understand that they are responsible for processes rather than activities. In order to do this, a bond must develop between the organization's leaders and employees. Leadership involves the sharing of power with every worker in the company in order for the business to succeed at accomplishing its major goals.

The leader who is gifted with charisma can communicate a vision of a workplace in such a way that workers are inspired to accomplish the goals inherent in that vision (Dubrin, 2007). The vision the leader articulates is capable of attracting others to want to be a part of it; it brings together workers who want to contribute to its successful realization.

Manning and Curtis (2007) point out that clarity of purpose can serve as a guide for a leader in making decisions that inspire others to follow the vision he or she puts forth. This clarity of purpose allows everyone the opportunity to understand the reasons for the decisions the business is making. Northouse (2007) argues that a transformational style of leadership is a necessity in getting workers motivated and involved in supporting the betterment of the company and the entire workforce, rather than only looking out for their own interests. The transformational leader works very hard to develop a supportive environment for listening to workers in an attempt to get them to self-actualize and become the best at what they do at work. This leader has a very clear vision of where he or she wants the organization to be in the future. Further, the vision the leader creates gives followers a sense of identity within the organization (Northouse, 2007). The followers are then capable of working together to ensure the successful realization of the vision. Strong team leadership most often manifests itself in the positive results the team achieves. Such positive outcomes are obtained as a result of the leader's constantly helping team members to keep their focus on goal achievement.

Individuals often become leaders in an organization after having the opportunity to be mentored by existing leaders. These mentoring relationships have been difficult to foster in health care facilities and more dangerous to develop in public health departments because of resistance to change. Such resistance often results from the fear of losing funding from the federal government because the program change is not included in the grant guidelines. This is another example of the problems with bureaucratic organizations. There is tremendous risk present when one attempts to deviate from the norm established by the bureaucracy holding the power in the health care system that includes public health departments. In an appointed leadership position in public health, your tenure can become extremely short if you try to be innovative in delivering health services. The reason for this tenure issue is found in the fact that politicians fear change and resist it to avoid alienating those who contribute to political campaigns. These politicians think that this risk is not worth the possible improvement in the public's health that might come from fostering innovative programs. Such resistance to change usually results in innovative public health leaders' leaving the public sector and taking their leadership skills to private agencies where they are appreciated. This results in there being very few leaders in public health who are willing to take a chance with innovation. It is simply not worth the risk.

Solving the many problems facing health care in the new century requires a shift from "I" to "we." This allows the leader to become humble, causing him or her to refocus on the development of others. It is the health care worker and not the leader who delivers health care services to the patient. The leader realizes that and attempts to empower the worker to improve the services delivered to that customer.

Incentives can be the catalyst to action when it comes to developing the necessary leadership to keep people healthy at a cost we can all afford. The problems in our health care system require the emergence of leaders in the medical care sector and in public health departments throughout our country. These leaders need to be able to recognize the value of partnerships in the attainment of better health for all Americans. For this to happen, there must be education programs offered that are capable of developing leadership in those responsible for both public health and medical care. There also should be an understanding by leaders of the value of the medical care system and public health departments working together.

The current incentives present in our medical care system and public health agencies encourage the development of power and the use of that power for personal gain. The medical care system uses the pursuit of quality as the excuse for completing wasteful tests in order to improve profits for both the system and those who complete the work. The same system does very little to encourage individuals to seek preventive care. This is where there is a need for public health leaders to assume the leadership role.

Public Health Leaders and Innovation

The skills that could come forth from public health departments have never been in greater demand than they are today because of the evolving epidemic of chronic diseases. As we have already discussed, however, public health departments are suffering from the legacy concept, looking to old successes to solve current problems. We need strong leaders with developed skills to face the major challenges presented by the chronic disease epidemic. This will require transformational leaders at the top of public health agencies who recognize the value of the true empowerment of all public health workers. Public health leaders are unequipped to deal with the challenges of chronic diseases without the complete support and creativity of all of their followers and the community.

One thing that most transformational leaders have in common is their propensity for taking risks through the development of innovative approaches to the challenges confronting them. Rather than attempting to use the same strategies that worked in the past with different challenges, these leaders will usually look to changing the way things are done in response to new problems. A transformational leader will also look outside of his or her discipline to find ways of dealing with new problems. This has never happened with public health departments because they believe that all of the solutions to contemporary health problems can be found within their own discipline and in their own past successes. It is time to broaden the search for solutions to other disciplines and, in the process, spark creativity and innovative approaches to health problems. In order to achieve success with new challenges, public health departments need to engage their employees and their community.

Christensen, Grossman, and Hwang (2009) argue that new ideas do not usually emerge from a specified discipline, but are spawned from other fields using their expertise to examine problems of another discipline. This interdisciplinary approach is being applied to solve the various problems in our current medical care system. It is now time for public health departments to incorporate this approach. Public health departments can only benefit from intense scrutiny by those from other disciplines who look at the way they attempt to solve problems—and from their own explorations of other disciplines. These other disciplines can then share their expertise, offering a different set of eyes for the sake of problem solution.

This is where the development of public health leaders is such a vital component of the solution to the health care crisis facing our country. There is clearly a need for public health departments to move past their previous successes and on to new and greater achievements, which in turn demands leaders who will motivate followers to higher levels of job satisfaction and commitment. The ability to inspire others to accomplish greater achievements is probably a leader's most important competency. It seems to be the one component of leadership that is absolutely necessary in order to motivate large groups to achieve virtually impossible tasks time and time again. Inspiration is the catalyst that helps to further develop the thick culture public health departments need in order to accomplish even greater successes in this century.

Zenger, Folkman, and Edinger (2009) found in their studies of leaders that there is a very strong link between inspiration and innovation. Followers are attracted to a leader who inspires them to become part of new and exciting possibilities. Followers enjoy working for leaders who bring excitement to the workplace with new and exciting ways for approaching problems. Public health departments also need inspiration and innovation in order to become the catalyst our health care system needs in order to do a better job at keeping people healthy at a reasonable cost.

Zenger et al. (2009) argue further that effective leaders are capable of instilling confidence in their followers. In fact, most research indicates that successful leaders spend a great deal of their time working very hard to instill the confidence employees need to take chances and assume risk. These confident followers challenge themselves to attempt new approaches at work because the leader has given them the signal that it is all right to fail as long as they try. They are very aware that the leader wants them to succeed and believes in their ability, which further boosts their confidence.

Public health employees need to develop this confidence in their ability to prevent disease. These individuals have suffered through years of neglect, reduced resources, and a feeling that they are not appreciated. This lack of confidence in their ability and lack of inspiration from their leaders have resulted in a loss of self-efficacy. I (Bernard) experienced low self-efficacy during my tenure as a public health employee. I met very few leaders during my twenty-five years in government employment, but I managed to develop leadership skills through formal education and perusal of research concerning leadership. I was able to practice these leadership skills when I was assigned supervisory authority over a public health office, at which point I became a leader by default. I grew as a leader by ignoring the appointed leader, and gained the respect of my followers by allowing them to work independently. As my self-confidence grew, my self-efficacy grew. The productivity of my office increased dramatically. When self-efficacy is low in public health departments they lose productivity, causing those who allocate health resources to question the need for continuation of several public health programs.

Brown (1997) argues that leadership in public health is a prerequisite for public health departments becoming more effective in achieving their goals and practicing innovation in the delivery of new public health programs. This is going to require collaboration with other agencies, especially businesses. In order to make partnerships work, however, there is a real need for exceptional leaders. These other agencies have experience, expertise, and of course resources that public health departments need if they are ever to resolve the tremendous health challenges facing this country in the next several years. Public health leaders must learn how to inspire these agencies to work together to achieve success.

Strong leadership skills are just starting to be appreciated as an absolute requirement for those who are charged with leading public health departments into the future. The challenges we face in this century—such as the epidemic of chronic diseases—are growing by the day, and they are incapable of being managed, requiring instead leaders with a vision for how to solve these public health problems.

According to Gallo (2011), for innovators to be successful they must follow their heart, as Steve Jobs has illustrated throughout his string of innovations for Apple over the last thirty years. Such passion should also drive those who truly believe in the enormous potential of public health departments. The secret to success for most leaders who are trying to make change happen seems to revolve around their passion not only to dream but also to spend the vast majority of their waking hours making their dream come true.

In order to truly become a change agent you have to follow your dream, that which is your passion—then you can work long hours, experience failures, and still follow the vision because you own it. The secret of successful innovation then becomes perseverance in striving toward the accomplishment of your dream.

People who work in public health usually love what they do or they would have abandoned the field many years ago. The compensation is low, promotions are rare, and frustration in meeting goals because of meager resources is a daily occurrence. Those who choose the field of public health as a career do so because they are passionate about trying to improve the health of the population. The problem is not the passion of public health workers; but quite often it is the dearth of credibility among leaders found in public health departments. This lack of credibility is not always a result of bad leadership, however, but rather stems from the short tenure that comes with being a political appointee with very little understanding of the goals of public health departments.

Credibility—that is, the leader and his or her vision are believable—remains one of the most important qualities of the leader, reinforced over years of research. A culture of credibility emerges when everyone in the organization is held accountable for high performance. This instills trust between the leader and all of the members of the public health team. These employees are then more likely to support risk taking and to become extremely interested in finding innovative ways to better serve their customers.

Gallo (2011) argues that the combination of passion and aptitude can truly change the world. Public health departments require such a combination among their workers to begin meeting today's health challenges, especially the current epidemic of chronic diseases and their complications. The development of Healthy People 2020 goals is fine, but meeting those goals requires unleashing the passion found in the vast majority of individuals who work in public health departments. These dedicated people need to experience empowerment in the workplace in order to devote their creativity toward innovation in finding solutions to complex population health problems.

According to Kouzes and Posner (2009), a culture of leadership is present when every person in the organization is thought to be credible and accountable to each other. In this type of working environment, risk taking is not only accepted but encouraged. Public health departments need this leadership environment if they are ever to repeat and expand on their past success stories. The problem lies in that bureaucratic government agencies do not support risk taking because of political dangers associated with risk. You cannot fully commit to something that is not important to you. This has been the major problem with public health departments—they are committed to population health but not to combating the inactivity associated with a bureaucracy. These dedicated employees want to make a difference in people's lives.

Gallo (2011) argues that real innovation is not the result of focus groups or expensive marketing research. It comes from knowing your customer and showing them products and services that will make their lives better. This is also true with programs that try to improve the health of the population. Americans do not know how much they want good health until they experience poor health, and then it may be too late to restore their health. Americans also do not realize the value of prevention begun at an early age.

A very good example of a company that makes things simple for the consumer is Apple computers. This company is exceptionally skilled at making very difficult tasks very simple. This is because the vision of the leader is capable of unleashing creativity and innovation in solving problems. This is the type of innovation public health departments require in order to deal with the epidemic of chronic diseases. Public health departments need to look at successful companies like Apple and make the process of delivering health education more successful through the use of disruptive innovation. They need to use innovative technology to deliver health education and health promotion activities to the entire population.

Summary

Leadership has replaced management as the component necessary to accomplish goals in most organizations in the United States. This is also very true for public health agencies as they respond to the many challenges to and opportunities for improving the health of the population as our health care system reorganizes.

The Institute of Medicine in 2002 called for tremendous change in the way we deliver public health services to the vast majority of Americans. These changes require leaders with well-developed skills who will provide direction to a workforce that encompasses a thick culture of caring workers who want to improve health. These workers are still using outdated approaches that were successful in the past in order to solve new problems. The old tools and skills of public health workers will not work in solving twenty-first-century health dilemmas. Therefore, there must be change in the way public health departments work.

Successful leaders in public health must receive formal leadership training to produce change. These leaders must then be empowered to use the newly acquired skills to improve the health of their community. This is not an easy task, but it can be accomplished.

Key Terms

Bureaucracies

Empowerment

Leadership

Leadership traits

Power

Transformational style of leadership

Discussion Questions

1. Why are individuals with strong leadership skills so important in solving the problems in the American health care system?
2. How does the thick culture found in public health departments relate to the achievement of public health goals?
3. Why is the transformational style of leadership considered to be optimal for leading those who work in service organizations?
4. Why are creativity and innovation so very important in solving the chronic disease epidemic our country faces?

CHAPTER 7

EMPOWERING PUBLIC HEALTH WORKERS

LEARNING OBJECTIVES

- Understand the need for a leader to appreciate the culture of public health employees in order to make change occur
- Acknowledge the need to instill trust in public health employees before attempting change
- Become aware of the opportunities available to improve community health through collaboration among the major players in the delivery of health care services in our country
- Identify the role of the public health leader and the empowered worker in improving quality in the health care system

There is something very different about working in a public health agency. Such an agency produces services whose proper delivery is dependent on the skill levels of the agency's public health workers. Working in a public health agency is an unbelievable experience that will stay with an employee for the rest of his or her life. An employee begins to feel the strong bond between workers and their profession very soon after beginning a career in public health. There is this overwhelming sense of achievement just by coming to work and answering questions from the public about the various diseases or programs associated with public health problems. There is a sense of privilege in being part of such an important occupation. It is the thick culture of the public health workplace that the employee feels when he or she first arrives.

As defined in Chapter Six, culture is a combination of learned beliefs, values, rules, and symbols that are common to a group of people. The members of an organization often take the culture for granted and usually are unaware of how important it is to their desire to remain or not remain with a particular organization. The culture in an organization encompasses the values that tend to rule the decision-making process of its members. This culture, which all members are encouraged to absorb, becomes the one thing that remains standard in the workplace. It is the way things are done on a daily basis. It is what can make the organization a special place to work or a place to which the workers do not want to go.

Managers often erroneously believe that they are responsible for building the culture of the organization. In reality, the culture is developed, nurtured, and thickened by the organization's workers. In fact, workers may very well develop a culture as a reaction to poor management and poor employee relations. Workers have their own way of accomplishing the goals of the organization, and worker unity becomes the culture that determines how things are done in the workplace. The best managers can do is try to accomplish goals by working with the existing culture. This is especially true of those who work in public health. These employees enjoy a unique bond that draws them to public health and convinces them that this is where they want to spend their career. It is nothing less than a feeling of family.

The public health leader must understand and respect the value of the organization's culture. If the leader avoids dealing with the culture, transforming the organization to react to the changing environment becomes virtually impossible. In order to be successful with public health employees, the transformational leader must become part of their culture, or positive change will not happen. I (Bernard) have witnessed so many unsuccessful attempts by public health leaders to make change happen. These leaders fail in their quest because of the rigid culture of the employees. The culture can actually work against the administration in leaders' efforts to produce change.

According to Hesselbein (2008), a leader is faced with a major problem when attempting to change a culture because the necessary first step in this change process is changing the organization itself. Workers, not the appointed leader, have the power to change the culture in the organization. This is where the political appointee in a public health department has a real problem. Newly appointed leaders think that they can bureaucratically order an existing culture to change. These individuals are so impressed by their newly acquired power that they fail to understand that just because they want the culture to change doesn't mean that it will.

The sad part about this failed change process is that the culture does not need to be changed. It is the organization and its performance that require the change. Public health departments have had tremendous success over the years that can be attributed to the dedication and thick culture of the workers found therein. Unfortunately, public health agencies have never been given the necessary resources to achieve their full potential. The thick culture is there, but the leadership has very often been lacking. No one has been available to nurture and continue to build on the public health culture, because government officials have never appreciated the true value of public health. It is ironic that in many instances tremendous successes have been achieved in spite of, rather than because of, leadership. In order for leaders to mobilize public health agencies to solve the multitude of problems found in our current health care system, they must understand and use the culture of the agency they are attempting to lead. This is going to be a very difficult task.

Leadership and Quality Improvement

There is no question that improving the quality of the product or service a business produces is an important responsibility of all leaders—including those who lead public health departments. The question becomes, then, What role should the public health leader play in the improvement of quality in the delivery of health care services? The answer is that the public health leader will be the catalyst in the improvement of the health of the community.

Quality in health care delivery is determined by comparing the desires of the health care consumer with the reality of the health care experience (Fottler, Ford, and Heaton, 2010). The health care experience and, therefore, the quality result of the health care interaction are considered negative for the consumer if his or her expectations are not met. The consumer does not, for example, expect to be injured when he or she enters the health care system. There is overwhelming evidence that many people are being hurt by the very system that is supposed to be curing their medical problems.

The following are the six major areas of action and change for public health departments proposed by the Institute of Medicine in 2003, p. 4:

1. Adopting a population health approach that considers the multiple determinants of health
2. Strengthening the governmental infrastructure, which forms the backbone of the public health system
3. Building a new generation of intersectoral partnerships that also draw on the perspectives and resources of diverse communities and actively engage them in health action
4. Developing systems of accountability to assure the quality and availability of public health services
5. Making evidence the foundation of decision making and the measure of success
6. Enhancing and facilitating communication within the public health system (for example, among all levels of the governmental public health infrastructure and between public health professionals and community members)

One of the most important areas found in this list deals with the development of accountability in order to ensure the quality and availability of public health services. It is quite obvious that in order to facilitate the improvement of public health—especially in regard to quality of services—there is a need for leadership development and the empowerment of public health workers.

On the one hand, physicians and hospitals provide us with a hope of curing illness and disease; on the other hand, medical care can be very dangerous and in some cases actually life threatening. There are medical mistakes made every day that could have been avoided had the medical care provider followed proper procedures. We must remember that ensuring conditions in which people can be healthy is the major responsibility of public health departments. Therefore, these health departments should be working closely with medical providers to ensure that the epidemic of medical errors is stopped.

The Institute of Medicine (IOM, 1999) released a study revealing that as many as ninety-eight thousand of the thirty-three million individuals hospitalized each year die, and many more receive secondary infections because of poor-quality health care while hospitalized. This quality issue needs to become a major concern of all public health departments in our country. Through public health surveillance and leadership, we should make medical errors a major priority, giving immediate attention to the causes of these errors, especially hospital-acquired infections.

The IOM (1999, p. 1) defines a medical error as "the failure of a planned action to be completed as intended or the use of a wrong plan to achieve an aim." Medical errors typically occur in operating rooms, emergency departments, and intensive care units. Mounting evidence suggests that entering the medical care system at any location increases the risk of adverse drug events, errors in care delivery, and hospital-acquired infections.

Medical errors, especially in hospitals, are a well-known problem that is given minimal attention by those in power (Sultz and Young, 2009). In many instances, physicians and hospitals actually receive reimbursement for treatments that contain an error, and then are reimbursed again for rectifying the error if the patient lives. The most common type of error in medical care involves administering drugs to patients (Brownlee, 2007). These drug errors include the administration of the wrong drug, giving the wrong dose of the right drug, or allowing drug interactions that harm the patient. Drug errors alone add five thousand dollars to the cost of every hospital admission (IOM, 1999). If the cost of drug errors is not enough to command national attention, the unnecessary disability and death following administration of the wrong drug should motivate those in charge of health care to take action.

According to the Centers for Disease Control and Prevention (CDC, 2009f), health care–associated infections, or nosocomial infections, are infections that patients acquire during the course of receiving treatment for another condition within a health care setting. They are secondary to a patient's original medical problem and usually appear shortly after admission to a hospital or health facility, or up to a month after discharge. According to the CDC, hospital-acquired infections affect over two million patients every year, with an annual cost of as much as $11 billion.

These infections are caused by housing together large numbers of individuals whose immune systems are often not functioning properly due to illness. In other words, hospital patients make up a large cohort of ill individuals who are susceptible to a secondary infection. Secondary infections can result from something as simple as providers' not washing their hands with soap and water between medical procedures.

The most common way to transmit microorganisms in a hospital setting is direct or indirect contact transmission, whereby the health care provider carries an organism and transmits it to another host, usually an ill patient. The vast majority of these infections can be prevented by adherence to good sanitation techniques, such as hand washing or having all medical personnel use alcohol rubs before and after each patient contact.

A very good example of a hospital-acquired infection is methicillin-resistant *Staphylococcal aureus*, better known as **MRSA**. Health care–associated infections are one of the top ten leading causes of death in the United States. They are quite often the result of poor sanitation practices, which are for the most part preventable when properly monitored. These infections need to be reported by health care providers to the local or state health department and dealt with immediately. They need to be considered unacceptable in a health care setting.

Several large medical facilities are using lean managerial tools and concepts, which require a checklist of important parts of the medical process and are designed to increase productivity in health care delivery. One of the lean concepts involves error proofing, an approach for ensuring quality and error-free manufacturing of products or services (Lighter, 2009). This method prevents defects in any medical process from being passed on to the next operation. It empowers the employee and the team to look for defects in process design and then correct the process in order to eliminate each defect at the earliest possible point. This empowerment of health care workers is a prerequisite for improving health care delivery in the United States.

The health care system must be better designed so that it is more difficult for practitioners to make mistakes. Brownlee (2007) argues that the system requires far too many people to do everything right every time in order to arrive at a successful patient outcome. This type of system is perfect for latent errors—mistakes in medical care that are waiting to happen. Even though they are quite often labeled as "never events," meaning that they should never happen, they are occurring all too frequently, causing the costs of health care to rise and patients to be hurt by the very system that is supposed to heal them.

According to Spear (2009), the old approaches to health care delivery must be replaced with more sophisticated methods that are improved when problems are revealed, and modified or dropped completely when the situation changes. This is clearly the case with medical errors, which we need to eliminate by dealing with the known flaws found in this complicated system. This can only be accomplished if medical staff do not attempt to work around medical errors but rather immediately redesign the process when problems arise. In order to eliminate system flaws, it is very helpful to look at other companies that have dealt with and solved the problem of errors in the workplace.

The only way to reduce and eventually eliminate medical errors and nosocomial infections is through better leadership and empowered followers in the public health sector. Ledlow and Coppola (2011) point out that there is no greater demand of a health care leader than to be able to define and ensure quality for the consumer of health care services. The public health leader needs to be able to address the quality issue for the entire population. Eliminating medical errors and outbreaks of nosocomial infections must become a major public health function.

The Public Health Employee

American businesses are beginning to understand the importance of their infrastructure in order to remain competitive in a global economy. Human resources are one of the most important parts of the infrastructure and need to be developed and retained in order for the business to grow and prosper. This is so very true for companies or agencies that provide services, because services are provided by people. Turnock (2009) argues that in order to improve public health services in this country we must come to better understand public health workers. Leaders are necessary, but it is the public health workers who provide public health services to the population. Successful public health leaders recognize that without dedicated public health workers there is no delivery of public health services to the population. These leaders go out of their way to develop and empower their staff.

Turnock (2009) points out that there are approximately four hundred thousand to five hundred thousand public health workers in this country, many of whom have a separate professional discipline (for example, nursing) in addition to being part of the public health workforce. There are more than thirty different job classifications in public health departments, with nursing and environmental specialists accounting for the largest number of employees. The vast majority of these employees are well educated but without any formal education in public health. They learn the craft through on-the-job training and practice.

Leaders have to recognize that providing specialized training in public health is a crucial step in preparing the workforce to reach the goals public health departments set for the future. Part of this training should include leadership development of all workers if they are to be empowered. Collins (2009) argues that exceptional companies must develop self-managed and motivated people in order to attain greatness. These individuals cannot work in a rules-based organization; they thrive when they are allowed to manage their own work. This is exactly what public health departments require in order to revitalize and improve their performance.

Transformational Leadership, Worker Empowerment, and Self-Managed Work Teams in Public Health

Experts believe that the transformational style of leadership will usually result in worker empowerment, but the worker must be prepared to become empowered. The public health workforce probably is not yet ready to become empowered, because all employees know is the bureaucratic style of management. This means we have to not only develop public health leaders who can successfully espouse the transformational style of leadership but also convince public health workers that they have been truly empowered. We need to build trust within public health departments. Never will this trust be more evident than when the leader starts to develop self-managed work teams dedicated to improving the health of the community. We have already discussed the need for leadership development of those charged with the day-to-day administration of public health departments. It is also important to concentrate our efforts on learning how to empower the entire public health workforce.

The new responsibilities for public health departments in this century will require the public health workforce to develop new **competencies.** Acquiring new skills is vital to improving workers' confidence levels and will be absolutely necessary in order to achieve the goals of public health departments. In order to gain a competency, an employee must be prepared for empowerment, and needs to learn this ability through advanced training and skill development programs.

The public health leader must learn to play a new role in the public health department, recognizing that public health workers are the most important part of the department because they are the ones who deliver public health services. These followers need the support of the leader in order to unleash their skills in service to the population. It seems that although leadership is important, good followership is the real catalyst for improving community health.

The public health leader will need to spend a great deal of time mentoring his or her employees. According to Spear (2009), leaders need to develop their followers so that public health departments can be self-correcting, self-improving, and self-innovating. In other words, the leader's most important function is to prepare and allow followers to continue accomplishing public health goals—a mentorship role. In fact, this is one of the areas that requires tremendous emphasis as the public health system attempts to focus on this century's daunting challenges.

Successful leaders are capable of providing energy and direction to both the organization and those who work for the organization—an important revelation for those in leadership positions in public health departments (Spitzer, 2008). Those who work in public health are looking for direction and want to see movement toward organizational goals. For too long, public health professionals have not witnessed great achievements from their work, in part because of dwindling budgets and reduced staffing. This must change because public health is too important in dealing with the current epidemic of chronic diseases, which is draining our country's resources.

The Role of Culture

Cultures have a very powerful effect on the performance of all organizations. A thick or strong culture is widespread; it takes years to build but very little time to destroy under certain conditions. It is interesting to note that culture is really built by the workers but can be either nurtured or torn apart by the leader, one of whose greatest responsibilities is caring for this culture. The major problem is that political appointees in leadership positions usually have very little concern for the long-term survival of an organization's culture. In fact, these temporary caretakers probably are not even aware that a thick public health culture exists.

The problems facing public health departments have increased in number and intensity in recent years. Public health departments are being asked to do more with reduced budgets and declining numbers in their workforce. The only way that they can address these public health issues is through collaboration. Kotter and Heskett (1992) argue that strong cultures can have powerful consequences because they enable groups to become proactive in the way they deal with problems confronting them. Public health challenges in the twenty-first century require collaborative solutions that can only materialize if the leader is absorbed into the thick culture found among public health workers. Kotter and Heskett also point out that strong cultures result in most leaders sharing with their followers a set of relatively consistent values and methods of completing work. This sharing of work values is a major prerequisite for organizational success and facilitates the entire organization's working together to accomplish common goals. This is exactly what is required for public health departments to remain successful today.

There is something special about working in the delivery of health care services to people, and there is something very satisfying about being involved in providing public health services to people in a community. These are the ultimate services that one person can provide to another. It requires a very special individual to want to work in health care delivery. The special nature of this profession fosters the growth of a very thick culture that has its own norms and nonmonetary reward system for recognizing excellent performance. Working in public health involves incentives for performance that are very different from those of most other businesses.

Public health workers like to help people and enjoy the internal satisfaction of assisting individuals to improve their health. It is certainly not for the money or the power that people become public health employees. In fact, job security is not even present in public health departments because there is always turmoil in the process of budgeting for public health. Public health seems to be a sector of government that is overlooked until an epidemic of disease is made public. In my (Bernard's) tenure in public health, every time the state budget was approved, the security of most public health employees was threatened. Even with the threat of unemployment, the culture of a public health department continues to grow stronger.

If you are an employee in a public health department, you have contributed to the formation of a thick culture around the strong values of service to people. These values grow stronger for you the longer you remain in the field of public health. They consume your life both at work and at home, becoming some of the most important motivators in your life. The public health leader must understand the culture among his or her staff and be able to respect their dedication to the public health tradition of helping people address their health issues. In order to truly lead these dedicated professionals, the leader of a public health department must absorb the culture of the individuals he or she is trying to lead and work to build the necessary trust that holds the organization together. Public health agencies are home to many long-term workers who have dedicated their lives to their profession. They will not easily accept this new person who has been assigned temporary leadership responsibilities in their strong culture. They have all been through this change of leadership in past years, and are quite capable of silently resisting it.

Hickman (1998) argues that companies with a corporate culture that pushes positive change understand the value of the individuals and the processes that create change. These companies truly believe in their workers and respect their customers, and it shows every day in the way top management acts in the workplace. These companies exhibit a **performance-enhancing culture,** taking pride in their workers and customers and never doing anything intentionally to hurt either group. Any leader must understand how to nurture the culture that has developed in his or her organization. This is certainly the case for those in public health agencies.

Special ingredients that can nurture culture include the following:

- Management and employee attitudes about the importance of their work
- Values, myths, and stories
- Leaders' priorities, responsibilities, and accountability concerning their vision
- Employee training and motivation
- Employee involvement

These factors have the ability to develop and nurture a thick culture that supports the goals of public health departments in this country. They also demonstrate the value of a leader's using a democratic and coaching style of leadership in pushing the organizational climate toward the achievement of departmental goals.

The **informal leader** plays a larger role in culture formation than does the formal leader. The formal leader has power that has been granted by the organization, whereas the informal leader has only the power generated by his or her own expertise and charisma. In order to accomplish the objectives of the organization, the formal leader needs to obtain the support of the informal leaders. For this to occur, the formal leader must first recognize the informal leaders' power. In order to make change happen in a public health department, the complete support of the informal leaders is absolutely mandatory. Obtaining informal leaders' support, too, will take the formal leader a very long time and require great deal of work.

When you work for a company that has developed a strong culture, you will notice a pervasive sense of purpose and trust. I (Bernard) found this type of culture when I began my employment with a state health department in 1972. This was my first professional job after completing college, and I immediately felt that this new workplace was very different from any that I had experienced up to that point in my career.

I was struck by the way fellow employees wanted to help me understand how fortunate I was to have gotten a position in a public health department. They were unaware of the fact that I had no idea what a public health department was or what was expected of me. Despite this fact, I was truly impressed as an outsider by how much they wanted me to become part of their work team. A thick, positive culture is defined by successes and even by failures. In reality, a culture becomes the unique way each organization responds to daily successes and failures in what it is trying to accomplish through the work of its employees.

Culture and Change

Public health departments not only have to accept change but actually must search out change opportunities to exploit. Employees will resist change that does not fit well within the boundaries of their thick culture. The strength of this resistance is something that is often overlooked by the new leader who is attempting to gain the trust of workers in a public health agency. Public health workers realize that their tenure will most likely be longer than that of the new leader, meaning that there is little risk in passively resisting the leader's requests for change in the goals and direction of the agency. The leader has thus lost power to the workers, making goal accomplishment much more difficult in the short term because there will probably be no long term for the leader. This fact alone makes the concept of empowerment that much more attractive to a new leader in a public health department. If public health workers are empowered to do what needs to be done, the leader is able to share in any success in the improvement of health that is achieved as a result of the employees' efforts.

One of the more obvious attributes of a thick culture is workers' resistance to leaders who attempt to change or even adjust that culture. The public health leader must understand that the culture found in a public health department is what keeps employees from moving to other organizations that pay higher wages and offer more employee benefits. Therefore, guiding cultural change is one of the leader's greatest challenges as he or she attempts to move the public health department to greater accomplishments in improving the health of the community. All organizations, including public health departments, face the need for change because forces in the environment that have an impact on these organizations have changed. Public health departments are not necessarily doing a poor job; rather, shifting environmental forces require a different response from public health departments as well as innovation in the way they attempt to meet new challenges. This means that the thick public health culture must also become more flexible and accommodating to change. Further, public health leaders need to provide the resources and training necessary to facilitate this change.

Public health departments usually are not considered to have a great vision and usually are not the birthplace of innovation and, therefore, spend very little time and effort marketing their accomplishments to the politicians. This is because they are limited to the guidelines that are included with their funding. The result is poorly funded, understaffed public health departments. Quite often legislators are completely unaware of the vast responsibilities of public health agencies, making it very easy for them to cut the public health budget.

Clark and Weist (2000) argue that change in the field of public health is demanding change in the way future public health professionals are educated. These individuals require training in community development in order to form partnerships with key community stakeholders. They need to develop and improve their communication skills in order to gain the respect of the community. The leader has to become the facilitator for this training and help prepare his or her followers for empowerment in the work they do on a daily basis.

Heifetz (2006) argues that cultural adaptation requires taking the best from an organization's past, leaving behind that which no longer works, and embracing innovation in order to rapidly respond to environmental change. This information is critical for public health departments confronting the changing world. The best of public health includes several skills that will work very well toward solving the problems in our current health care system. For example, epidemiological investigators can uncover the real causes of many of the chronic diseases that are currently epidemic in this country; and expanded health education programs can prevent high-risk behaviors from ever beginning. The old notion of controlling diseases has to be left behind as a task that never should have been considered to be a goal of public health departments. If you are only trying to control and not eliminate a public health problem, you will never achieve any real success.

Public health departments are having a great deal of difficulty handling new disease threats because the field of public health resists alternative methods of coping with disease occurrence and intervening in the disease state. Many of the older public health employees are still living on past successes that involved eliminating communicable diseases through immunization programs. They do not want to accept that the new epidemic of chronic diseases requires a change in the way things are done in public health.

This is the case with the strong culture found in public health departments. Many of the long-term employees in these departments are still seeing their future value in terms of their past successes. The leader needs to gently guide followers to acceptance of the new challenges facing public health departments. This will require a cultural shift that will never occur when employees think that they are already doing things correctly. Public health departments need to spend the vast majority of their time and resources attempting to develop programs and methodologies to prevent diseases entirely rather than designing elaborate strategies to control diseases and epidemics. This represents the new world of public health and will require public health agencies to change what they do on a daily basis. It will also require leaders to empower all public health professionals to become innovative in their approaches to solving public health problems.

There is a growing body of research demonstrating that a strong culture does not always support excellent performance. If the norms and behaviors found in an organization with a strong culture do not lead to expected performance and goal accomplishment, the culture can actually be destructive to the future of the organization. Kotter and Heskett (1992) argue that a culture must also be adaptive to the changing environment that supports the continuation and expansion of the organization. Public health workers have to change by adapting to their new roles and receiving additional training in new approaches for dealing with the problems affecting community health. The starting point for the public health leader in strengthening the culture is to complete a culture audit of the department that he or she is attempting to lead.

Culture Audit

The leader's task in a public health agency is to achieve the goals put forth by elected government officials. These goals may be the result of new laws passed by the state legislature, federal mandates, or personal preferences concerning public health departments that these political appointees bring to the job. This is why it is so important for the new leader to have a solid understanding of the culture of the agency or department for which he or she is responsible.

In order to understand the culture of an organization, the leader must devote substantial time to studying that culture. This cannot be done by gathering only primary data through a questionnaire or reading books or journals about the topic of public health. The leader needs instead to analyze the qualitative data that can only be gathered through observing what people do in the organization. This is called a **culture audit,** and it requires a great deal of time and understanding but is worth the effort.

The public health leader has to understand that he or she is never going to accomplish twenty-first century public health goals without the complete agreement of the entire department—which he or she can only secure by truly understanding the culture that has developed in this agency over the years. The leader needs to focus on surprises in the workplace, things that seem different to him or her. These may very well be the foundations of the employee culture. The leader then needs to share such data about the cultural practices he or she has observed with some of the employees to discover if these behaviors are widespread and why they happen. This is the starting point for uncovering the real culture and determining why it exists in this particular agency.

Performance-Based Culture

An editorial by Stover and Bassett in the November 2003 edition of the *American Journal of Public Health* discussed practice—which might involve something as simple as granting a birth certificate or something as complicated as investigating an outbreak of communicable disease affecting an entire community—as the purpose of public health. The article explored the definition and the roles of public health practitioners—those who conduct the practice of public health on a daily basis. These workers form the culture or soul of a public health department. Their credo involves the prevention of disease and the promotion of good health for all Americans. They have been responsible for unbelievable past success stories involving the reduction of morbidity and mortality in this country. But public health departments can do better. Despite the tremendous success that our prevention efforts have achieved, our country is still burdened by epidemics of preventable illnesses, injuries, and disabilities. In order to improve public health departments, the workers have to change the way they do business.

The Future of Public Health (IOM, 1988, p. 159) offered an in-depth analysis of the condition of public health in the United States. The report concluded with the following statement: "Public health in the United States has been taken for granted, many public health issues have become inappropriately politicized, and public health responsibilities have become so fragmented that deliberate action is often difficult if not impossible." In order for continued success in meeting old and new public health challenges, public health departments have to develop and maintain a performance-based culture that includes the goals of public health and a method of measurement. This is not an easy thing to do when resources are continually being reduced.

The public health culture in America today is strong because of the type of individual who devotes his or her life to serving others by accepting a position in a public health department. Public health employees are motivated and achieve great success in dealing with all kinds of public health problems, despite the limited availability of resources. They remain dedicated to core values that make a public health department such a special place to work and grow. They can be successful in changing their methods to accomplish even greater goals, but their talent needs to be unleashed and expanded by the leader. The leader must empower these valuable workers so that they can use their creativity to discover innovative solutions to current public health challenges.

Kotter and Heskett (1992) argue that a strong culture has a positive effect on the performance of an organization's members because culture contributes to goal alignment, unusual levels of motivation, and a strong desire for goal achievement. The leader needs to understand the value of these attributes of a strong culture as they relate to enhanced organizational performance. Public health workers usually exhibit an understanding of universal goals, accompanied by motivation and self-imposed control to reach these goals.

One of the most visible signs of a performance-based culture is public health workers' ownership of the work process. These workers take personal responsibility for preventing disease and keeping people healthy. They are working to achieve the goals set forth by Healthy People 2010 and help in developing greater goals for Healthy People 2020. In effect they collectively own the future obligations of public health departments. This is not a culture that can be easily changed by temporary public health leaders who are political appointees, usually with a short tenure and quite often with little if any personal power.

Zenger, Folkman, and Edinger (2009) point out that one of the biggest differences between managers and leaders is found in the way the leader approaches the process of change. Managers normally block change because it can lead to conflict, and conflict is usually not allowed in a bureaucratic organization. In an organic organization that prides itself on leadership, however, change becomes the norm even if it causes conflict.

Public health departments need to become more organic and experiment with change in the way they approach population-based health problems. It is clear that public health departments have become very insulated in recent years while continuing to dwell on their past achievements. The success stories of the past reside in the past, and it is now time for public health departments to work toward the future. They have to develop partnerships with community agencies, businesses, and schools to expand prevention programs for the community. They need to realize that the resources they need so very badly are actually available from the population that they serve. In order to attract these resources, the public health sector needs leaders and workers who will exploit change and turn it into an opportunity.

Empowerment of Workers in Public Health

The many professionals working together in public health agencies, and the collegial culture that develops among them, make worker empowerment an absolute necessity. The strong culture in public health departments throughout this country pushes employees to take chances by looking for change and living innovation, and encouragement of change and innovation becomes part of doing business on a daily basis in these agencies. The workers are empowered to make decisions and become leaders in their own right. In fact, leaders of public health agencies believe that their most important function is to develop their followers into leaders themselves by inspiring them to grow and take chances. This is a very good approach for the public health leader to follow. It helps to build the trust that is necessary to make change become the norm for the organization. The process of change requires the support of all followers.

Pierce and Newstrom (2006) argue that worker empowerment is a multidimensional concept that usually increases workers' ability and motivation. This empowerment also can increase workers' self-efficacy, giving them more confidence in their own ability to perform their tasks. Also, because the leader holds very high expectations for his or her workers, their self-esteem increases and they come to believe that they have a real impact on goal accomplishment. The only way we are ever going to achieve the enormous goals of public health is through empowering public health professionals and allowing them to be creative.

Lussier and Achua (2004) discuss the concept of the self-managed work team, which relates closely to worker empowerment. Self-managed work teams are not without external guidance, but they do subscribe to self-responsibility and self-accountability. In order to be successful in achieving their goals, these teams require leadership rather than management. The team leader gradually relinquishes power to the team members, therefore empowering them to get the job done.

Public health administrators often attempt to manage their public health department using bureaucratic management styles that do not work very well with educated, experienced public health employees. This type of supervision will not work, for example, with public health employees who know more about public health than do those who are charged with overseeing them. The more these managers attempt to control their employees, the more the employees resist the supervision. It is time to recognize that workers in public health departments require a different type of supervision if they are ever to meet their goals. They need a leader to inspire them to accomplish their goals, and they need the freedom or empowerment to be innovative in this process.

The public health leader must understand that lower-level employees are the ones who actually deliver public health services designed to keep people healthy. These are the people who investigate disease outbreaks, offer screening programs for chronic illnesses, and deliver education programs to help individuals understand the value of healthy behaviors and the dangers associated with high-risk behaviors. These employees are dedicated to their profession and do not require direct supervision in order to do their work. In fact, I (Bernard) would argue that public health employees cannot be supervised because of their advanced levels of expertise in their respective disciplines. Attempting to manage these employees only leads them to passively resist the change that is so necessary for public health departments today. It is a much better strategy for the leader to share power equally among followers—in the long run this will make change the normal course for the organization to follow.

As discussed in Chapter Six, there are generally five types of power—legitimate, reward, coercive, charisma, and expertise—that leaders may possess. The sharing of any of these forms of power with followers generally improves their commitment to the task at hand. Dubrin (2007) argues that the power the leader holds can only increase when he or she shares it with others in the workplace. It is interesting to note that the greatest source of power is personal power, which resides in the individual and usually takes the form of expertise and charisma, both of which are found in the majority of public health workers. Leaders only need to set this personal power free by empowering public health professionals to work toward even greater successes in the future.

Dubrin (2007) defines true employee empowerment as the process in which a leader shares decision-making authority and responsibility for production with employees. In order for this sharing of power to work for the employee, the employee must want the power and the power must be real. Many leaders talk about empowerment of employees but hesitate to release real power to others because they fear that followers will make mistakes that will threaten their leadership role. Sharing power with others seems very risky to a leader who does not trust his or her followers or is frightened of losing power to them. This fear and lack of trust force the public health leader to refrain from practicing leadership skills and to revert instead to management principles. This results in the institution of rules and regulations that block change and destroy any incentives for innovation in the delivery of public health services.

One of the most important forms of power is expertise concerning the work process. Public health employees enjoy this form of power from their education and their experience. Therefore, they are already empowered on their own, a fact that a leader would be rather foolish to ignore. The leader needs to take advantage of the tremendous experiences that have marked a number of his or her followers' tenure. Expertise is an especially important form of power for professionals attempting to identify potential public health issues and developing strategies to deal with them. This power is usually already present in the workers and just needs to be activated by the leader. There are several ways in which the workplace leader can empower workers to make their community healthier. According to Dubrin (2007), the easiest way to accomplish this task is by requesting greater initiative and responsibility concerning program development and evaluation from all workers. Another way to empower employees is to incorporate their suggestions for improvement into the organization's strategic goals.

Bossidy and Charan (2002) argue that for the leader's vision to materialize, he or she must build and sustain employees' momentum, which is critical to the attainment of public health goals. The leader needs to consistently search for people who want to win and empower them to translate short-term achievements into long-term successes. If the ventures turn out to be successful, it will increase the followers' self-confidence and motivate them to look for more change. The result will be the development of a culture in public health that seeks out change on a daily basis—which is so very important when trying to accomplish public health goals with limited resources. It is evident that being able to further develop a public health culture is becoming one of the public health leader's most critical competencies in working to achieve the lofty goals set forth by Healthy People 2010 and 2020 (Koh. H., 2010). The leader's starting point for success in this task is to find out more about the culture in his or her department. Again, learning more about the culture is going to take a great deal of the leader's time, but it will be time well spent.

Disappearance of the Public Health Worker

There is yet another looming crisis facing our public health system that we must address in the very near future. According to an article in *The Nation's Health* (Johnson, 2008), there will be a shortage of 250,000 public health workers over the next few years due to retirements of the aging public health workforce. Further, it is becoming more difficult to recruit replacements for those who are leaving public health service. This critical shortage of public health workers will make our country susceptible to the threats of epidemics of disease, bioterrorism, and natural disasters. Now more than ever we need our young, bright college graduates to seek a career in public health.

The U.S. population continues to grow while the number of workers available to tend to their health continues to dwindle. As already stated, this shortage is the result of retiring public health employees and is not due to a mass exodus of workers leaving for other employment opportunities. The projected shortage does, however, draw attention to the fact that younger workers are not choosing a public health career. This should worry public health leaders, who need to actively seek solutions to this encroaching problem in the not-too-distant future.

The skills that served public health professionals so well in the infectious and even the current chronic disease period are becoming less useful in dealing with the emerging public health issues of the twenty-first century. Public health departments are at a crossroads that requires new approaches to disease prevention. These approaches in turn demand new leaders with the skills necessary to become the change agents that mold the public health culture for the sake of achieving new success stories. A public health career must become exciting and rewarding, and public health departments must become places where young people want to work. This is not the case with public health departments today, which is a large part of why recruiting new employees is so difficult.

Public health activities are usually specified by legislation that includes laws, codes, and regulations. This legislation usually deals with the reporting of disease by health facilities, quarantining of those who are infected with a disease by public health departments, and conducting mandatory surveillance of and providing treatment for communicable diseases. These laws are quite specific, and health professionals usually follow them in a very bureaucratic way. There is little or no room for innovation in dealing with reportable diseases, and there is very little emphasis on the prevention of disease. This too must change as public health agencies lobby for their legislators to pass laws that will support the accomplishment of public health goals.

Summary

Public health successes in the past were often accomplished in spite of bureaucratic management. It is an awesome thought to imagine what could have been accomplished had public health professionals been empowered by their administrators. There are many opportunities, as our health care system is reformed, for public health agencies to take a leadership role in the improvement of the health of the population. The leader cannot exploit these opportunities without the help of his or her dedicated employees. In order to obtain the support of these professionals, the leader must work with their thick culture.

Culture is a combination of learned beliefs, values, rules, and symbols that are common to a group of people, in this case public health employees. Most public health employees have made a career of delivering public health services to the community, and over the course of their work they have formed a thick culture. In order to gain followers' trust, the leader must learn about their culture and actually become part of it.

The thick culture found in public health departments has primed employees for even greater accomplishments in the area of prevention in the future. The only thing missing is for public health leaders to take advantage of the opportunities present in the current health care system, which is struggling to reduce costs. These leaders must realize that public health employees are the most important component of health care reform. These workers know what to do and how to do it, but they must be empowered to use their creativity in solving our health care problems, doing what they think is right without fear of getting in trouble. This is where the inspirational leader's guidance is so important.

Leaders should understand clearly the role culture plays in bringing all employees together in preparation for future challenges to public health departments in the United States. In order for agencies to face future challenges, the entire workforce must embrace the mission of public health and accept new strategies to accomplish that mission. This will require trust, dedication, incentives, empowered workers, and leadership. If any of these components is absent, the mission may not be attainable.

Key Terms

Competencies

Culture audit

Informal leader

Performance-enhancing culture

Discussion Questions

1. Why is a complete understanding of the public health culture so important to a leader's success or failure in achieving public health goals?
2. What is the leader's role in maintaining a thick culture in his or her public health agency? Explain.
3. How can the leader better understand the employee culture that he or she is responsible for nurturing?
4. Why is a performance-based culture so necessary for the new roles that will be required of public health departments?

CHAPTER 8

PARTNERSHIPS TO IMPROVE THE PUBLIC'S HEALTH

LEARNING OBJECTIVES
- Describe the ecological model of health
- List partners based on the ecological model of health
- Discuss strategies for sustaining partnerships
- Define the key elements for assessing partnerships

Public Health Partners

Health is created at the intersection of multiple factors that contribute to or hinder the healthiness of populations. Health depends not just on access to medical care but also on such factors as individual makeup, social settings, and environmental conditions (Institute of Medicine [IOM], 1997). The Institute of Medicine defines health as the "state of well-being and the capability to function in the face of changing circumstances" (IOM, 1997, p. 41). The factors contributing to a healthy state, the determinants of health, occur across many parts of life and include individuals' lifestyle and genetic makeup, the communities in which we live, the local economy and employment options, opportunities for recreation, social support, the built environment, government and policy, the natural environment, and the global ecosystem. Collaboratives, coalitions, and partnerships have long played important roles in the history of public health. For our readers, we will make some distinctions among these commonly used terms. Collaboratives are formed by groups and individuals working toward a common purpose and sharing power. Coalitions primarily involve groups working together to reach an agreed-upon goal. Partnerships embody efforts to include the representation of individuals and groups from a wide array of organizations and sectors found in a given community (Padgett, Bekemeier, and Berkowitz, 2004).

The role of partners from the array of sectors of society affecting health is an essential area for exploration and development in achieving good health outcomes, broadening participation in policymaking, planning for public health interventions, and ensuring accountability to the communities that are served. **Public health partnerships** include community-based, grassroots groups and stakeholders from major sectors of society, such as business, the media, government, schools and academia, and the health care system (IOM, 2002). As opposed to coalitions, which are generally viewed as time- and resource-intensive and occasionally experience conflicts around coalition goals, processes, and areas of work, most partnerships are organized at the community level and are often characterized as having face-to-face connections that reach across traditional boundaries found in community-wide organizations (Padgett et al., 2004). Coalitions typically involve groups, rather than individuals, working together. In Florida during the past twenty years, Healthy Start Coalitions were mandated by law to convene an array of health organizations that shared a mission to provide quality maternal and child health (MCH) services. A major function of this coalition was the awarding and accounting of public revenues for MCH services. The engagement of representative community members—for instance, mothers who were or would one day be recipients of public health MCH services—has been difficult to achieve across the thirty-plus Healthy Start Coalitions organized to oversee funding and services by contracted public health organizations around the state of Florida. Alternately, public health community-wide partnerships are formed by individual stakeholders and community groups; are organized locally; and tend to focus on health promotion, community health assessment, and disease prevention. Building capacity to improve community health and empowering community members are also goals of community-wide partnerships. Mobilizing for Action through Planning and Partnerships (MAPP), a comprehensive process for improving community health, is an example of a community-wide partnership initiative (National Association of County and City Health Officials, 2011). Community partnerships, with their diverse makeup and shared responsibilities, might be especially useful as we work toward significant system changes to address the complex health problems of modernity.

The term **collaborative partnerships** was coined during the Turning Point initiative, a joint venture of the Robert Wood Johnson Foundation (RWJF) and the W. K. Kellogg Foundation from 1996 to 2006 to support the work of partnerships in creating more effective, community-based, and collaborating public health systems (Padgett et al., 2004). Collaborative partnerships are practices that include cooperative work across multiple private, public, and community partners at the state and local levels, and as such combine elements of two traditions in public health—collaborative decision making and community partnerships. An evaluation of the Turning Point project found that collaborative partnerships at the state level demonstrated an ability to transform the public health infrastructure and foster change (Padgett et al., 2004). The study was unique in that partnerships involving local, state, and national partners in pursuit of effective local public health systems rarely appear in the literature, an unfortunate gap when you consider that many important and far-reaching policy and program decisions are made at the state and national levels.

Value of Partnerships for Public Health Organizations

In the United States, private foundations and government entities have invested hundreds of millions of dollars to promote coalitions and partnerships around health issues (Lasker, Weiss, and Miller, 2001). As a result, thousands of coalitions, alliances, collaboratives, and other health partnerships have been formed. The common, underlying theme in this massive effort to foster partnerships is the belief that the complex problems of today are just too monumental for any one group or sector to address alone. The socioeconomic and environmental components of many health issues have not responded to top-down or single-solution programs (for example, abstinence-only adolescent pregnancy prevention programs). Partnerships offer great potential to engage other people and their organizations or community groups to work together in a supportive atmosphere in which strengths and resources are maximized (Lasker et al.). Partnerships can also be very frustrating, in part due to their formal procedures and structure—and in a number of cases because some organizations providing health and human services are required to work together in "forced partnerships" in order to qualify for funding. Coalitions or partnerships have become common requirements in many federal, state, and private foundation grants and may be partnerships on paper only. Some estimates indicate that half of all partnerships fail within the first year—although the reasons are not well established (Lasker et al.). Telltale signs of a partnership on the brink of failure include a history of conflict, manipulation, or domination by one partner; the absence of a clear purpose; a lack of communication; an imbalance of power; hidden agendas; and philosophical differences. One striking characteristic of weak partnerships is their noticeable lack of group efforts to incorporate community voices into their plans and actions (Shortell et al., 2002). Conversely, a successful partnership experiences trust, a shared interest in maintaining the partnership and building a vision together, collaborative decision making, and shared mandates and agendas (Wilcox, 2000).

Effective public health programs engage individuals and organizations knowledgeable about or active in every level of the public health system to create and sustain conditions that produce health. The practice of partnering with groups or organizations that operate within a specific area of the ecological model of health (environmental protection agencies promoting ecosystem health, county building and zoning offices affecting the built environment, and so on) is a recognized strategy for achieving health outcomes. Although public health experts are fairly united in their beliefs about engaging community partners in improving public health system and agency performance, local public health agencies typically involve their community partners when community support is needed for priorities that have already been identified by officials for targeted community populations (Lewin Group, 2002). Without a system-wide understanding of the components of effective partnerships, agencies are often defining and developing partnerships according to their own standards. Such variation in the use of the term *partnerships* complicates the process of establishing an evidence base concerning partnerships. A systematic review of available research on the effect of partnerships on public health outcomes in England from 1997 to 2008 reveals limited evidence about the impact of partnerships on health outcomes (Smith et al., 2009). The primary explanation for the lack of evidence is the absence of rigorous evaluation research on the connection between partnerships and improvements in population health. In the absence of evidence, the benefits of partnerships in public health are primarily presumed (Smith et al., 2009). The lack of evidence has not diminished the strong belief that partnerships and community engagement are important public health activities endorsed by national public health groups, including the National Association of County and City Health Officials (NACCHO), the Public Health Leadership Society, the U.S. Department of Health and Human Services, and the American Public Health Association.

Two examples illustrate some of the evidence that is building in support of the value of partnerships. First, an evaluation of community substance abuse programs and the active presence of community partnerships showed a weak but statistically significant difference in substance abuse prevalence rates between programs with partnerships and those with none (Yin, Kaftarian, Yu, and Jansen, 1997). Second, the Mectizan Donation Program (MDP) has been instrumental in controlling onchocerciasis, or river blindness, in Africa and Latin America, and has been described as one of the greatest miracles of the twentieth century (Peters and Phillips, 2004). The success of the program is attributed, in great part, to MDP partnerships involving twenty-five different international organizations. In a self-assessment survey of the partners, members rated highly the partnership's governance and management, identifying few problems. An analysis of results determined that members gave high ratings based on the perceptions of the program by external organizations. Partners believed that their opinions mattered and resulted in action. The program was also ranked highly in the area of performance evaluation and accountability. As the relatively new field of research into public health systems evolves, it will be important to study the degree of partnership involvement in public health efforts along with the effect of such involvement on process and outcomes.

Many different models of partnerships have emerged over the past decades, including strategic alliances and partnerships of a few stakeholders; coalitions of ten or more organizations; and community-wide initiatives that engage many people, groups, and organizations. This chapter explores the logic behind community-wide partnerships as a strategy for public health practitioners, presents the ecological model of health to guide the formation of valuable public health partnerships, and suggests methods for assessing the role of partnerships in achieving the mission of public health.

Building Community-Wide Partnerships Using an Ecological Model of Health

Creating conditions for people to be healthy and contributing to the well-being of family, friends, neighbors, and people across a region, state, and nation—and the world—are shared responsibilities. Health is a primary public good because so much of what humans are able to accomplish in the areas of employment, social relationships, and participation in civic activities depends on health status. Because health is important for employers, government entities, communities, and society, maintaining and improving conditions in which people can be healthy are shared tasks that are best achieved through strong and broadly based partnerships.

The task force on community preventive services that developed the Guide to Community Preventive Services recommended evidence-based interventions for improving the public's health, to be implemented through public and private partnerships (Community Guide Branch, n.d.). The Community Guide includes interventions in which community-wide partners are essential participants in decision making and capacity building, such as in the development and promotion of walking trails to increase physical activity. Further, the Institute of Medicine, an independent organization that provides unbiased, expert advice on health to decision makers and the public, recommends far-reaching, population-centered health strategies to address the behavioral and lifestyle interventions needed to reduce hypertension rates across the nation (IOM, 2010b). The IOM identified community-wide public and private partnerships that include businesses and community health workers as essential actors in the efforts to increase adherence to medications. Hypertension is one of the leading causes of death in the United States—one in six people who die each year do so as a result of this disease. The scope of the interventions the IOM has identified to significantly reduce and control hypertension in the population reflects the broad range of factors influencing an entire nation's health and indicates the need for action and partnerships across many sectors of society, involving both private and public resources and efforts.

In Chapter One we presented an expanded **ecological model of health** showing the major domains of the determinants of health and well-being and including the additional domains of the global ecosystem and the built and natural environments. The areas of the model highlight the many factors that affect a community's health and help us consider the different types of partners that could work together toward improving health outcomes for community populations. Because health is a product of factors and interrelationships between and across the multiple domains that contribute to health status, organized efforts to improve community health outcomes require the participation of representatives from multiple domains of the ecological model of health. Engaging partners from all areas affecting health ensures a consideration of relevant risk and protective factors when assessing, planning, and implementing community health improvement initiatives.

A recent study on the risk of injection drug use (IDU) conducted by faculty in the Department of Epidemiology at the University of Michigan School of Public Health provides an example of the interactive effects of different domains of the ecological model of health (Roberts et al., 2010). Researchers found that the risk of IDU was greater for metropolitan statistical areas in the study with worse local environmental conditions and economic circumstances. This finding underscores the importance of sociopolitical and economic factors as determinants of IDU for the metropolitan areas in the study and supports the concept of partnering with groups and individuals experienced in environmental and economic research and services.

Table 8.1 describes each component of the ecological model of health and offers examples of likely partners. The contributions of some organizations occur in multiple domains of the model, and it would be important to monitor overrepresentation of such organizations during community health improvement initiatives. Diversity in partnerships is a valuable asset, especially when addressing the great health disparities present in communities, and encourages a broader input of advice and expertise. By directly involving members of communities experiencing excessive health disparities, the likelihood of creating and maintaining sustainable and culturally appropriate strategies increases significantly (Mensah, 2005).

Community organizations, such as hospitals and other health care provider groups, are knowledgeable about the patient populations they serve and provide

Table 8.1 Examples of Partners for Each Domain of the Ecological Model of Health

Domain of the ecological model of health	Examples of partners
Individuals—biology (age, sex, hereditary factors) and behavior	Community representatives, including youths, older persons, persons from minority populations, and members from impoverished neighborhoods
Social relations—family, friends, neighbors, and coworkers	Neighborhood groups and leaders; support groups; religious organizations; and youth groups
Community—social capital and networks	Parent-teacher organizations; local public health agencies; community coalitions; health care providers; homeowner associations; police and sheriff departments; schools, colleges, and universities; local transportation groups; domestic violence coalitions and homes; juvenile crime organizations; probation and parole staff; substance abuse programs; the local housing authority; community development, building, and zoning programs; YMCAs and YWCAs; libraries; and local assemblies of national organizations (for example, the National Association for the Advancement of Colored People, United Way, and Red Cross)
Local economy—businesses, market opportunities, economic policy	Business owners; advertising companies; government and academic economic institutes; rural and urban development councils; chambers of commerce; art councils; banks; major community employers; mass media outlets (newspapers, radio); extension services; ecotourism centers; pharmaceutical companies; veterinarians; and health care providers
Government and policy—local, state, national, and international governance	Elected and appointed officials; the military, the national guard, and the coast guard; and government-funded organizations
Built environment—human-made surroundings in which daily activities and development occur that affect ecosystem quality and services, habitat protection, water resources, energy consumption, and indoor and outdoor air quality	Planning and zoning staff; academic and nonprofit organizations working on sustainability and the reduction of pollutants; building and landscape architects; recreation departments; housing authorities; building inspectors; and local public health agencies
Natural environment—an environment as close as possible to its natural state, unaffected by human activity; includes climate, weather, and natural resources that affect human survival and economic activity	Environmental protection agencies, businesses, and nonprofits with a mission to protect the natural environment; conservationists; and park services

(Continued)

Table 8.1   (*Continued*)

Domain of the ecological model of health	Examples of partners
Global ecosystem—millions of species of organisms in complex patterns created by many interacting physical environmental factors, chemical reactions, competition among organisms, predation, human disturbance, and other biotic and abiotic interrelationships	Experts in climate change, agriculture, fisheries, forestry, biodiversity and habitat, water, and air pollution, and ecologists.

valuable information on a variety of factors influencing health. Health care providers are represented in the community domain as well as in the local economy area of the ecological model of health. For many private health care providers, improving the bottom line of profit for the business is the primary force behind the types of services they offer and the charges they bill to the consumers of those services. Another group of private health care providers is classified as nonprofit, including organizations that do not share their profits with shareholders or owners and instead reinvest the surplus in pursuit of organizational goals. Recent changes in tax law require health care providers who are classified as being *not for profit* to report the costs of the activities in which they engaged during a tax year to protect or improve the community's health or safety, the community benefit requirement. Recently, the group for Advancing the State of the Art in Community Benefit (ASACB) developed uniform standards that focus on better alignment of nonprofit hospitals' governance, management, and operations as well as the strategic allocation of resources at the program level. Nonprofit hospitals are now exploring a range of primary care and community-based prevention programs to meet new tax requirements. The development of these programs involves engaging a wide array of stakeholders as ongoing partners in promoting healthy behaviors and building healthy environments (Association for Community Health Improvement, 2006). Historically, nonprofit hospitals have written off the debt of unpaid charges to meet the monetary obligations of a *not for profit* organization.

These changes in tax law increase opportunities for strategic partnerships between the local public health sector and nonprofit health care providers, potentially adding notable capacity to the efforts for improving community health. Strategic partnerships involve partners' working together and planning to achieve specific objectives by maximizing the efficient and effective use of their resources. Local public health agencies have engaged in strategic partnerships with community organizations that share the public health mission. For example, federally qualified health centers receive federal funding to promote health in the community by providing primary care services, outreach programs, and health education for vulnerable populations. Strategic partnerships between local public health agencies and federally qualified health centers are common in many parts of the nation. LPHAs have also partnered with not-for-profit hospitals to provide services that benefit the community.

Communication and collaboration across the wide array of community health organizations have the potential to increase coordinated efforts for providing the services and products with the highest likelihood of improving community health status—and may reduce costs associated with redundant and ineffective programs. The Centers for Disease Control and Prevention (CDC, 2010a) reported an example of a strategic partnership between private and public entities in 2010. A community-level partnership between the New York City Department of Health and Mental Hygiene, municipal hospitals, and the New York Business Group on Health resulted in increased depression screening and management as standard practice and secured coverage for this service in all primary care settings in New York City. Partners collaboratively managed resources to increase access to mental health services in primary care settings and minimize duplication of their efforts.

Employers are important and strategic partners in the interest of public health, as their business decisions have wide-ranging effects. For example, businesses can stimulate the local economy by creating jobs, increasing demand for housing and services, and improving the overall quality of life. If we consider the high correlation between poverty and poor health outcomes, working on bolstering the local economy by creating sustainable jobs is a logical part of improving community health status. Forging strong partnerships between public health and local businesses increases the potential of both partners to recognize and address the determinants of health, thereby improving community health status and increasing the benefits of this primary social good. Businesses are also major contributors to the pollution of the natural environment, endangering life in the community and disrupting the local ecosystem. Engaging business leaders and their employees in promoting health and protecting the local ecosystem seems to be a high-leverage strategic activity when we consider both the positive and the negative effects of industry on health. Galvanizing the participation and responsibility of public and institutional stakeholders (businesses and employers) is expected to increase the quality of information necessary for effective decision making (Committee on Public Health Strategies to Improve Health, 2010).

Health and quality of life information, obtained largely through surveillance systems, is a primary tool for public health agencies. This information must be translated into messages to influence policy and decisions made by local governments and individuals. Public health professionals, for the most part, are not skilled at using surveillance information to communicate, market, and advocate for sound public health policies (Teutsch and Churchill, 2000). **Communication** in the field of public health is an important strategy of informing the public about health in their communities and around the world; this strategy helps to keep vital health data in the public domain and involves mass and multimedia techniques (World Health Organization, 1998). Because relationships with the mass media can either help or hinder communication, a strong and ongoing partnership with local and regional newspapers, local marketing groups, and television and radio stations can help local public health agencies plan and select communication strategies, identify appropriate media and materials for presenting those strategies, evaluate communication efforts, and use feedback to continuously improve health policies and messages. An example of an effective partnership can be found in the global Public-Private Partnership for Hand Washing with Soap for developing nations (Curtis, Garbrah-Aidoo, and Scott, 2007). This public health organization learned from commercial marketers how to understand consumer motivation; employ a single, unifying idea; plan for efficient outreach; and ensure its message was effective on a national scale. After the organization's first marketing program, 71 percent of the target audience knew the television ad, and rates of reported hand washing increased.

Partnerships with academia create the interface for increasing awareness and communication around translating academic research into actionable strategies for public health agencies and others working to improve the quality of life for various community populations. At the national level, the Council on Linkages Between Academia and Public Health Practice, a coalition of representatives from seventeen national public health organizations, has worked since 1992 to further academic and practice collaboration in order to develop a well-trained, competent workforce and a strong, evidence-based public health infrastructure (http://www.phf.org/link/index.htm). Collaborators are well known for their win-win philosophies and a sharing or leveraging of resources. Partnerships between universities and colleges and the public health sector at the community level can also serve to increase local workforce competencies, creating pathways to promotion as well as ensuring the practice of evidence-based public health services. Public health agencies working with academic partners can foster continuous quality improvement as the different entities share skills and experience to achieve the common goal of improved community health. Over the last decade, in multiple states, state and local health departments have partnered with universities to plan and evaluate the tobacco settlement projects, demonstrating the effectiveness of tobacco use prevention programs. Finally, evaluating the interventions of public health organizations contributes to the evidence base for public health practice and increases the likelihood of services and products that will improve the public's health. Partnering with local or regional universities and colleges helps to ensure that the skills and knowledge of evaluation science and models of continuous quality improvement are embedded in the practice of public health.

Successful Partnerships

Successful partnership efforts are those that conform to a few basic principles. Effective partnerships are open, inclusive, and diverse (Johnson, Grossman, and Cassidy, 1996). Partnerships that work well empower stakeholders and promote the development of leadership at multiple stages of the process, allowing leadership to emerge from the ongoing interactions of different and multiple persons engaged in addressing and solving complex health issues. Successful partnerships develop key strategies to reach and engage members of the target group whose health requires some population-centered prevention initiative. Shortell et al. (2002) provide an example of a rural site that supported two special councils—an interagency council and a community health council—to successfully ensure the participation of community agencies and the broader community. The partnership's steering committee was made up of members from both councils, along with important members of the business and health sectors. An urban community partnership in the Southwest with an aim to improve children's access to health care through school-based services provides another example of a successful partnership. The partnership represented a community advisory committee with three subcommittees: (1) a group of corporate and community organization members; (2) a resident group comprising parents and family members; and (3) a clinical group made up of school nurses, dental staff, nurse practitioners, and a physician. The subcommittees met routinely to respond to stakeholders and address the needs and concerns of all (Shortell et al., 2002). A compelling and shared vision often evolves from this partnership process and forms the basis for selecting the strategies and tactics designed to achieve the overall aim of improving community health status.

Using the ecological model of health helps to expand the list of potential partners. Once possible partners, with their varying levels of resources and value, are identified by public health agencies, community leaders will need strategies for engaging them (IOM, 1997). The likelihood of sustaining these key community partnerships increases when partners measure progress and communicate successes to the community at large. To that end, partners need goals for monitoring performance to ensure that changes are being implemented, improvements are under way, and outcomes are getting better.

Assessing the Role of Partnerships in Improving Community Health

Forming partnerships between and among multiple groups and organizations appears to be a logical strategy to address public health challenges when we consider the variety of factors and different sectors in society and nature that affect health. However, relatively little evaluation research has been conducted to assess the effectiveness and performance of community-wide partnerships. People enter into partnerships with some basic assumptions about their power, including partnerships' ability to enhance outcomes at a rate that is greater than any individual partner's contribution (Brinkerhoff, 2002).

An assessment of community-wide partnerships has two aims: (1) ensuring good partnership practice, and (2) determining the effect of partnerships on the performance of activities to achieve a common good. Within the health field, the following criteria for effective partnerships have been identified: "willingness to share ideas and resolve conflicts, improved access to resources, shared responsibility for decisions and implementation, achievement of mutual and independent goals, shared accountability of outcomes, satisfaction with relationship between organizations, and cost effectiveness" (Leonard, 1998, p. 148). Further, a 2002 research project to evaluate partnerships for community health improvement programs found six components of partnership management that distinguished between successful and unsuccessful partnerships: managing partnership size and diversity, developing multiple approaches to leadership, maintaining focus, managing conflict, recognizing life cycles or the different stages of partnership development and knowing when to "hand off the baton," and having the ability to redeploy and blend funds easily to focus on local community needs (Shortell et al., 2002). Also, extensive empirical research and the work to produce the World Health Organization's *Verona Benchmark* led to the identification of six dimensions of partnerships (Watson, Speller, Markwell, and Platt):

- Recognizing and accepting the need for partnership
- Developing clarity and realism of purpose
- Ensuring commitment and ownership
- Developing and maintaining trust
- Creating clear and robust partnership arrangements
- Monitoring, measuring, and learning

Incorporating many of these concepts into an assessment tool enables stakeholders to reflect on the effectiveness of their partnership, benchmark their current status, and focus on identified strengths and weaknesses and areas for improvement. The use of such a self-assessment tool and the analysis of data generated about partnerships have the potential to inform the partnership process and to significantly increase learning and development for partnership members (Halliday, Asthana, and Richardson, 2004). Finally, Web-based partnership assessment tools are proliferating and demonstrate the need for and value of benchmarking quickly and easily for the purpose of partnership development.

Summary

Partnerships between local public health systems and community members, groups, and organizations help engage communities in the work of improving their health outcomes. The effectiveness of public institutions, including local public health agencies, depends to a large degree on the public's trust. Building and keeping trust involve communication and reciprocity, which are enhanced by effective and efficient partnering skills. Collaboration is vital for the implementation of successful public health efforts, given the number and range of organizations that work to keep the public healthy. As the public health challenges grow, so will the need for new or evolving partnerships. Public health departments are called upon to achieve positive health outcomes in a way that respects the rights of the individuals and of the community as a whole. This principle is achievable only when people and organizations have an opportunity to participate or be represented as partners in decisions about public health priorities, programs, and policy. Challenges facing public health practitioners include developing processes for building and sustaining partnerships, and assessing the functioning of each partnership in terms of trust, mutual support, and the leveraging or combining of resources that results in expanded capacity and sustainability.

Key Terms

Collaborative partnership

Communication

Ecological model of health

Public health partnerships

Discussion Questions

1. Describe the differences between coalitions, collaboratives, and partnerships. Can you provide examples of each type of group?
2. Explain how the use of the ecological model of health can assist public health practitioners in forming partnerships that are broadly representative. What key partners from your community or state would you engage in a partnership to improve health outcomes?
3. What are the characteristics of a successful partnership? A failed partnership?
4. How would you assess the success of a partnership?

CHAPTER 9

LEADING AND MANAGING CHANGE IN PUBLIC HEALTH ORGANIZATIONS

LEARNING OBJECTIVES

- Identify characteristics of complexity and servant leadership
- Describe the public health system's need for change
- Articulate the need for public health leaders to achieve the Millennium Development Goals
- List the elements of the Model for Improvement
- Discuss system models of health

Public Health and the Urgent Need for Change

Public health is "the science and art of preventing disease, prolonging life, and promoting health" through organized efforts of society (Charles-Edward A. Winslow, quoted in Turnock, 2009, p. 10). The mission of public health organizations is to fulfill society's interest in ensuring conditions in which people can be healthy (Institute of Medicine [IOM], 1988). The broad spectrum of issues that public health must address to accomplish its mission calls for public health leaders throughout an organization who are capable of adapting to a world in which economic, social, environmental, political, and health challenges are ever changing. Unprecedented rates of emerging diseases pose substantial threats to planet Earth and can be attributed in great part to population growth, intensive farming, environmental devastation, climate change, and the misuse of antimicrobials. Our environment is contaminated with chemicals that threaten the health of all plants and animals inhabiting Earth. The increased mobility of the world's populations and growing economic interdependence facilitate the rapid spread of dangerous diseases and contaminated products. These complex threats require action by public health organizations that moves beyond the types of programs and services traditionally offered to improve population health. Public health organizations must now lead efforts to assure the public's health through broader initiatives involving numerous stakeholders and partners and addressing multiple determinants of health. For example, the World Health Organization (WHO, 2007) leads a campaign to promote **global public health security,** a call to reduce the vulnerability of populations to acute threats to health. WHO recommends the integration of public health into economic and social policies and systems, global cooperation in surveillance and alerts and response for disease outbreaks, and cross-sector collaboration (agriculture, commerce, tourism, and health) within governments. Another example can be found in the work of local public health agencies (LPHAs) located in counties and cities across the United States who work with partners to conduct surveillance of communicable diseases and prevent the spread of these diseases across community populations. The efforts to prevent and contain the spread of H1N1 also exemplify the work of public health agencies to monitor and control disease. This chapter explores the opportunities for public health practitioners to lead and manage changes in the delivery of public health services that are most likely to produce improved health outcomes for communities in the twenty-first century.

Challenges Facing Local Public Health Leaders

The challenges a public health leader will face in his or her career are too numerous to list. In spite of this overwhelming prospect, public health leaders can be found at different levels of government, within community-based organizations, and in nonprofit nongovernmental organizations (NGOs). Much has been written about the qualities of a successful leader—able to catch the crest of a wave and ride it with strategies in hand, value driven, technically competent, tenacious, personally credible, self-aware in regard to strengths and weaknesses, persuasive, and politically savvy (Grainger and Griffiths, 1998). Add to this the qualities that are deemed essential for a leader—visionary; ethical; having a sense of mission; being an effective change agent, political navigator, negotiator, mediator, power broker, collaborator, capacity builder, forecaster, marketer, team builder—and it is stunning that so many professionals sign on to direct their community public health efforts. Courage and a thirst for knowledge would seem to be the essential and initial traits for any person seeking greatness in public health leadership.

Public health organizations face a world that has become more interconnected and more interdependent, and in which the rate of change is unprecedented. As so aptly stated by the scientific leader and luminary Stephen W. Hawking, the twenty-first century will be the century of complexity (Sanders, 2003). Studying **complex adaptive systems,** or systems in which the parts are strongly interrelated, self-organizing, and dynamic, is an endeavor within the larger field of complexity science (Sanders). Rain forests, societies, human immune systems, and the world economy are all considered complex adaptive systems. Certainly the field of public health practice falls into this category as well. In order for public health organizations to thrive, they must be responsive to community needs, which are intrinsically affected by local, state, national, and global economies; emerging and reemerging diseases; and environmental pollution. To thrive, public health agencies must adapt to changes that occur in the larger environment in which they operate—locally, nationally, and globally. These are the types of adaptations that public health agencies must make to remain a relevant part of a broad effort to improve global health, which includes the health of all nations, through health care and public health services.

In this chapter we discuss the skills that our public health leaders require to assure conditions that protect and promote health in this era of complexity, and we offer recommendations to advance global public health security. Better security means stronger global, national, and regional partnerships that perform surveillance, continuously learn about emerging events and risk factors, develop processes and changes that address problems early on, and conduct primary prevention efforts by reducing exposure to risks and promoting well-being on a broad scale.

Millennium Development Goals

In 2005 members of the United Nations established goals and commitments to work together to promote the economic and social advancement of all peoples (United Nations [UN] General Assembly, 2010a). Noteworthy is this group's dedication to achieving these noble **Millennium Development Goals** by 2015 (UN General Assembly, 2010b):

- Eradicate extreme poverty and hunger
- Achieve universal primary education
- Promote gender equality and empower women
- Reduce child mortality

- Improve maternal health
- Combat HIV/AIDS, malaria and other diseases
- Ensure environmental sustainability
- Develop a global partnership for development

Achieving these wide-reaching goals means intensifying national responsibility and leadership. The problems they identified and their proposed solutions require leaders with the following (UN General Assembly, 2010b):

- Skills to communicate and to transform the current public health systems at the local, state, and national levels into active partners in assessing the broad settings in which our health and social issues reside
- Courage, compassion, and spirit to reignite new and old partnerships to help redesign the current system of public health

The authors of the Millennium Development Goals report acknowledge that each nation must define its own social and economic policies and resources, and especially work on building the political will for achieving the 2015 targets. However, in such an interconnected global economic system, finding ways to effectively lead and develop partnerships to leverage the world's trading and investment opportunities has great potential to reduce and eventually eliminate the poverty that plagues many nations around the globe and disrupts their opportunities for improving the health of countless people.

Urgent Need for System Change

Today's public health practitioners not only are concerned, as were their predecessors, with controlling communicable diseases and epidemics but also must recognize and address the health effects of a vast array of new health problems associated with the built environment, climate change, pandemics, natural disasters, bioterrorism, and poverty. U.S. public health practitioners must also focus on the relatively poor health of Americans when compared to inhabitants of other developed countries. Ironically, while the overall health of Americans declines, the nation grapples with excessive health expenditures, a warning sign for other developing countries to keep an eye on the evolution of their health care systems and the associated costs.

The United States ranks highest in per capita spending for health care among all countries in the world. However, in recent reviews of health care systems, the United States ranked thirty-seventh in preventable deaths, forty-third in mortality for adult females, and forty-second in adult male mortality (Murray and Frenk, 2010). The U.S. population has a shorter life expectancy, a shorter *quality* of life expectancy, and a higher infant mortality rate when compared with other developed Western countries (RAND, 2006). Evidence also establishes that health performance in the United States not only is poor but also is improving at a slower rate than that of other developed countries (Murray and Frenk). The U.S. rates of obesity, a known risk factor for diabetes and cardiovascular disease, are among the highest in the world. In 2009 adult obesity rates increased in twenty-three states and did not decrease in a single state, an obvious indication that public health policies and services are not addressing a clear and present danger for the American populace (Trust for America's Health, 2010a). A recent analysis of the effect of obesity on longevity predicts that the steady rise in life expectancy in the United States over the past two decades will soon come to an end, and today's generation may not live as long as their parents (Olshanksy et al., 2005).

This information should be an alarming wake-up call to public health agencies who are just now beginning to address the problem, while at the same time the skills of the public health workforce remain focused on the provision of personal health care services and not on population-centered primary prevention services. The U.S. health care system is adept at treating particular diseases and illnesses, such as cancer and cardiovascular disease. We spend over $2 trillion each year to pay the costs of health care (Urban Institute, 2009). Almost 80 percent of these health care costs are attributed to treating preventable chronic diseases. The health care system is made up of health care providers and institutions, such as hospitals, that treat sick or injured patients and provide clinically based preventive services. Less progress has been made to prevent risk factors and promote policies and behaviors that reduce the rates of chronic diseases, which are linked to the smoking and obesity that are widespread throughout the nation (United Health Foundation, 2009). Local public health systems continue to emphasize personal health care services over population-centered health services. **Personal health care services** involve the treatment of disease and the provision of clinical services to individuals or families to address and resolve their individual health problems. The lack of knowledge about population-centered health services on the part of key public health practitioners, as well as the current mandates for public health agencies to provide personal care services, such as maternal and child health care, are barriers for a needed redesign of the public health system.

Investing in public health services that seek to reduce tobacco use through education, regulations, and taxes, or that involve communities in campaigns to promote physical activity by increasing access to safe recreational areas, are highly effective when compared to the curative model predominant in the U.S.

The curative model has as its primary function the treatment of illnesses, such as lung disease or diabetes, and it costs more than $3 trillion annually (Trust for America's Health, 2010b). Millions of Americans suffer from such preventable diseases as cancer and diabetes. Their quality of life is diminished, and for some their retirement years become a nonstop series of visits to various providers of health care. Underinvesting in preventive care and population health is the norm, although evidence continues to show that the nation's health would improve with such investments (Kindig and Stoddart, 2003; McGinnis, Williams-Russo, and Knickman, 2002). The 2009 Trust for America's Health report determined that an investment of 10 dollars per person in evidence-based community health programs to promote physical activity, improve nutrition, and expand smoking cessation would amount to a savings of $16 billion annually in health care costs within five years.

Most public health agencies have changed little over the past decades. Among the ten most frequent services LPHAs offer, according to a review conducted by the National Association of County and City Health Officials (NACCHO, 2008), are adult immunizations provision, communicable disease surveillance, childhood immunizations provision, tuberculosis (TB) screening, food service inspections, environmental health surveillance, food safety education, tuberculosis treatment, tobacco use prevention, and inspections of schools and day care programs. Tobacco use prevention is the only new program added to the top ten list during the past decade, a result of the master settlement of a class action suit in which tobacco companies agreed to pay $365.8 billion over twenty years to compensate states for treating smoke-related illnesses as well as to finance anti-tobacco programs.

NACCHO's profile (2008) of LPHAs, based on agency-reported data, states that most primary prevention services, including programs to address tobacco use, nutrition, chronic disease, unintended pregnancy, physical activity, injury, substance abuse, violence, and mental illness, are being provided by NGOs, not by LPHAs. In a comparison of providers of primary prevention services in various communities, just fewer than 40 percent of LPHAs, some in partnership with NGOs, were shown to provide chronic disease prevention services. The report does not specify the amount or type of primary prevention services offered by LPHAs or LPHAs in partnership with NGOs. Twenty-five percent of LPHAs deliver home health care, and 11 percent offer comprehensive primary care services. When LPHAs provide primary prevention services, they mainly focus on tobacco use, nutrition, chronic disease, and physical activity. Nutritional services are largely organized around the federal program Women, Infants, and Children (WIC) to ensure access to healthy foods for low-income mothers and their young children up to age five. LPHAs serving smaller populations generally offer a smaller percentage of primary prevention services than do their larger counterparts. NACCHO also reports that although a large percentage of LPHAs conduct surveillance and epidemiological services for communicable diseases, fewer than half of LPHAs apply these skills in the area of chronic illness.

Because every system is perfectly designed to achieve exactly the results it gets (Berwick, James, and Coye, 2003), the current public health system is a prime candidate for change that redesigns the system to support public health services that are population-centered, address the principle causes of disease through primary prevention, and incorporate a global health focus. Much work remains to be done to reduce the occurrence of preventable diseases. Experts in the field of cancer, for example, maintain that 40 percent of cancer cases worldwide could be prevented. Relatively simple population-centered strategies shown to be effective at reducing cancer cases include policies and campaigns that lower the rates of tobacco use, limit exposure to secondhand smoke, and decrease alcohol consumption; that encourage people to avoid getting too much sun and maintain a healthy weight through good nutrition and exercise; and that seek to protect against infections that cause cancer through vaccines (Union for International Cancer Control, 2010).

A number of public health agencies are engaged in quality improvement projects to address gaps in performance. Some use standards to identify gaps, such as the Centers for Disease Control and Prevention (CDC) National Public Health Performance Standards Program (www.cdc.gov/od/ocphp/nphpsp/) or public health accreditation criteria (for example, the Public Health Accreditation Board standards, www.phaboard.org/index.php/accreditation/standards/). Often the scope of changes undertaken to improve the performance of local public health agencies is limited. Efforts by LPHAs trying to improve current services, such as by reducing clinic wait times or reworking billing practices, amount to more of the same. Although these endeavors can achieve some improvements in organizational performance and community health outcomes, the resulting improvements generally do not accomplish the level of change that is fundamentally necessary for the public health system to grapple with today's complex and global health problems. What is needed is change *of* the system, not changes *in* the system. Producing great health outcomes requires great systems of care for health, including public health, and a will to improve, along with methods for systematic change (Berwick, 1996). An interesting exercise for most LPHAs would be for each one to check the alignment of its community health assessment priorities, established in partnership with community stakeholders, with its strategic plan, a current report of its services over the past two years, and the agency's strategic budget. Our recent review of a rural local public health agency revealed significant misalignments among the community health assessment priorities, the organization's strategic plan, its report on current activities, and financial documents about funded programs. The vision for local public health agencies involves community partnerships that guide the selection of priority health outcomes and the budgeting of and advocacy for adequate resources to meet community expectations for health improvement—known as customer service in other industries.

Visioning the New Public Health

The ultimate concern of public health practitioners is with the underlying structures that create the society in which we live and that have an impact on whether we are a healthy or unhealthy community, state, or nation. "Because fundamental social structures affect many aspects of health, addressing the fundamental causes rather than more proximal causes is more truly preventive" (Public Health Leadership Society [PHLS], 2002, p. 4). Whether protecting the public during a disaster or epidemic or reducing exposure to risk factors that lead to chronic illness and suffering, public health leaders must work collaboratively across community groups to form partnerships, as well as taking stock of state, national, and global health perspectives to identify and promote the fundamental requirements for health that contribute to global public health security. These requirements extend beyond access to quality health care and include the effects on health that originate from lifestyles, social relationships, economies, policies, and the built and natural environments—components of the ecological model of health.

The **vision for public health** reaches beyond the traditional provision of personal services and community health education, and includes advocacy and actions at the local, state, national, and global levels to encourage the sustainable use of finite resources; to reduce the impact of climate change; to protect the world's natural resources; to create built environments that promote and sustain healthy lifestyles and reduce the spread of chronic diseases; to sponsor policies that foster healthy local economies, reducing the impact of poverty on health and the social dimensions of life; and to update and expand regulations and controls that reduce the opportunities for the spread of toxic threats and infectious and chronic diseases.

The public health services of the future will routinely incorporate a system model of health with the major determinants of health for addressing the profound changes in the way we inhabit our planet, such as the growing use of intensive farming practices or rapid urbanization in parts of the world. Models incorporating the determinants of health, such as the ecological model of health, are valuable tools for action by local, national, and global public health leaders (Centers for Disease Control and Prevention [CDC], 1999a; IOM, 1996;

Schneider, 2006). Employing such models facilitates thinking about and working simultaneously on the multiple dimensions of the system that create the incredible threats to all forms of life on our planet today. Newer versions of the ecological model of health are more expansive and include the global ecosystem, acknowledging problems associated with climate change and biodiversity, and with the macroeconomy, politics, and global forces that represent the significant interrelationships and interdependence among societies across the globe. An example of the interdependence of societies around the world can be found in the financial crisis in the U.S. banking system in 2007, which created significant risks for world economies, many of whom experienced decreasing economic growth, recessions, and growing unemployment and poverty. Earlier versions of the ecological model of health included individual characteristics (such as age, sex, race, and hereditary factors); lifestyles; community (social capital); the local economy (wealth creation and markets); activities (such as walking, shopping, moving); the built environment (buildings, places, roads, and so on); and the natural environment. Developing local strategies for reducing health inequalities and merging that work with sustainable environmental and economic determinants of health included in current models of health can be part of a global effort to improve the health consequences of poverty, crime, wars and conflicts, climate change, natural catastrophes, and man-made disasters. Preventing infectious disease epidemics and pandemics and avoiding other acute health events are equally critical areas for emerging public health leaders.

Leadership for the New Public Health

Modern day problems are just too complex for traditional leadership thinking formed during the Industrial Age and based on top-down management principles. The multifaceted challenges facing human organizations today call for a range of new skills among public health leaders that transcend the conventional view of leadership in which one person, the leader, exerts sufficient influence over another, the subordinate, to achieve an intended outcome. The traditional view of leadership is based on a role rather than a behavior, a role occupied by a person with the responsibility of regulating the behavior of others toward the achievement of some end.

Conventional views of leadership conceptualize the leader as a visionary who is charting the course for the future. The traditional view of leadership implies certainty, influence, and control. Leading an organization, according to the conventional view, requires a leader's vision and direction to create the necessary changes, removing any and all obstacles until the goal is met. The emphasis is on one individual's skills and capabilities. Further, the vision for the organization is created based on one leader's ability to scan the external environment and his or her adeptness at making changes, motivating employees, and including strategic partners (Uhl-Bien and Marion, 2008). A public health leader formed by the teachings of these traditional leadership models would have a vision and a story, and would be an able communicator and formidable strategic planner. These conventional models of leadership maintain that effective leaders control organizations and direct employee behaviors to achieve specific outcomes.

Alternatively, we can think of leadership as a behavior that emerges from the continuing interactions of different and multiple persons engaged in a wide variety of activities, a "roving leadership" (Max De Pree, quoted in Plowman and Duchon, 2008, p. 131). This emerging view expands the concept of leadership beyond one person, a formal leader, and considers the manifestation of leadership behavior across multiple persons in an organization. "Leaders emerge, not from self-assertion, but because they make sense" (Plowman and Duchon, 2008, p. 131). Fostering teamwork, engaging communities in decision making, and being ethical and authentic are additional competencies of leaders who help to get the right things done.

Complexity Leadership

The theory of **complexity leadership** is based, in part, on the uncertainty of events and the nonlinearity of relationships, which affect our ability to predict or even fully understand outcomes. This view of leadership is also based on the observation that most actions, regardless of how well they are directed and targeted, will have multiple effects. Complexity leadership theory asserts that ongoing interactions among entities at lower levels of an organization (front-line employees, information system personnel managers, and so on) result in emergent order at the higher levels of that organization (organizational outcomes), creating a new order, an emergent state of the organization. Proponents of complexity leadership believe that traditional leadership based on control and regulation to reduce conflict or disorder drains the energy from leaders and their followers. The challenges for today's public health system under these conditions of uncertainty and unintended effects are beyond the capabilities of a handful of people at the top who are "in control." Leaders alone cannot direct all the changes, because they do not know what changes are necessary. The questions we face as a society are too big for any one discipline alone to answer. The key to solving complex issues is the emergence of leadership throughout and across the organization and the different disciplines within the organization, allowing the whole system to adapt to the myriad of changes that occur routinely in the organization and the surrounding environment. Leadership is specifically concerned with adapting organizations and employees to change, creating the capacity to thrive.

Complexity leadership theory helps answer the question of how leaders participate in developing an organization that can thrive in a complex environment (Uhl-Bien and Marion, 2008). The nonlinear, dynamic, and emergent aspects of ensuring conditions that keep people safe and healthy create challenges for public health leaders who are concerned with organizational structure and processes. Leadership is necessary to develop and guide processes by which public health solutions emerge to address complex issues, enabling rather than controlling fundamental change. To illustrate, controlling increasing rates of tuberculosis among migrant farmworkers is possible through leadership across an LPHA to accomplish

- Adherence to evidence-based practices that address the multiple determinants of health
- Continual assessment of farmworkers' living conditions and travel
- Cultivation of trust and engagement of the farmworker community leaders
- An understanding of transmission paths that include domestic and foreign travel
- A willingness to extend case finding and treatment across borders
- Attention to nutrition and safe living conditions
- Empowering staff to plan, perform, refine, and develop policies for managing the multiple services required of community members exposed to or with an active case of TB
- Employing information systems to track and report on each patient's risks, care, and contacts with possible exposure to the disease

The complex nature of the disease as well as the migrating characteristics of population members, many of whom travel between countries, are best addressed when leadership is shared and barriers to controlling the disease are removed by those who work successfully with the population and are most knowledgeable about their needs and assets.

In the complexity leadership model, the leader's role is one of making sense of a variety of factors and being a catalyst for change, altering the functioning of the entire system by introducing or removing elements, thereby loosening up the system to be adaptive. This is accomplished by integrating three key leadership functions: **adaptive, enabling, and administrative leadership** (Uhl-Bien and Marion, 2008). Adaptive leadership is the source of change in an organization. Adaptive leaders scan across disciplines and industries to see emerging conditions, paradigm shifts, and opportunities for innovation. Enabling leadership fosters or supports adaptive leadership, and adaptive and enabling leadership can be found at multiple levels of an organization. Administrative leadership is the function of administering, planning, and organizing the bureaucracy toward flexibility and allocation of the resources needed for the organization to adapt to and implement the changes. Administrative leadership is found in formal managerial roles within an organization. The tendency for an organization to become stagnant and nonresponsive to events due to leadership by a handful of people can be offset by the distribution of leadership across an organization. The emergence of such talent is termed *collective intelligence*, or *distributed intelligence*, and is a cornerstone of complexity leadership (Uhl-Bien, Marion, and McKelvey, 2008).

In this environment, leadership development shifts from a sole focus on individual development to an emphasis on fostering leadership capacity throughout the organization. This broadened approach to leadership development enhances the ability of the organization to practice emergent and collective leadership. For example, one way to foster emergent or collective leadership is to coach leaders to shift their thinking away from a controlling role and toward a catalytic or facilitative role. Another key principle of complexity leadership theory is the deliberate creation of aggregates, small groups or teams with a shared identity who interact with other groups or teams in the organization, creating networks of teams. Leadership capacity increases as opportunities for leaders to emerge multiply based on the expanded interaction of individuals within and across teams. A primary goal of leadership development in complexity theory is to promote more interaction and leadership across various roles, organizations, and locales, which inevitably leads to new connections and innovative relationships for solving complex problems (Van Velsor, 2008). Improving these connections increases the social assets and learning potential of an organization. In this modern era, organizational IQ and learning capacity have become more important than physical assets because they generate flexibility and the necessary knowledge to adapt to new conditions.

Tension is an accepted characteristic of the complex organization and its leadership, given the dynamics of multiple and diverse groups working together on common problems. The diversity and number of organizations that could potentially form a public health partnership to tackle one or more major health issues would no doubt result in many voices, not always harmonious, defining the health problems to be resolved and identifying solutions to be implemented (Gray, 2009). This tension or disequilibrium is not necessarily viewed as a bad thing within the framework of complexity leadership. In this state, a system is injected with energy and information that spread throughout the system and break up existing patterns, creating disturbances and presenting opportunities for new, emergent system order and solutions (Plowman and Duchon, 2008). Some claim that it is only in such conditions that emergent ideas surface, new adaptations are possible, and innovation and creativity arise. Leaders in this instance must support and facilitate the environment for adapting to such changes, busting up the equilibrium now and again to allow for continual innovation.

Leading and Serving

The tenets of **servant leadership** blend well with many of those of complexity leadership, and also embody the principles laid out in the *Principles of the Ethical Practice of Public Health* (PHLS, 2002). Servant leaders have a strong desire to serve, and they achieve organizational results by placing high priority on the needs of their colleagues and the customers of the organization (Greenleaf and Spears, 2002). Successful public health practitioners who serve their communities and fellow employees possess many of the competencies of the servant leader: listening, empathy, healing, awareness, persuasion, conceptualization, foresight, stewardship, commitment to the growth of people, and building community. A servant leader is one who promotes the growth of other persons in areas including health, wisdom, freedom, autonomy, self-worth, and willingness to serve (Greenleaf and Spears, 2002).

The servant leader works to clarify the thoughts and will of a group, listening to as well as reflecting on those thoughts through the experience of body, spirit, and mind, becoming an empathetic listener (Greenleaf and Spears, 2002). The ability to heal oneself as well as others is a strength found in servant leaders. Servant leaders rely on persuasion rather than command-and-control models of leading. They nurture great dreams, and they are able to think beyond day-to-day tasks; they can see the whole of the organization and the dynamic nature of the organization and the environment that surrounds it, as opposed to seeing only the parts. The servant leader is skilled at foreseeing potential outcomes or likely consequences of decisions, and makes decisions based on the commitment to serve the needs of others. Such a leader is committed to the development of others—professionally, personally, and spiritually—and creates real opportunities for people to grow. Lastly, the servant leader creates the culture that supports a sense of community among employees and engages the larger community with the work of the organization.

Similar to proponents of the emerging and collective intelligence tenets of complexity leadership, servant leaders are strong believers in the power of a group-oriented approach to decision making. In the case of public health, this type of approach strengthens organizations through a process that ensures wide participation and commitment to solving problems and improving community health. Leaders have a responsibility to build socially responsible products, progress, and services for the betterment of their community and ultimately the world. Engaging multiple partners and disciplines provides the knowledge—the system IQ—to do just that. The interconnectedness of today's global societies requires that leaders make informed decisions, undertaking an ecological or systems approach to monitoring events and detecting problems early on. Leaders derive such knowledge from diverse sources or groups of individuals working on the same, related, or even different perspectives of the system. The successful public health leaders for the twenty-first century are developers and facilitators of processes that promote interaction across units within and beyond their organization. In this way they promote service and increase the organization's flexibility to adapt to the ever-emerging complexities of improving the public's health.

Changing the Public Health System for the Future

We have celebrated ten great accomplishments of public health from 1900 to 1990: vaccinations, motor vehicle safety, safer workplaces, the control of infectious diseases, a decline in deaths from coronary heart disease and stroke, safer and healthier food, healthier mothers and babies, family planning, fluoridation of drinking water, and recognition of tobacco use as a health hazard (CDC, 1999b). Looking forward, what will be our top achievements? How will our public health agencies and leaders help communities stay healthy in the midst of major changes emanating from a world undergoing climate change; reeling from an international economic meltdown; facing threats from terrorists; and experiencing ongoing poverty, hunger, and increased rates of disease? What role can local public health systems plan to take in promoting local and global public health security?

In the United States, the governmental arm of public health at the local level, the local public health agency, is frequently referred to as the backbone of the public health system (see, for example, IOM, 1988; IOM, 2002). The limited research on local public health agency performance indicates that the bulk of public health expenditures continue to be related to personal health care services and treatments for preventable diseases, and not population-centered services (Brooks, Beitsch, Street, and Chukmaitov, 2009). The obesity epidemic is an indicator that the public health system must become more alert to new risk factors and undertake changes to prevent new diseases and epidemics, adapting to emerging health events. Public health agencies do this by conducting surveillance to monitor health status for community health problems; informing, educating, and empowering people about health issues; and engaging community members and organizations to address the primary causes of disease, thereby improving health and preventing excessive health care costs. Public health officials alert to the growing rates of obesity and informed about the emerging determinants contributing to this epidemic have broad community support, committed funding streams, and evidence-based interventions under way (see the Guide to Community Preventive Services, www.thecommunityguide.org/index.html). Public health agencies must transform into providers of population-centered health services, supporting interventions aimed at disease prevention and health promotion. Ideal public health services have an effect on entire community populations, for example by reducing exposure to risk factors with a negative impact on health (such as alcohol and tobacco use); supporting policies and services for promoting healthy diets and active lifestyles (such as workplace wellness programs); and reducing environmental pollution and degradation (such as by supporting small and local farming efforts).

The primary services found in most LPHAs are inadequate to address the expanded determinants of health and the threats to the public's health. Changes are needed in the current public health system to improve the health status of communities and to make progress toward global public health security. Theories of complexity and servant leadership offer guidance for creating processes that will help organizations thrive in today's complex environments.

Managing Change

Strong public health leaders are effective change agents, developing their creative capacities as well as expanding opportunities and support for other practitioners of public health to assume leadership roles. Leadership is primarily about managing change and creating processes that facilitate change. Complexity leadership concepts offer a dynamic means of understanding and explaining social phenomena and methods by which public health officials may improve organizational IQ. Complexity leadership concepts are aimed at enhancing motivation through employee empowerment, and they create ways to speed up the emergence of distributed intelligence across an organization (McKelvey, 2008). Accelerating the emergence of organizational IQ is accomplished through the deliberate creation of small groups or teams interacting with other teams and establishing networks of human capital—the knowledge, skills, health, and values of individuals. The goal is to increase the presence of these interacting groups throughout the organization, rather than confining such knowledge networks to upper management alone. Employees then become responsible agents for adaptive capability rather than individuals who merely carry out orders.

Improving the process by which we identify and undertake changes is a catalyst for loosening up the system to be more adaptive, introducing elements, methods, and new processes that move the system closer to its goals (Dodder, 2000). The obvious purpose of improving organizational processes is to increase the quality of operations and services. In the field of public health, quality is defined as "the degree to which policies, programs, services, and research for the population increase desired health outcomes and conditions in which the population can be healthy" (U.S. Department of Health and Human Services, 2008).

As mentioned earlier, the efforts to improve quality in public health agencies have focused on fairly specific goals, changes *within* the system, rather than undertaking a change *of* the system. Programs to change the public health system, including standards promoted by the CDC based primarily on the ten essential services, have not brought about such a shift. Change of the system is desirable if we are determined to contain the threats present today as well as achieve greater improvements in health outcomes, reducing health and environmental inequalities.

Within the field of health care, Don Berwick is the Administrator of the Center for Medicare and Medicaid Services, past president and CEO of the Institute for Healthcare Improvement (IHI) and national leader in and authority on health care quality and improvement. IHI is an example of an organization that operates primarily through the development of networks, which in this instance comprise IHI professionals partnering with motivated groups within organizations and applying the scientific method to build knowledge—with an ultimate goal of spreading changes that result in improvement across the health care system. To accomplish their goals for improving health care, a simple and elegant model for achieving changes that lead to improvement was devised—the Model for Improvement (Berwick, 1996). In addition to the Model for Improvement, those seeking credible improvements in their system of care are introduced to a system model for considering change, the Chronic Care Model, which is aimed at assuring fundamental change of the system, not only changes in one program or one division. The Chronic Care Model identifies the essential components of a quality system of chronic care, which include the community, the health care system, self-management support, delivery system design, decision support, and clinical information systems. Each component of the model incorporates evidence-based change concepts to improve the quality of care and the patient's interaction with the health care provider and the larger health care system (Improving Chronic Illness Care, n.d.). The ecological model of health is a comparable model for ensuring quality public health services. Both models identify the essential areas of the system in which work is needed to ensure high-quality services that lead to improved health outcomes. Improving the organizational performance of an LPHA also requires the identification of major components of the organization. We suggest the following categories, which represent common organizational domains: the customer (community and employee), financial management (stewardship of public funds and adequacy of resources for community and global priority health issues), internal processes (evidence-based services and quality improvement), and learning and growth (employee education and widespread opportunities for leadership) (Kaplan and Norton, 2001).

Using the Model for Improvement is a method for undertaking change that has the highest likelihood of achieving organizational goals. The initial step is establishing an aim. The aim should be measurable, time-specific, and clear in regard to the community or other population to be served. The model requires measures to establish that changes made result in improvements—measures that have value beyond focusing on the past. Reported measures create focus for the future because they communicate what is important to the organization. Reports on the performance of changes through the use of measures become a management tool, providing ongoing information about whether or not the change process is progressing and allowing the organization to adapt to the changes' resulting effects. Selecting changes that are the most likely to result in improvement will increase the likelihood of progress toward the organization's goals. Evidence-based practices are new to LPHAs, and their use must be emphasized by developing workforce skills, by linking evidence-based practice with funding for current and future public health programs, and through leadership.

Effective leaders of improvement maintain that frequent challenges to the status quo are needed by actively testing promising changes to the organization—an argument supported by complexity leadership theory (Berwick, 1996). The process for testing changes in real work settings is the Plan-Do-Study-Act (PDSA) cycle. Using the PDSA cycle, ideas for changes in work settings are planned, tried, studied, and acted on based on what is learned. Metrics are an important part of the study process, helping to inform the leader of any progress that is being made. The PDSA cycle is designed to allow a leader to swiftly test a change in a real work setting before fully implementing that change across an entire department or organization.

Summary

Public health organizations addressing current and future complex health issues understand that change is a basic principle of public health work. Systems and cultures that support and adapt to the shifting environment and cope with the uncertainty of events are needed. The following conditions should be present in the new world of public health practice:

- The network of groups working both independently and collaboratively on overlapping public health issues set the mission, vision, and strategy of public health.

- Leaders throughout an organization have an active willingness to foster change for improvement by establishing a plan for improvement, setting aims and allocating resources, employing a performance measurement system, and fostering leadership at various levels of the organization.
- Leaders encourage ideas for positive change throughout the organization, employing evidence or the best available knowledge attained through listening to community members and stakeholders.
- Employees throughout the organization contribute to a culture of emerging knowledge that is managed and shared.
- Such methods as using the Model for Improvement are employed to manage change, study results of initiatives, spread ideas, and sustain levels of performance improvement.
- Values surrounding the empowerment of employees, the development of knowledge and organizational IQ, relationship building, and broadly based leadership development are evident.

Theories of complexity and servant leadership offer new strategies for public health practitioners leading change *of* the public health system. Solving complex problems relies on the development of collective intelligence; the ability of practitioners to study and adapt to the changing environment while challenging the status quo and listening to the thoughts and will of groups created throughout the organization and community; the linking of groups to create networks that share knowledge as they work on common public health issues; and the ongoing practice of applying system models.

Key Terms

Adaptive, enabling, and administrative leadership

Complex adaptive systems

Complexity leadership

Global public health security

Millennium Development Goals

Personal health care services

Servant leadership

Vision for public health

Discussion Questions

1. What are the challenges facing today's public health leaders, and what are some of the skills they will need to address them?
2. Describe two types of leadership models, and explain why you think they are important to consider given today's complex health problems.
3. Explain the distinction between health care and public health. What does this mean for public health leaders?
4. Do you think public health leaders need to consider fundamental change *of* the public health system versus changes *within* the public health system? Please explain.
5. How likely are we to see achievement of the Millennium Development Goals by the predicted year of 2015? Please explain.
6. How can public health leaders use the Model for Improvement to change the health care system?

CHAPTER 10

DEVELOPING AN OUTCOMES ORIENTATION IN PUBLIC HEALTH ORGANIZATIONS

The quality of public health organizations has become an essential part of a national effort to reduce health care expenditures and improve the health outcomes of individuals and community populations in the United States. **Quality public health** involves the degree to which policies, programs, services, and research increase desired population health outcomes and assure conditions in which people can be healthy (U.S. Department of Health and Human Services [HHS], 2008). **Health outcomes** are indicators of how healthy an individual or a community is. Two types of health outcomes are frequently used to report on health: how long people live (mortality) and how healthy people feel while they are alive (morbidity). Access to quality and affordable health care has proven to be inadequate when addressing the health problems plaguing the U.S. population. The current status and impending onslaught of chronic diseases will result in tremendous suffering and erode the quality of life for many. This may be the greatest challenge for public health during the next decade. Members of minority populations and groups that have been marginalized based on socioeconomic status will continue to bear the burden of early death due to chronic diseases. Public health organizations can prevent many incidences of disease, injury, and early death by addressing the underlying causes of diseases. Tobacco use, obesity, alcohol and substance abuse, a lack of physical activity, poor nutrition, and risky sexual behavior are commonly known risk factors that contribute to morbidity and early mortality.

In addition to providing adequate public funding to quality public health organizations and supporting policies that are proven effective in reducing risks and improving rates of mortality and morbidity, supporting quality experts and advocates in the role of assisting public health organizations with methods that are aimed at improving community health outcomes is an important strategy to ensure a healthy nation. Good stewardship of public health funds by public health leaders is guaranteed when public health organizations make progress toward improving community and national health outcomes. The use of proven continuous quality improvement methods that require public health professionals to measure performance, link changes in services and operations to desired outputs and outcomes, assess intervention results, and design and redesign the public health system on an ongoing basis are all part of the journey to transform U.S. public health organizations into outcomes-based service providers. This chapter is about refocusing local public health organizations, particularly governmental local public health agencies (LPHAs), also known as county or city public health departments, on outcomes by implementing continuous quality improvement processes.

Quality Nexus of Public Health and Health Care

The nation spends over $2 trillion annually to treat Americans suffering from preventable injuries, infectious diseases, and such chronic diseases as cancer, diabetes, and Alzheimer's (Trust for America's Health, 2009). Transforming the U.S. system of health care and public health into a system that not only treats diseases and injuries but also addresses their principle causes is a crucial part of solving the current health care crisis. Although the United States has the highest per capita health care spending in the world, its health care system is far from the best in a number of measures of healthiness (for example, infant mortality and obesity rates), and is far behind its peers in developed countries.

During the past two decades, quality improvement experts and organizations have led efforts to increase the benefit to patients from health care services and to reduce the harm that patients experience. The Institute of Medicine (IOM, n.d.) defines quality in health care as "the degree to which health services for individuals and populations increase the likelihood of desired health outcomes and are consistent with current professional knowledge." The IOM's publication (1999) of *To Err Is Human,* a report on the serious flaws in the U.S. health care system that result in deaths and injuries to hospital patients, placed the U.S. health care system under the microscope. What followed was an expansive effort to improve health care, guided by six areas for improvement: safety, effectiveness, patient centeredness, timeliness, efficiency, and equity. Recently, public health agencies in a number of states, for example Florida and North Carolina, have adopted, studied, and adapted quality improvement methods, such as Six Sigma and the Institute for Healthcare Improvement's Breakthrough Series (IHI, 2003; Six Sigma Online, n.d.).

Today a number of health care organizations throughout the United States can point to improved health outcomes as a direct result of implementing and evaluating changes to improve their systems of care with the highest likelihood of success. The Northern New England Cardiovascular Disease Study Group (NNECDSG, 2009) is a regional interinstitutional organization that provides information about the management of cardiovascular disease in Maine, New Hampshire, and Vermont. The group maintains and studies patient data from all coronary artery bypass grafting (CABG), percutaneous coronary intervention, and heart valve replacement surgeries. The NNECDSG also monitors and studies clinical outcomes from these procedures, tracks outcomes by region, and develops prediction models to assist patients and their doctors with making the best decisions about cardiovascular health care. Finally, the group compares and uses outcomes from each participating hospital, such as CABG mortality rates, cerebrovascular accidents, and returns to the operating room for bleeding, to continuously improve institutional and regional cardiovascular disease treatment across the northern New England region.

The goals and tools for quality improvement in the health care industry have been developed through the combined efforts of multiple public and private organizations, including the Joint Commission on Accreditation of Healthcare Organizations, the National Committee for Quality Assurance, the Agency for Healthcare Research and Quality, National Quality Forum for Health Care Measurement, the Institute for Healthcare Improvement, and a number of hospitals and provider groups. In the process, health care has been evolving away from a disease-centered model toward a patient-centered model (Agency for Healthcare Research and Quality, 2002).

Notwithstanding this massive effort, most consumers are still dissatisfied with the U.S. health care system. A random survey conducted on behalf of The Commonwealth Fund Commission on a High Performance Health System found that 80 percent of consumers agreed that the U.S. health care system needed fundamental change or a complete rebuilding (How, Shih, Lau, and Schoen, 2008). A report by the National Committee on Quality Assurance (2008) indicates that the quality of health care in the United States reached a standstill in 2008 after years of steady improvement. It will no doubt take decades to remedy the quality issues associated with the vastness of the American health care system. Instituting quality public health services that "principally address the fundamental causes of disease and requirements for health, aiming to prevent adverse health outcomes," will help to accelerate the goals of improving population health and reducing the ever-increasing and excessive costs of health care (Public Health Leadership Society, 2002, p. 4).

Quality improvement efforts in the public health system have taken a somewhat different path than those in the health care system. During the past twenty years, the public health sector has been clarifying its mission, vision, core functions, and essential services to a nation that has "lost sight of its public health goals and has allowed the system of public health activities to fall into disarray" (IOM, 1988, p. 19). In 2008 the Public Health Quality Forum was established and organized under the leadership of the U.S. Department of Health and Human Services (HHS). This forum developed the *Consensus Statement on Quality in the Public Health System* (HHS, 2008), which clearly stated, for the first time, a uniform definition of quality in the public health system, modeled after the IOM's definition (n.d.) of quality in health care. Quality in the public health system was defined as "the degree to which policies, programs, services, and research for the population increase the desired health outcomes and conditions in which the population can be healthy" (HHS, 2008, p. 2). The *Consensus Statement* identifies the optimization of population health as the ultimate goal of quality improvement by public health organizations. Optimizing the health of the population is an outcomes-based approach and is aligned with the mission of public health put forward by the IOM: "Public health is what we, as a society, do collectively to assure the conditions in which people can be healthy" (IOM, 1988, p. 1).

Focusing on Core Functions and Essential Public Health Services

Gaps in performance that threaten the public's health and security continue to exist within the public health system, according to the IOM and other analysts (IOM, 2002; Turnock, 2009). Developments that clarified mission, core functions, essential services, and the definition of a public health agency have brought changes to local public health systems. However, minimal evidence exists to demonstrate whether these changes have resulted in improvements in the organizational performance of local public health systems or whether population health outcomes have improved. Paul Juran, a prominent leader in the field of quality improvement, declared that every system is perfectly designed to achieve exactly the results it gets (cited in Berwick, James, and Coye, 2003). The current U.S. public health system is designed to achieve exactly the results that are in existence today. Improving performance and outcomes requires changing the practice of public health professionals and the organizations that support the delivery of public health services.

Public health experts and analysts have promoted a variety of methods to change the public health system and improve performance. The American Medical Association (AMA) completed the first reported review of public health practice in 1914. The goal of the review was to describe services of state agencies. Findings by the AMA indicated a lack of focus on preventive health services. A scorecard was developed to rate state agencies according to their performance of preventive health services, a method the American Public Health Association (APHA) adopted in the 1920s in its appraisal form, a self-assessment tool designed to obtain information about official and unofficial public health services within metropolitan areas. The evaluation schedule for local public health followed in 1943 was also voluntary. APHA's Emerson Report of 1945 listed six basic public health services: vital statistics collection, communicable disease control, environmental sanitation, public health laboratory services, maternal and child health services, and public health education (cited in Turnock and Handler, 1997). During the late 1980s and early 1990s the National Association of County and City Health Officials (NACCHO) helped to identify local public health services and infrastructure measures in its *National Profile of Local Health Departments* (cited in Corso, Wiesner, Halverson, and Brown, 2000). NACCHO continues to conduct national periodic studies of governmental local public health agencies, establishing a comprehensive description of infrastructure and practice (National Association of County and City Health Officials [NACCHO], 2005a).

The Institute of Medicine's 1988 report on the future of public health was the impetus for a new round of performance reviews for public health organizations and instituted the core functions of assessment, policy development, and assurance as major components of public health practice. Public health experts around the nation believed that operationalizing the core functions in order to assess their performance across local public health systems was an important step in changing the practice of public health. The Public Health Practice Program Office of the Centers for Disease Control and Prevention (CDC) assembled a group of public health professionals from a number of national public health organizations and the Health Resources and Services Administration of the federal government to identify the tasks associated with each of the three core functions (Corso et al., 2000). The ten organizational practices (Exhibit 10.1) they identified "describe a continuum of problem solving activity, cycling from problem identification to evaluation in order to redirect interventions" (Turnock et al., 1994, p. 479). A number of LPHAs used the ten organizational practices intermittently to evaluate their performance of the core functions. In 1990 the Assessment Protocol for Excellence in Public Health (APEXPH), sponsored by

EXHIBIT 10.1

TEN ORGANIZATIONAL PRACTICES

Assessment

1. Assess the health needs of the community

2. Investigate the occurrence of health effects and health hazards in the community

3. Analyze the determinants of identified health needs

Policy Development

4. Advocate for public health, build constituencies, and identify resources in the community

5. Set priorities among health needs

6. Develop plans and policies to address priority health needs

Assurance

7. Manage resources and develop organizational structure

8. Implement programs

9. Evaluate programs and provide quality assurance

10. Inform and educate the public

Source: Turnock et al., 1994, p. 480.

NACCHO, was the first self-assessment tool to incorporate the core public health functions identified by the IOM in 1988 as well as a community health improvement process that assessed community partnerships (CDC, 1991).

A public health researcher and endowed chair of health services research at the University of North Carolina at Charlotte, James Studnicki, found that almost 75 percent of local health department resources in Florida were being spent on communicable disease programs and primary care (Studnicki et al., 1994). Today, public health agencies continue to focus a substantial portion of their resources on providing medical care to vulnerable populations, including women and children living at or near poverty levels and HIV/AIDS patients with limited access to medical services. The emphasis on direct delivery of health care services can be attributed to the era following Word War II when concern over the lack of health care for many resulted in local public health agencies' becoming safety net providers. Controversy continues over the emphasis by local public health systems on ensuring health services for the uninsured or poor while assessment and policy development activities remain limited. Turnock et al. (1994) observed similar results when they assessed LPHAs using the ten organizational practices framework. A surveillance tool with eighty-four performance measures built around the core functions was developed in the early 1990s to assess public health system performance around core functions (Miller, Moore, McKaig, and Richards, 1994). Subsequent studies showed that results from a set of four, twenty-six, or eighty-four performance indicators coincided, and each could be used successfully to predict effective LPHA performance. The four questions to predict the performance of LPHAs are as follow (Miller et al., p. 660):

1. In the past three years in your jurisdiction, have there been age-specific surveys to assess participation in preventive and screening services? [Assessment]
2. In the past year, has there been a formal attempt to inform candidates for elective office about health priorities in your jurisdiction? [Policy development]
3. In the past year in your jurisdiction, has a community health action plan, developed with public participation, been used? [Policy development]
4. In the past year in your jurisdiction, has there been any evaluation of the effect that public health services have on community health? [Assurance]

Studies conducted by Richards and colleagues report results very similar to Studnicki's—assessment ranked lowest in frequency of occurrence, and assurance ranked highest. Richards and colleagues also found that of the organizational practices in Exhibit 10.1, "Develop plans and policies to address priority health needs" and "Investigate the occurrence of health effects and health hazards in the community" had the lowest ranking, and "Inform and educate the public" had the highest (cited in Corso et al., 2000).

By the mid-1990s the leadership within public health adopted the ten **essential services** of public health (see Exhibit 10.2), with the following organizations playing predominant roles: the IOM, the CDC, APHA, and NACCHO. The three core functions of public health the IOM identified in 1988 are well addressed in the ten essential services, along with all of the activities from the earlier frameworks for identifying and evaluating public health performance. In addition, the task of developing a trained and competent public health and personal health workforce makes its first appearance.

The National Public Health Performance Standards Program (NPHPSP), in collaboration with NACCHO, developed performance standards and a self-assessment tool using the framework of the ten essential services in Exhibit 10.2 for local public health systems. The NPHPSP is a voluntary effort led primarily by LPHAs to assess the performance of all key community partners in the local public health system who work to improve the public's health, including LPHAs, health care providers, academic institutions, businesses, government entities, and the media (Corso et al., 2000). The self-assessment tool asks state and local public health practitioners how well their organizations are meeting the standards.

EXHIBIT 10.2
TEN ESSENTIAL PUBLIC HEALTH SERVICES

1. Monitor health status to identify community health problems.
2. Diagnose and investigate health problems and health hazards in the community.
3. Inform, educate, and empower people about health issues.
4. Mobilize community partnerships to identify and solve health problems.
5. Develop policies and plans that support individual and community health efforts.
6. Enforce laws and regulations that protect health and ensure safety.
7. Link people to needed personal health services and assure the provision of health care when otherwise unavailable.
8. Assure a competent public health and personal health care workforce.
9. Evaluate effectiveness, accessibility, and quality of personal and population-based health services.
10. Research for new insights and innovative solutions to health problems.

Source: CDC, n.d., p. 2.

This local public health agency assessment tool includes over sixty pages of questions related to the performance of the ten essential services. The assessment process is designed to support quality improvement initiatives by identifying gaps in achieving optimal performance by state and local public health systems and local boards of health, which govern LPHAs in many states. To date, twenty-two states have used the state-level instrument. The use of the local public health system performance assessment instrument (see Figure 10.1) has varied throughout the United States: ten states report significant use, six states indicate moderate use, and the remaining thirty-four states have minimal or no use reported (Centers for Disease Control and Prevention [CDC], 2008a).

Although the conceptual frameworks developed during the 1990s around public health practice have some merits, "none provide a well-defined theoretical framework concerning the elements that constitute and influence effective public

FIGURE 10.1 NPHPSP Local Instrument Use, Through August 2007

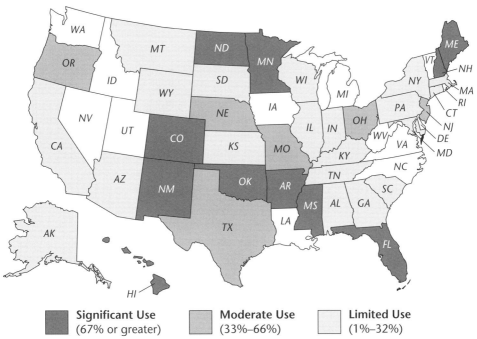

| Significant Use (67% or greater) | Moderate Use (33%–66%) | Limited Use (1%–32%) |

*Also includes sites using field test versions of the NPHPSP Local Public Health System Performance Assessment.

Source: CDC, 2008c, slide 19.

health practice" (Roper and Mays, 2000, p. 71). Public health practitioners will need to know with some certainty that the decisions they make concerning public health services for their respective communities and regions and the resources expended to produce those services will have an impact. Public health work in motor vehicle safety, immunizations, workplace safety, promotion of safer and healthier food, and control of infectious diseases has been credited with extending life expectancy and improving health status in past decades. However, newly emerging health problems and threats, generated by the effects of chronic diseases and unhealthy environments, raise concerns about the ability of public health to have an ongoing impact in the future. The limited funding currently allocated to public health in the United States makes these decisions even more critical if we expect to see ongoing improvements in the health status of the U.S. population. Public health experts continue to refine their definitions of the essential services of LPHAs. Linking these services to improved community health outcomes will help practitioners employ evidence-based practices that are tied to the content of their work, such as increasing the percent of the population with a healthy weight and reducing health care–associated infections. A well-defined theoretical framework not only must include the services or processes necessary for great performance but also should identify expected outcomes.

Attempts to assess effective public health practice were hindered by the design of the assessment tools. The inclusion of all system partners (governmental public health departments, health care, the media, academia, businesses, and communities) in the assessment of the local public health system, although a valuable attempt to bring all key players to the table, led to some confusion as governmental public health agencies tried to identify what areas their particular organizations needed to improve. Additionally, many local public health agencies considered the essential services to be too broadly defined to describe their individual work. NACCHO recognized this dilemma, and by 2005, working collaboratively with public health experts, leaders, and practitioners around the nation, created the *Operational Definition of a Functional Local Health Department* (NACCHO, 2005a). This effort was considered a major step in creating a shared understanding of what any community member might expect from his or her local public health agency and was designed to foster a climate of accountability (Lenihan et al., 2007). The operational definition is based on the ten essential services and includes forty-five standards that define public health practice and community health improvement efforts. Local public health agencies that are assessing their ability to perform, for example, the first essential service (monitor health status and understand health issues facing the nation) are asked to respond to questions about obtaining and maintaining such community health data as immunization rates, hospital discharges, environmental health hazards, and rates of uninsured. In addition, a LPHA is required to assess the development of relationships with local providers and other community partners, its contributions to the community health assessment process, and its ability to integrate data from multiple sources and analyze trends and health problems that adversely affect the public's health. Little has been reported on the use of these standards by LPHAs.

Current Quality Improvement Efforts in Public Health Organizations

The disarray in the public health system's performance of services to improve the health of community populations continues across many governmental public health agencies. Evidence mounts concerning the wide variation in availability and quality of public health services in U.S. communities, such as in regard to the following (Mays et al., 2009, p. 256):

- Population-wide strategies to investigate threats to the public's health,
- Promotion of healthy life styles that prevent many diseases and injuries,
- Preparedness for man-made and natural disasters, and
- Assuring environmental conditions that reduce exposure to risks such as unsafe water, pollution, and climate change.

The establishment of core functions, essential services, and standards for local public health systems and agencies has helped public health organizations clarify their roles to the community, engage partners in an assessment process, and evaluate to some degree the performance of the local public health system and agency. From a national perspective, however, a large proportion of local public health agencies have made limited use of the national process to assess their performance of the essential services. A **continuous quality improvement (CQI)** process requires ongoing assessment of performance, measurement of processes to achieve goals, and a diligent review of implemented strategies and their effect on improving health outcomes. Until recently, the emphasis on improving quality in public health organizations has been primarily based on providing the ten essential services, establishing standards of performance, and instituting a quality assurance process that compares current performance levels to the standards. This approach is based primarily on improving processes. Achieving the mission of public health to ensure conditions in which people can be healthy is possible by identifying gaps in performance, selecting priority community health outcomes to be improved, choosing evidence-based strategies that address the priority outcomes, and measuring performance of the public health mission to see that changes are implemented and outcomes are improving. Improving health outcomes is the primary focus.

In 2004 momentum picked up for establishing a process to accredit public health organizations. The Robert Wood Johnson Foundation (RWJF) convened a group of stakeholders who created a set of guiding principles for an accreditation process for local public health organizations and developed recommendations addressing the desire for and ability to implement a voluntary national model for local public health agencies (Russo, 2007). Proponents of the process believed that it would promote greater accountability and prompt more quality improvement initiatives by local public health agencies. Others worried it would be a meaningless bureaucratic exercise that would absorb resources for public health services and label organizations as malfunctioning while offering little or no help to improve (Russo).

The Robert Wood Johnson Foundation launched a three-year Multi-State Learning Collaborative (MLC I, II, and III) in 2007 to explore standards in public health organizations. The goals of the MLC projects were to prepare state and local health departments for accreditation, contribute findings from the grantee projects to the voluntary national accreditation process, and foster the application and institutionalization of quality improvement methods in local public health agencies (NACCHO, 2009). RWJF believed that the processes associated with QI would help local public health agencies become more effective and efficient in delivering services and producing better health outcomes for communities (Robert Wood Johnson Foundation, 2009). MLC III participants were asked to select at least two target areas for improvement, one from the "process" list and the second from the "outcomes" list below. The lists were developed by the MLC program team and its partners for the third year of the MLC initiative (National Network of Public Health Institutes, 2010, slide 48):

Process Target Areas

- Community Health Profiles
- Culturally Appropriate Services
- Health Improvement Planning
- Assure Competent Workforce
- Customer Service

Outcome Target Areas

- Vaccine Preventable Disease
- Reducing Preventable Risk Factors That Predispose to Chronic Disease
- Reducing Infant Mortality
- Reducing the Burden of Tobacco-Related Illness
- Reducing the Burden of Alcohol-Related Disease and Injury

Sixteen states were involved in the MLC initiative. Preliminary results from the MLC III initiative indicate that the sixteen states are using a variety of quality improvement methods, and most of the states are providing training to LPHA staff on quality improvement methods and tools. Some of the states are adding quality improvement standards to their current assessment process. All sixteen states have selected one or more of the target areas for improvement and are learning to work collaboratively across jurisdictions as they implement QI techniques. Working on common goals while learning from a variety of approaches to improving quality are core principles of the MLC III initiative.

Standards for a voluntary program for the national accreditation of governmental local public health agencies were developed by the Public Health Accreditation Board in partnership with a number of public health leaders and organizations (PHAB, 2009). Following an alpha test of the standards with two state agencies and six local health departments, a beta version of the standards for state and local health departments was launched in 2009 with two major sections (Parts A and B) identified for review and assessment of performance. Thirty public health departments are participating in the beta test. Part A includes standards for the administration and governance of public health agencies. Public health agencies applying for accreditation would be reviewed by PHAB site teams to assess their operational infrastructure, financial management systems, and engagement of the governing entity. Part B of the review is built around the ten essential services and operational definition of a functional local public health agency. To help local public health agencies prepare for the accreditation process, NACCHO developed a self-assessment tool based on its *Operational Definition of a Functional Local Health Department*.

Public health agencies have been exposed to many standards and performance expectations since the 1988 IOM report *The Future of Public Health*. In spite of all the attention given the governmental public health infrastructure by a variety of public health policymakers, researchers, experts, and leaders, little evidence exists to suggest improvement in the delivery of public health services and associated health outcomes. Wholey, White, and Kader (2009) raise questions about the wisdom of emphasizing the ten essential services framework instead of goals for specific health outcomes, such as those found in Healthy People 2010, to drive quality improvement in public health agencies. These authors express concern about whether the strong emphasis on function and services is the best method for creating effective and accountable local public health agencies. They advocate instead for a focus on content—which is the actual work of public health professionals—defined according to outcomes they seek to achieve, such as reducing tuberculosis rates or increasing rates of physical activity. Public health professionals need knowledge about evidence-based practice and CQI methods that link process to outcomes to help them achieve their public health goals of improving health outcomes. The following are some concerns about a public health initiative that is primarily focused on process—in other words, on the ten essential services (Wholey et al., 2009):

- The absence of a body of evidence to be employed as a vehicle for improving population health outcomes
- Limited research supporting the ten essential services framework as a driver of quality for public health agencies
- The use of scarce public health resources for accreditation in place of well-established quality improvement methods focused on achieving specific aims

Gaps in the Quality of Public Health Services

Conceptually and in reality, the use of the ten essential services as standards to improve the practice of public health at the local level is under scrutiny. The conceptualization of standards to guide public health performance has taken place during the past twenty years, and many in the field have expressed a strong predilection for the ten essential services. In addition to questions about the choice of the ten essential services as the basis for accreditation of LPHAs and the seemingly lackluster acceptance of the ten essential services by LPHAs around the nation, LPHAs have to face growing challenges in order to maintain their positive effects on community health. A 2004 study concluded that the percentage of adults ages fifty to sixty-five receiving routine and recommended cancer screenings and influenza vaccinations in our nation's capital was low, with less than 25 percent of the scientific sample being up-to-date (Shenson, Adams, and Bolen, 2008). In Florida, researchers found that a majority of resources within local public health agencies were used for individual health care services, even as demand for improved population-centered services increased (Brooks, Beitsch, Street, and Chukmaitov, 2009). Further, an assessment of public health practice in Georgia determined that the core business of public health in the state was not aligned with the essential services, demonstrating that "the primary drivers or determinants of public health practice were finance related rather than based in need or strategy" (Smith et al., 2007, p. 1). Lastly, a growing body of evidence reveals that public health services around the nation vary greatly in terms of availability and quality (Mays, Smith, et al., 2009). The financing of public health services along with staff characteristics contribute to this observed variation.

Following the HHS announcement on April 26, 2009, of a public health emergency caused by the swine flu (H1N1) epidemic, the ability of local health departments to communicate about the risk of H1N1 within twenty-four hours of a declaration of an emergency was analyzed by researchers at RAND, a nonprofit institution conducting research to improve policymaking and decision making for public and private organizations (Ringel, Trentacost, and Lurie, 2009). The assessment of a sample of state and local health departments' success in providing online information about H1N1 within the specified time frame revealed that forty-nine states and the District of Columbia had some information about H1N1 on their Web sites. Out of the sampled local health department Web sites, 34 percent provided some type of information or link to information related to swine flu within the required twenty-four-hour time frame. The study was limited by the absence of any in-depth review of the quality of messages on the studied Web sites. As of 2009, state preparedness funding was tied to performance on a preselected set of performance measures and standards, including risk communication. The threat of funding loss does not appear to have resulted in improved risk communication for a number of local health departments based on the RAND study. Risk communication is a critical public health responsibility and works toward fulfilling the public health mission of ensuring conditions in which people can be healthy. A possible explanation about the variability in performance found in this study may be the lack of consensus among those who are employed by local public health agencies, including agency leaders, about what public health departments do. After thirty years of defining public health and its essential services, questions remain about LPHAs' responsibilities.

In spite of the tremendous effort to define the mission and functions of public health, quality issues persist. What is becoming more apparent is that the U.S. public health system, despite a twenty-year period of increasing awareness of the importance of improving population health outcomes and public health agency performance, has neither the organization nor the incentive to comprehensively address population-centered, primary prevention health services that are evidence based or linked to improved health outcomes.

Federal Leadership of Quality Improvement in Public Health

The Office of Public Health and Science in HHS, using a consensus-building process with multiple public health system partners, released in 2008 its *Consensus Statement on Quality in the Public Health System*, which included a set of nine quality aims similar to the quality characteristics identified for the delivery of health care to patients by the IOM in 2001. Universal aims and indicators for improving the quality of public health services are not commonplace in public health practice. The goal for creating this set of quality aims was to promote consistency in quality improvement initiatives across all organizations providing public health services, not only governmental public health departments. The provision of a national framework for quality was deemed necessary to facilitate consistent implementation of quality improvement methods in the daily routine of public health practitioners and their organizations. All or some of the aims may apply to a single public health service or function when public health researchers evaluate current and future public health services for quality, or the degree to which policies, programs, services and research increase desired population health outcomes (HHS, 2008).

The *Consensus Statement on Quality in the Public Health System* (HHS, 2008) is the most recent effort to enhance and guide the goals of public health programs by defining quality for public health and identifying a list of nine characteristics of a quality public health service (see Exhibit 10.3). The statement was created under the direction of the assistant secretary for health, the U.S. Department of Health and Human Services, and the Public Health Quality Forum in partnership with multiple public health associations and leaders. The goal is to provide a national framework for quality that can be used to inform quality improvement efforts in the everyday practice of public health in LPHAs. Identifying the characteristics of a quality public health service is a first step in a national effort led by HHS to focus the governmental local public health agencies on areas to improve in order to achieve a high quality public health service (HHS, 2008). A number of professions apply quality characteristics to their industries, including education, software engineering, and air travel.

Another purpose of this federal initiative is to demonstrate a national commitment to providing leadership and steering a course of action that results in the routine use of CQI techniques throughout all parts of the public health system, including finance, programs, management, governing, and education (Honoré, 2009). Table 10.1 depicts a proposed method for applying the national aims to identify potential gaps in quality characteristics of existing or planned public health programs. Improving the quality of services in a state office of HIV/AIDS includes a population-centered approach that routinely studies HIV/AIDS data to detect emerging trends in case rates and risk factors. Obtaining current epidemiological data from such studies is a proactive health practice that ensures any emerging risk factors are incorporated into current program design. Epidemiological studies are also important to detect trends in case and infection rates by race, gender, and age and promote equity by focusing resources on health disparities as they emerge. Planning and implementing the ABC Program (see Table 10.1) can prevent the spread of disease and promote health. Instituting a culture of CQI with the state office will help guarantee that changes are implemented to ensure success and that progress is measured and outcomes are achieved.

EXHIBIT 10.3
HHS CHARACTERISTICS OF QUALITY IN PUBLIC HEALTH

Population-centered—protecting and promoting healthy conditions and the health for the entire population

Equitable—working to achieve health equity

Proactive—formulating policies and sustainable practices in a timely manner, while mobilizing rapidly to address new and emerging threats and vulnerabilities

Health promoting—assuring policies and strategies that advance safe practices by providers and the population and increase the probability of positive health behaviors and outcomes

Risk-reducing—diminishing adverse environmental and social events by implementing policies and strategies to reduce the probability of preventable injuries and illness or other negative outcomes

Vigilant—intensifying practices and enacting policies to support enhancements to surveillance activities (e.g., technology, standardization, systems thinking/modeling)

Transparent—ensuring openness in the delivery of services and practices with particular emphasis on valid, reliable, accessible, timely, and meaningful data that is readily available to stakeholders, including the public

Effective—justifying investments by utilizing evidence, science, and best practice to achieve optimal results in areas of greatest need

Efficient—understanding costs and benefits of public health interventions and to facilitate optimal utilization of resources to achieve desired outcomes

Source: HHS, 2008.

The next steps for this national initiative on quality are the development of economic and financial indicators of quality and the identification of priority areas for CQI in public health, including a core set of quality indicators and measures. HHS (2010b) published *Priority Areas for Improvement of Quality in Public Health* in 2010, a call to action for public health practitioners to build public health quality by focusing "on building better systems to give all people what they need to reach their full potential for health" (p. v). This report reiterates the importance of connecting the overall health of the nation to the health of individuals and health conditions in the communities in which they live (Koh

Table 10.1   Application of National Quality Aims for Public Health

National AIMS for Improvement of Quality	PROGRAM: State Office of HIV/AIDS (Gage of conformity to meeting National Aims)
Population Centered	Routine Epidemiological studies
Equitable	Stratify data by race, gender, age and build programs accordingly
Proactive	Implementation of the HERR Program—Health Education and Risk Reducing Program Disease Investigation Specialist Program
Health Promoting	Implementation of the "ABC" Program (Abstain, Be Faithful, Use Condoms)
Risk Reducing	Implementation of the HERR Program—Health Education and Risk Reducing Program Offering of Partner Services (notifications, testing, suspect interviews, etc)
Vigilant	State-wide surveillance systems
Transparent	Reporting of data to funders
Effective	Implementation of national evidence-based programs
Efficient	Document and justify costs to identify new cases of disease

Source: Honoré, 2009, p. 2.

and Sebelius, 2010). Accomplishing better health of individuals and communities is best achieved, according to the broad array of public health experts involved with the HHS report, by focusing on six priority areas for improving the quality of our local public health systems. The priority areas in which local public health systems are called upon to make changes for improvement include population health metrics and information technology; evidence-based practice, research, and evaluation; systems thinking; sustainability and stewardship; policy; and workforce and education. Further, HHS (2010b, p. 6) and its strategic partners have identified specific recommendations for improvement:

- Improve the analysis of population health and move toward achieving health equity
- Improve program effectiveness
- Improve methods to foster integration among all sectors that impact health (i.e., public health, health care, and others)
- Increase transparency and efficiencies to become better stewards of resources
- Improve surveillance and other vigilant processes to identify health risks and become proactive in advocacy and advancement of policy agendas that focus on risk reduction
- Implement processes to advance professional competence in the public health workforce

FIGURE 10.2   Criteria Used to Establish Priority Areas (Processes) for Improvement

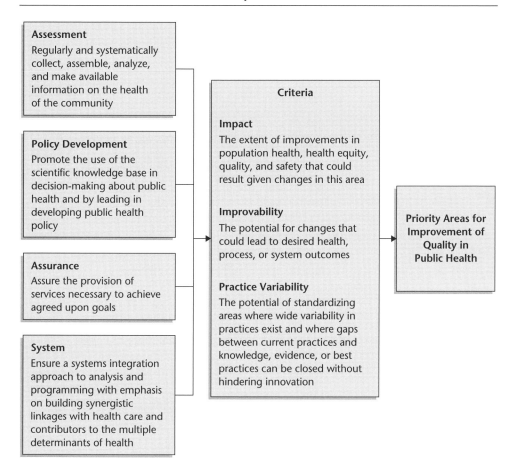

Source: HHS, 2010b, p. 14.

Figure 10.2 outlines the criteria HHS (2010b) used to establish the priority areas for improving public health processes and outcomes, and demonstrates the linkages between current efforts to concretely identify areas for improvement in public health using criteria and the core functions of public health established by the Institute of Medicine in 1988. The impact of these changes, the likelihood of improvements occurring, and the degree of practice variability are the three criteria that HHS applied to develop the priority areas for improvement of public health services.

The three outcome areas identified for improvement as part of this national initiative include reducing the incidence of health care associated infections, reducing the national incidence of HIV infections, and increasing the percentage of Americans with a healthy weight (HHS, 2010b). Figure 10.3 demonstrates an example of how these priority areas for outcomes and processes can be

FIGURE 10.3 Outcomes and Primary and Secondary Drivers

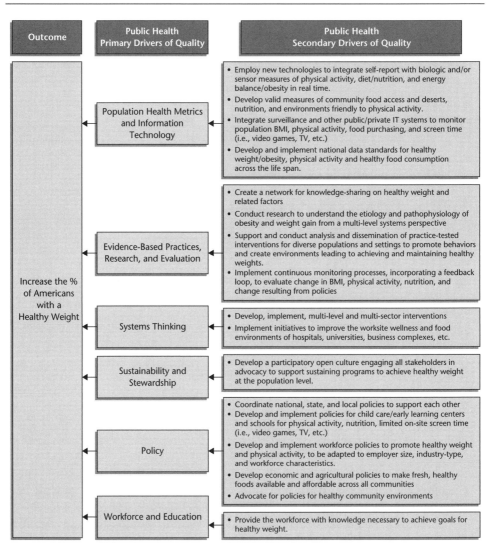

Source: HHS, 2010b, p. 89.

operationalized. Primary drivers are key categories of change that have the greatest likelihood of helping us achieve our goals. Secondary drivers are collections of key processes that are highly recommended for implementation within each priority category, and they must occur reliably to achieve progress (IHI, n.d.). Figure 10.3 offers a look at the key processes within the secondary drivers of public health quality that an agency can undertake to ensure the implementation of the primary drivers of quality that ultimately lead to improvement in outcomes. In this figure we see that a primary driver for increasing the percentage of Americans with a healthy weight is the use of population health metrics and information technology. Public health professionals require data and information systems to conduct accurate surveillance of community indicators related to community food access and environments supportive of physical activity. This allows them to monitor current and future community conditions associated with evidence-based public health services in order to increase healthy weight rates in a community population. Another primary driver of quality to aid in reaching the goal, the use of evidence-based practices, includes the creation of a network for knowledge sharing as a secondary driver.

Road Map to Improve Public Health Outcomes

The leading causes of death in America are heart disease, cancer, stroke, chronic lower respiratory disease, accidents, diabetes, Alzheimer's disease, influenza and pneumonia, nephritis or nephritic syndrome, and septicemia (CDC, 2009e). Healthy People 2010 and 2020 are the nation's health promotion and disease prevention agendas developed to monitor and improve quality and years of healthy life and reduce the rates of the leading causes of death. Leading indicators, listed below, were chosen as sentinel measures of the public's health, with the goal of reducing exposure to risk factors that result in mortality (CDC, 2010b):

- Physical activity
- Overweight and obesity
- Substance abuse
- Responsible sexual behavior
- Mental health
- Injury and violence
- Environmental quality
- Immunization
- Access to health care

Quality improvement in the health care world has much to offer the burgeoning CQI efforts of public health agencies and organizations. The 2008 *Consensus Statement on Quality in the Public Health System* (HHS) defined quality for public health systems and listed the characteristics of quality public health services, similar to the early efforts at quality improvement in health care. An expanded definition of quality in health care has been proposed to include the "unceasing efforts of everyone—healthcare professionals, patients and their families, researchers, payers, planners and educators—to make changes that will lead to better patient outcomes (health), better system performance (care) and better professional development (learning)" (Batalden and Davidoff, 2008, p. 1). Quality public health services will need a similar cultural change across local public health agencies to reach the full potential of public health. Achieving improvement in community health outcomes requires change making and is an "essential part of everyone's job, everyday, and in all parts of the system" (Batalden and Davidoff, p. 1).

Health care data are being used in multiple ways, every day, and in all parts of the system to improve patient outcomes and health. A good example of data use, mentioned earlier in this chapter, is found in the efforts of the Northern New England Cardiovascular Disease Study Group, which uses patient registries to collect patient and procedural data, monitor outcomes in a region, and compare, for example, the practice of cardiopulmonary bypass operations in affiliated hospitals to recently published recommendations (DioData et al., 2008). When gaps are identified, hospital staff members employ CQI methods to improve patient outcomes, system performance, and professional learning and growth.

Public health agencies can follow a similar path. As already discussed, a number of tools, such as NACCHO's *Operational Definition of a Functional Local Health Department* (2005b) and the accompanying local health department standards, have been developed to assess performance of essential services and key administrative responsibilities. Data on health status, including those pertaining to mortality, morbidity, life expectancy, and quality of life, are generally available at the state and local levels. Data on the determinants of health found in the natural environment; the built environment; the social, political, and economic environment; biological composition (genetics, age, and gender); and individual behavior (for example, diet and nutrition or physical activity rates) are also available to some extent at the state and local levels through periodic surveys, such as the Behavioral Risk Factors Surveillance System; the Youth Behaviors Risk Survey; and state information systems such as the North Carolina Comprehensive Assessment for Tracking Community Health (NC-CATCH), a collaborative effort between University of North Carolina at Charlotte and state and local public health agencies in the state. The NC-CATCH system provides easy access to profiles of all one hundred NC counties, including a wide array of demographic and community health data sets, along with comparisons with peer counties in the state. In addition, the NC-CATCH "Indicator Fact Sheets" supply users with trends in indicators over time, as well as breakdowns by race and ethnicity for many health measures (www.ncpublichealthcatch.com/ReportPortal/design/view.aspx).

Deciding on an aim to improve a community health outcome, one in which a gap has been identified, is a critical first step in developing a health-outcome-focused improvement project. The gap may exist between current rates and goals set locally or by a national initiative, such as Healthy People 2010 or 2020, or it may become obvious when one county's health outcome is significantly different from that of another similar public health system and community. Considering the following questions is helpful in selecting the area for improvement, the aim:

- Is this an important health outcome for the community?
- Does a gap exist between the evidence and practice?
- Are there examples of better performance?
- What is the potential for increasing the value of public health services for the stakeholders?
- Will the benefit exceed the cost of the service?

The "aim statement" includes the intent of the project, the target population, the goals to be achieved, and the date by which goals will be attained. Engaging community members in the process of selecting the aim, as well as in developing the plan for implementing and evaluating change, promotes broader support for the CQI effort. As stated in the *Principles of the Ethical Practice of Public Health*, "Public health should achieve community health in a way that respects the rights of individuals in the community, . . . [and] policies, programs, and priorities should be developed and evaluated through processes that ensure an opportunity for input from community members" (Public Health Leadership Society, 2002, p. 4).

Selecting the changes based on evidence or the best available knowledge is vital to achieving goals for community health outcomes. CQI projects in the world of health care commonly use Wagner's Chronic Care Model (www.ihi.org/IHI/Topics/ChronicConditions/AllConditions/Changes) to maintain a systems focus when identifying areas for improvement. The use of the ecological model of health, including strategies that address intrapersonal, interpersonal, institutional, community, public policy, and ecosystem factors, will ensure a systems approach for public health interventions that incorporates changes across multiple levels of the system rather than focusing solely on one part of the system. For example, a public health intervention not only would focus on changing individual behavior but also would explore evidence-based strategies that would have a positive impact on the social realm (establishing buddy systems to encourage physical exercise), the physical environment (developing walking trails), and policy issues (requiring food service establishments to post nutrition information on menus) affecting the CQI aim.

Planning effective programs, ones that achieve intended outcomes and account for the acquisition and use of public health revenues, follows the selection of the project's aim. Although all improvements involve change, not all changes lead to improvement. Addressing the tough issues of climate change or high obesity rates will involve systematic planning and measurement to know which interventions produce the best outcomes.

The process of improving health outcomes involves selecting changes that are based on evidence, expert opinions, consensus statements, or successful CQI initiatives. Using evidence-based programs increases the likelihood of achieving the goals to improve priority community health outcomes. Local public health agencies that proceed with services that have not been researched or reviewed for compliance with the most recent recommendations are at odds with the definition of quality that calls for "increas[ing] the desired health outcomes and conditions in which the population can be healthy" (HHS, 2008, p. 2).

Measurements of the process and outcomes are formed as part of the planning phase. Such measures serve two primary purposes: they ensure that the desired changes are undertaken appropriately (process measures) and that the program is achieving the desired results (outcome measures). Funders and stakeholders require more accountability for the use of the revenues they provide, both private and public, by insisting on quality outcome data that establishes whether a program has been successful. Developing accurate measures of the changes being implemented (the process) and the community health outcomes that form the aim statement's intent requires teamwork and expert guidance. Using criteria to develop a balanced set of measures that are reflective of changes across the system helps confine the number of metrics to a manageable and easily understood set.

Public health practitioners embracing CQI methods routinely report on the metrics through the use of tables or graphs (trend charts) in support of the goals of continuous quality improvement. CQI is only possible by ongoing review and analysis of the data. Positive and negative trends in the data reports afford the public health practitioner opportunities to ask questions about how changes are being implemented, whether planned changes are actually occurring, and how those changes are affecting the health outcome or aim of the project. Review of the data provides opportunities to improve on the work already under way or to redirect efforts toward an alternate evidence-based practice. The principal focus

FIGURE 10.4   Cycle of Continuous Quality Improvement
for Public Health

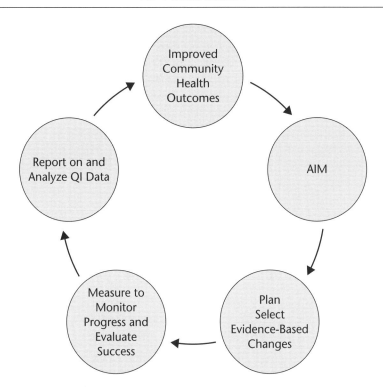

Source: Adapted from Shewhart, 1986.

of local public health agency and system efforts is always on improving health outcomes in the community. Figure 10.4 is a modified version of the Shewhart cycle, commonly referred to as the Plan-Do-Study-Act cycle, which is part of an important strategy for testing changes on a small scale before implementing them fully on a grander scale.

Summary

In 2008 quality in public health was defined for the first time as "the degree to which policies, programs, services, and research for the population increase the desired health outcomes and conditions in which the population can be healthy" (HHS, 2008, p. 2). Achieving quality in public health requires a commitment to and accountability in public health programs that will improve the length and quality of life for all people. The historic emphasis on services that define the core functions of public health and the associated standards have helped identify gaps in the performance of local public health agencies and systems. The link between the performance of essential services and the achievement of community health goals is very weak, some would say nonexistent. The epidemic of obesity in our nation is some indication of the lack of attention to the determinants of health and health status by public health leaders, local public health systems, and those in charge of allocating the resources available for public health services. Developing an outcomes-focused public health initiative to address one or more of the complex public health problems of modernity at the local, state, and national levels, following the concepts of CQI, will undoubtedly help reduce the costs associated with health care and restore credibility and, ideally, funding to the U.S. public health system.

Key Terms

Continuous quality improvement (CQI)

Essential Services

Health outcomes

Quality public health

Discussion Questions

1. What lessons have been learned in improving health care that can be applied to the field of public health?
2. What strategies have public health departments undertaken in the United States to improve the quality of public health services?
3. Discuss the disarray of the public health system in the United States, identified by the Institute of Medicine in 1988. What evidence exists about the current state of the U.S. public health system?
4. Describe the current efforts of the U.S. Department of Health and Human Services to address the quality of public health services.
5. Review Figure 10.3 and explain how the primary and secondary drivers are designed to affect the health outcome found in the figure.

CHAPTER 11

OPPORTUNITIES FOR IMPROVEMENT IN PUBLIC HEALTH PRACTICE

LEARNING OBJECTIVES

- Understand the major opportunities that are present for public health as the health care industry is being reformed
- Become aware of the need for a shift in the goals of the U.S. public health system to expand health education programs
- Comprehend the value of risk communication in preventing the development of chronic diseases and their complications
- Understand the value of developing technology to improve the health of the population
- Recognize the need for innovation in the development of health education and health promotion programs
- Be able to explain how health education and health promotion programs can offer solutions to the various problems found in the delivery of health care services in this country

Our system for delivering health care services to over three hundred million individuals in this country is in a state of chaos. The media reports high health care costs, problems related to countless uninsured Americans, low-quality services, and bankruptcy resulting from concentrating scarce health resources on curative rather than preventive efforts. Lee and Mongan (2009) argue that the real cause of chaos is the tremendous progress in health care every day thanks to advances in technology. A great deal of this use of technology is wasteful, and with these advances also come new dangers for many patients: costs are soaring for health services, and there is an epidemic of medical errors with no end in sight. Every time a patient is subjected to the use of medical technology there is always the possibility of medical errors in the procedure. In many cases the new procedures were not even necessary but were still completed because they represented profits to some.

The older paradigm of health care services delivery is becoming unsustainable, resulting in a revolution in the delivery of health care services (Lee and Mongan, 2009). The curative model of disease cannot work once a chronic disease becomes present in an individual. The epidemic of chronic diseases in our country is causing the medical care system and the public health system to undergo tremendous change in the way they do business, disrupting all of the components that make up health care services delivery.

This change may also produce great opportunities for improving the health of the U.S. population. As the nation deals with the problems associated with uninsured and underinsured Americans, policymakers are gaining a greater appreciation for the benefits of preventing rather than curing disease. This reform of our health care system presents opportunities for public health departments to provide real leadership in improving the health of the population. Because the vast majority of U.S. health care expenditures are for chronic disease complications, it seems logical for the medical care system and public health system to focus their attention on the increasing epidemic of chronic diseases.

Although the United States is ranked number one in spending for health care, it is ranked thirty-ninth for infant mortality, forty-third for adult female mortality, and forty-second for adult male mortality (Murray and Frenk, 2010). The United States is falling further behind other countries every year, even though the percentage of gross domestic product (GDP) devoted to health care continues to rise. The majority of policymakers cite the lack of health insurance for millions of Americans as the cause of this growing problem, but this is not the cause of the poor health. Rather, the high-risk health behaviors Americans practice, such as using tobacco, eating unhealthy food, and maintaining a sedentary lifestyle, result in chronic diseases, which are the real culprits. More health insurance is not going to solve this problem; reducing the incidence of chronic diseases and their complications will.

According to How, Shih, Lau, and Schoen (2008), a survey conducted on behalf of The Commonwealth Fund Commission on a High Performance Health System investigated the general public's perspectives of and experiences with the nation's health care system. The results from this representative sample of 1,004 adults revealed great dissatisfaction with the health care system, as well as problems associated with accessing care, poor coordination of care, and great inefficiency in the delivery of care. These problems are real and must be dealt with in the near future, but they are too complicated to be solved by any one part of this very large health care industry. It is going to take all segments working together—including an educated patient, or customer—to discover solutions to these very complex problems. There needs to be a catalyst, however, to get the reform process started in the right direction toward focusing on the health of the population rather than that of the individual patient. Public health departments can drive the change from an emphasis on expensive cures for individuals' diseases to a focus on investment in prevention programs for the entire population, which in turn will improve the quality of life for millions of Americans.

Quality in public health requires a commitment and accountability to public health programs that will improve the length and quality of life for all people. Maintaining this quality entails the promotion of healthy lifestyles that prevent diseases and injuries. The problem is that the current financing system including government and other third-party payers in health care delivery does not pay for outcomes or prevention programs. In fact, health care providers make more money by allowing the population to become sicker. Those paying the bills for health services have consistently designed payment mechanisms that reimburse for activities rather than patient outcomes. Public health departments, however, concentrate on the health of the population, which requires them to focus on population health outcomes.

Shi and Singh (2010) point out that even though public health is about protecting the population's health, public health agencies have been relegated to a level of unimportance by the medical care system. The medical complex in this country resents a government-funded public health system interfering with the health decisions for its patients. And yet public health has many of the answers to questions of how to control or even reduce the costs of health care.

In order to make a collaboration between the public health and medical care systems work, everyone must agree that keeping the patient healthy should be the most important goal of a reformed health care system. Such an attitude toward the need for preventive health care is growing as more policymakers recognize that the current desire to cure disease entirely is not working. It is one of the factors contributing to chaos in health care delivery, and creativity and innovation are required to produce a new model of health care services delivery.

This chapter is about pursuing innovation in the delivery of public health services to the population of the United States. It is also about making creativity and innovation a large part of public health departments in order to achieve the goals of those organizations. In order for public health departments to become innovative in responding to the chronic disease epidemic, they have to first ask and then answer two very important questions:

1. Do people really want to develop life-threatening and disability-producing chronic diseases as they grow older?
2. How does a public health agency make preventing these diseases as easy as possible for the population?

Disruption and Change in Public Health

Public health departments in America have received neither a great deal of credit for their many accomplishments nor an appropriate budget for their various mandates. In recent years there has been renewed interest in the public health sector of health care. Shi and Singh (2010) argue that the war against bioterrorism has elevated public health departments to a new level of respect in this country. These departments have also received a great deal of media attention in response to the threat of an H1N1 influenza epidemic. The increased need for public health expertise has also given these departments an infusion of monetary resources. Public health departments seem to gain respect and increased funding every time there is a health emergency, but then both the interest in public health and the funding for its operations disappear as health threats facing the population recede.

In order to retain respect and funding, public health departments are forced to rethink how they do business. Public health leaders have never been able to command respect (supported by a reasonable budget) for long. This is because many such leaders are political appointees concerned only with keeping their job and are usually not interested in the long-term success of public health programs. It is time for this situation to change, because our health care system needs public health expertise. Public health departments have the opportunity to lead the way in system reform as the United States faces the epidemic of chronic diseases and their complications.

Lee and Mongan (2009) point out that in order to improve the health care system in this country there must be greater coordination between physicians and their patients. This is going to require a better understanding of health by each patient, who will need up-to-date health information, especially concerning the potential complications from chronic diseases. Public health departments can take on the new task of using technology to provide this health information and education for the patient, which can go a long way toward helping the patient become an active participant in his or her own prevention or treatment of chronic diseases. In order to prevent the long-term complications from chronic diseases, patients must understand the serious complications that usually result from continuing to practice high-risk health behaviors. They must assume an active role in the long-term chronic disease prevention and treatment process.

Such health education delivery by public health departments is an example of a population-based community intervention effort. Turnock (2009) points out that enhancing community health status in this way is really an investment that will eventually pay off by reducing future health care expenditures. This is exactly the education strategy and behavior change that can lead to longer life—and better quality of life—and can solve the vast majority of health problems our country currently faces. Investing in health education programs that have been shown to work is mandatory for any reform of our health care system to be successful. Unfortunately, Americans have never had a real understanding of the true value of well-developed and adequately funded health education and health promotion programs.

The implementation of change has become so vital to an organization's survival that change management skills must be found in all layers of management (Balogun and Hailey, 2008). The ability to respond to change and deal with the disruption it causes has become a very important and desirable managerial skill. Change management is necessary in the evolving health care system and will require public health departments to modify how they operate in order to seize the opportunities the changing system presents. This calls for leaders who will seek out change and turn it into opportunities for public health departments. Helping to change Americans' high-risk health behaviors, for example, is one such opportunity, which public health departments must exploit by using innovative and creative approaches to share important health information with large segments of the population.

The Institute of Medicine (2002) argues that because of the failure of government reform efforts in 1993, when the federal government attempted to pass a single-payer health care system similar to that found in Canada, the medical care system does not interact effectively with the largely government-financed public health system in this country. Therefore, the medical care system does not allow time for external relationship building, which is so very necessary for the development and expansion of disease prevention and health promotion programs. For example, public health education programs and medical care system resources should be combined in order to end the epidemic of chronic diseases in this country. This has not happened because of distrust of government involvement among medical care professionals and the failure of many public health leaders to seize the opportunity for collaboration.

This is very sad because the medical care system in this country for the most part does a poor job of providing clinically appropriate and cost-effective care for the millions of Americans suffering from chronic diseases. This clearly represents a missed opportunity for successful collaboration between public health and the medical care system. Public health departments must assume a leadership role in the reduction of chronic diseases. This has not happened for a variety of reasons, but it is clear that without the public health system's help our medical care system will continue to fail in its attempt to solve the problem of chronic diseases. We cannot afford to lose this war against chronic diseases.

According to Christensen, Grossman, and Hwang (2009), the transformational force that works well when a business is seeking to lower costs and increase the availability of a product or service has been labeled **disruptive innovation,** which entails making products and services simpler and more affordable. According to these authors, health care is ripe for this type of innovation, the catalyst for which could very well be the work of public health departments and the preventive strategies that they have developed. The process of disruptive innovation should occur not only in the medical care system but also in public health agencies at the federal, state, and local levels. In order to respond to the opportunities that are present because of this disruption, there will need to be strong leaders and empowered workers in public health departments.

Disruptive innovation allows the combining of resources in the production process in new and innovative ways that usually result in greater value produced by the process. This is exactly what our health care system needs to survive and to deliver better-quality services at lower prices, because both the medical care system and the public health system are faced with limited resources and demands for improved value in health care services. Professionals in our public health and medical care systems have had many tremendous successes in improving the health and life expectancy of most Americans. They need to come together again as the country faces its greatest health challenge in the form of the expanding epidemic of chronic diseases—diseases that are increasing rates of morbidity and mortality, reducing health quality, and escalating the costs of health care. This chaos in health care delivery presents an opportunity for disruptive innovation by public health departments, which can form partnerships with other health care providers to produce a new system of health care delivery that is capable of keeping people healthy rather than allowing them to become ill.

Public Health Education and Health Promotion Programs

Although the major goal of the health care system should be to keep people healthy, the majority of its resources are focused on curing diseases after they have occurred rather than preventing them in the first place. Those in charge of the U.S. medical care system care very little about the prevention of disease because current financing approaches reward interventions that are aimed at curing disease. Instead, prevention of disease is relegated to public health departments with a limited staff and an even more limited budget. This has resulted in public health agencies' being reduced to performing activities like case finding and counseling individuals with disease rather than focusing on the outcomes, such as preventing disease from ever occurring, that they desire; and well-developed health education and health promotion programs have not been as successful as they could have been. The problem is that health care providers do not get paid if individuals remain well, but they are reimbursed when individuals become ill. This is a substantial loss because these programs, armed with the requisite resources, could achieve great success in the war against chronic diseases and their complications.

The vast majority of the costs of health care delivery in this country are a direct result of chronic diseases and their complications. Currently, almost 80 percent of health care costs are for chronic diseases, and these costs are expected to rise rapidly as a result of high-risk health problems like obesity and the increase in diabetes and other diseases with no cure. Although these diseases cannot be cured, however, they could be prevented with well-funded, population-based education programs developed and implemented by public health agencies.

Individuals with chronic diseases require care that is continuous, collaborative, informative, reliable, safe, and proactive (Lee and Mongan, 2009). Our medical care system does not offer the vast majority of these components to individuals diagnosed with chronic illnesses. The patient with one or more chronic diseases is instead left in many cases to fall victim to the very expensive and life-threatening complications that may result from having a chronic disease for a long period of time—complications that could have been prevented with better information. Individuals need information about the causes of and prevention approaches for chronic diseases before they develop them so that they can prevent these diseases' occurrence. Healey and Zimmerman (2010) argue that the individual should have a primary role in determining his or her level of wellness. In order to fulfill this role, the individual requires accurate health information to make health-related decisions.

The major focus of most health promotion efforts is on high-risk health behaviors and individual lifestyle choices. Barton (2010) argues that the medical care system is not organized to systematically deliver comprehensive health promotion programs to the population, leaving a very real opportunity for public health departments to provide leadership in this area. The major goal of public health has always been the prevention of disease and the prevention of complications from disease if it occurs. This goal will only be met by the development of health promotion programs that can be delivered to large numbers of people in innovative ways.

Health education and health promotion initiatives can be expensive and produce only limited outcomes in the short term. They have to be looked at as long-term investments that will only pay dividends over time. Health behaviors develop gradually, and changing high-risk health behaviors will take a great deal of time and effort by many dedicated health education professionals. If the nation is willing to invest in health education and health promotion programs, the health of the U.S. population can be improved, ultimately reducing health care costs. This change in health care delivery will take a long time and consume many resources before yielding a healthier population, but it is well worth the investment.

Because health education programs have been almost nonexistent in most school districts, most Americans are unaware of the threat of disease as they grow older. They do not realize that they are developing and practicing high-risk health behaviors that can shorten their life. They believe that they are invincible and that they do not have to worry about potentially life-threatening diseases. They are also unaware that chronic diseases, once acquired, cannot be cured. They have generally not received any education concerning the risk of chronic diseases from the medical community, other than being told that it is not a good idea to use tobacco products.

The development of chronic diseases is also a serious concern for people in the workplace. A large number of businesses in the United States are beginning to realize the value of workplace disease prevention and wellness programs. Baicker, Cutler, and Song (2010) argue that disease prevention programs can improve health while lowering the costs of medical care. In a meta-analysis of the literature, these authors found that medical costs fell by $3.27 for every dollar invested in wellness programs and absenteeism costs dropped by $2.73 for every dollar spent. This study supports the assertion that the prevention of chronic diseases represents a long-term investment with substantial returns.

Risk communication has become a critical public health function and fulfills the public health mission of ensuring conditions in which individuals can remain healthy. This function has never received the credit that it deserves because the payment system in health care does not reward the prevention of disease, instead reimbursing for activities in medicine that are in response to the occurrence of disease. It pays for activities rather than outcomes. Unfortunately, the vast majority of the activities in health care today deal with chronic diseases that cannot be cured, but that could have been prevented with health education.

Major improvements cannot occur in health care until physicians move from paper data to computer medical records (Lee and Mongan, 2009). This is also true for public health departments, which in order to improve their services need to embrace and exploit technology. A real opportunity exists for health promotion and chronic disease education programs to be delivered in a format similar to an electronic medical record for easy patient access. Information technology can go a long way toward helping public health departments disseminate vital information to the population in order to prevent the development of chronic diseases or postpone their complications.

Optimum Health, a division of UnitedHealth Group, the nation's largest insurer, is going to offer a type of virtual doctor-patient visit using video chat in 2012 (Miller, 2008). This method of delivering health care has been developed to eliminate travel and waiting time for the patient because of the shortage of primary care physicians. This method of communication could also represent an inexpensive way to deliver highly important chronic disease information to large numbers of people.

Our health care system is not doing a very good job of dealing with chronic diseases and their possible complications (Halvorson, 2009). The good news is that the care of those with chronic diseases can be improved by providing them with better information. Halvorson calls for care registries as an important tool in the improvement of chronic disease care. These registries would include specific protocols for the data, care tracking that would include interventions and outcomes, and linkages among the various physicians dealing with the patient with comorbidities. There is also a very important role for public health departments in the improvement of chronic disease care because these departments have the necessary information concerning the prevention of chronic diseases.

The Need for a Chronic Care Model

Morewitz (2006) points out that every year three chronic diseases, heart disease (including stroke), cancer, and diabetes, account for about $700 billion in direct and indirect health care costs. These costs continue to escalate because of chronic disease complications and comorbidities. The only way to prevent these diseases is by educating the population and supplying them with information about the prevention of chronic diseases from a reliable source on a consistent basis. Creativity and innovation are clearly required to develop a mechanism for providing such population-based health information.

The major goal of chronic disease control programs in this country should be the reduction of the incidence of these diseases through prevention initiatives (Brownson, Remington, and Davis, 1998). For those who already have a chronic disease, the goals would also include the reduction of disability and prevention of premature death. These goals are nothing new, but the large number of individuals affected by these diseases is requiring immediate intervention with innovative education programs. It has become evident that the current health care system is failing to deal appropriately with the chronic disease epidemic facing America. Therefore, we need to change our strategy and use population-based health education programs available from public health departments.

Primary care doctors in our country need to implement a Chronic Care Model designed to reduce the incidence of chronic diseases and their complications. One of the most popular models of helping individuals with chronic diseases was developed by Edward Wagner at Group Health Cooperative in Seattle. The important aspects of this model include patient self-management, delivery system design, decision support, and clinical information systems, all of which are designed to improve the outcomes for chronic diseases in this country. According to Bodenheimer, Wagner, and Grumbach (2002), the Chronic Care Model has shown evidence of quality improvement and cost reduction in the management of chronic diseases. The model is expensive to totally integrate throughout the health care system but much easier to implement in any primary care practice. Public health departments can play a leadership role in the development of a Chronic Care Model for primary care practice.

Chronic diseases, unlike communicable diseases, present the patient with deferred consequences. There is a need for a definitive protocol to deal with these diseases before the expensive complications develop. Although compelling research suggests that a form of evidence-based medicine is appropriate for the treatment of chronic diseases, more research needs to be completed, and comprehensive education programs seem to offer more value at the present time. Dlugacz (2010) argues that physicians practice evidence-based medicine by heeding expert advice about best practices in dealing with the treatment of diseases, instead of relying solely on their individual, independent decisions. It has rapidly become the gold standard of modern medicine, and may represent one method for reducing the rates of complications resulting from chronic diseases.

Another important component of a Chronic Care Model involves the way patients pay for health care. Christensen et al. (2009) argue that chronically ill patients require a payment system that profits by wellness and not illness. The payment system currently pays for provider activities and not for health outcomes. It is interesting that our health insurance system has no billing code for wellness, even though creating incentives for wellness would reduce health care costs. The focus of the payment mechanism has to shift from activities to outcomes.

Minimal Political Appreciation of Public Health Activities

The vast majority of our elected representatives at the federal, state, and local levels know very little about the value and accomplishments of public health departments. This is a critical issue for public health departments because most of their funding comes from the government. Public health leaders need to become more political by sharing their successes, along with their current efforts to deal with chronic diseases, with their local, state, and federal representatives. This would allow them to demonstrate the need for their expertise in health reform by concentrating on the change necessary to defeat the epidemic of chronic diseases. It is a fact that anything can be marketed, including impressions of what well-funded public health departments could do if just given the chance. Leaders of public health departments thus need to receive education about the marketing process.

Although the vast majority of marketing activities are found in the for-profit sector, marketing is also an acceptable process in the nonprofit realm. For example, public health departments can use marketing strategies as a tool for conveying to policymakers their true value and accomplishments. In the last few decades government agencies have started using marketing techniques to improve their budget allotments and obtain better relationships with their clients and their suppliers of resources, usually government entities. Professionals in the medical sector have increasingly begun to understand the value of developing a marketing orientation as they go about delivering health services to their patients. In recent years, public health practitioners have also begun to recognize how to use marketing techniques to more effectively and efficiently deliver health-related information to community audiences.

Health services, especially public health services, include the components of individual and community needs and wants that require an exchange process in order to be satisfied. In this type of exchange there may be a nonmonetary price, such as effort or time. The marketing concept is useful in several aspects of the provision of health promotion programs, including the development, implementation, and evaluation of new health promotion efforts.

Marketing tools can help combat the rapid escalation in the occurrence of chronic diseases in our country. Many public health professionals are convinced that acquiring marketing skills can be greatly useful to public health practitioners. The use of marketing skills offers public health workers a way to better understand and motivate behavioral change in individuals (Novick, Morrow, and Mays, 2008). Therefore, the development of marketing skills in public health agencies may contribute to innovative approaches to improve effectiveness in changing high-risk behaviors in the community. These skills would include the ability to understand their market, segment their market, and develop a marketing plan to change behaviors. These new strategies involving the use of marketing skills need to be better developed, organized, and evaluated—and then expanded.

The use of marketing skills can be thought of as a series of steps that are directed at satisfying the needs and wants of the consumer through an exchange process. A need involves a condition in which there is a deficiency of something, whereas a want entails a wish or desire for something perceived to be useful (Berkowitz, 2006). Gaining a better understanding of what individuals desire from health care can be helpful in marketing the concept of good health to consumers while also advocating for practicing healthy behaviors. The key here is to make certain that a need (good health) is being satisfied in exchange for something of value (practicing healthy behaviors).

Public health departments have largely ignored marketing, most likely because very few of the directors of public health departments (or any other public health workers) have ever received any formal education in the marketing process. This is probably due to public health programs' having been considered too important for public health departments to use the marketing approach to improve their funding stream. However, when public health workers encourage changes in individual behaviors and lifestyles they are actually in the business of marketing (Siegel and Lotenberg, 2006). Many people think of marketing as only advertising, not realizing that advertising is just one component of marketing. The marketing approach to doing business has produced successful results for businesses and government agencies for many years, and it can certainly be applied to public health departments' efforts to increase their funding stream and accomplish goals.

Use of Technology in Risk Communication

The use of technology also can help in the battle against the growing epidemic of chronic diseases. Technology is available to improve the communication of the dangers of high-risk behaviors to large portions of our population. Although public health departments have the information that is necessary to help individuals prevent chronic diseases from developing in the first place, the problem has been that the money these departments receive is never enough to develop, implement, and evaluate massive efforts at dissemination of chronic disease information to the entire population. This is not to say that there have not been chronic disease education efforts by health departments—there have been many successful programs developed and implemented in schools, workplaces, and the community, but the funding stream has not been dependable because of budget reductions. Public health departments need to make greater use of technology to get more information to the population consistently and innovatively. Mukherjee (2009) argues that in a crisis situation, companies need technology that allows for intelligent adjustment to major environmental shifts and that supports their prior principles. This recommendation rings true for public health departments. The chronic disease epidemic in America is causing an environmental shift for these departments, which now must use information technology in innovative ways to resolve this disease crisis.

According to Mukherjee (2009), certain drivers will cause the bureaucratic organization to become more flexible and increase worker productivity and the quality of the products or services delivered. These drivers include the transformation of systems and the nature of work, worker skills, and the structure of organizations. He was referring to an adaptive business strategy that is applicable to making things and producing services. These drivers are also extremely important in the improvement of the health of the individual and the community, and they need to become a functional part of the new world of public health. This is going to require public health workers to develop and apply many new skills in delivering population-based preventive services that are driven by health education programs.

The public health leader needs to change the nature of work, improve workers' skills, and allow structural change, with an ultimate goal of improving the health of the population. Computers and electronic communication have improved their ability to gather, analyze, and disseminate disease surveillance data (Turnock, 2009). Public health departments have to expand their use of this technology to deal with the chronic disease epidemic by providing a continuous stream of information about chronic diseases to the entire population. The CDC (2011b) offers several examples of success stories concerning the innovative use of technology that include Epi-X and Health-e-Cards, discussed in the paragraphs that follow. On a local level, I (Bernard) have had success using voice-narrated PowerPoint slides to educate large numbers of people about colorectal cancer and H1N1 influenza.

One of the best examples of a public health surveillance and information system is Epi-X, which offers Web-based communication for public health professionals. State and local health departments and poison control centers are currently using this system to access preliminary health surveillance information and share it with large numbers of health care professionals. This system supports postings of up-to-date medical information and discussions about disease outbreaks and other public health events that involve various parts of the nation and the world. Epi-X provides rapid communication whenever there is a need, and its staff is available twenty-four hours a day, seven days a week to provide consultation. I have personally been part of this excellent public health communication system and have grown in my knowledge of communicable and chronic disease information as a consequence. This system was created to provide public health officials with current information and alerts involving the health of the public, and its primary goal is to inform health officials about important events that can affect the public's health and help them respond to public health emergencies. This type of system would be excellent for rapid sharing of chronic disease information with the U.S. population.

As another example of the innovative use of technology, the CDC currently has available over one hundred free Health-e-Cards (electronic greeting cards). These colorful cards encourage healthy living, promote safety, and can even celebrate a health-and-safety-related event. They are currently available from the CDC and many local and state health departments. This concept could be extended to address the prevention of chronic diseases and to communicate ways of avoiding the complications that can develop later in life as a result of having a chronic disease.

Public Health Leadership Required

Prevention of chronic diseases and their complications should be a major component of any health reform endeavor. Success in the effort to become proactive with the epidemic of chronic diseases requires intensive public education programs that individuals first encounter in grade school and that continue into the workplace, and the implementation of such programs is going to require the development of public health leadership. As it stands, however, the chronic disease epidemic continues to expand despite public health efforts. Many dedicated public health workers find the limitations of conventional public health practice very hard to accept—in particular the fact that they are unable to use their creativity to develop innovative programs to deal with the chronic disease epidemic (Turnock, 2009). In order to exploit the opportunities present in the current chaotic health care system, public health departments will need strong leaders. This is especially true when it comes to pursuing innovations in health education and health promotion programs for dealing with the epidemic of chronic diseases. Halvorson (2009) argues that America needs leadership from public health that will focus on chronic disease care. The tools needed to improve the care for individuals with chronic diseases in this country include electronic medical records that will also act as connectors to all of the providers required to improve the quality of life for those with chronic diseases. In order to achieve this improvement, however, there is a need for better use of available data and of the various connectors.

The vast majority of Americans are not satisfied with the system of health care in this country. They want much more than they are currently receiving from the providers of medical services. According to Lee and Mongan (2009), there are only two ways for patients to improve the health care they receive: they can demand quality from their current providers or change providers, or they can take charge of their own health care. In order to participate in their own care they will require up-to-date health information that is available when they need it and that they can understand. This is where public health departments can help the individual patient and the community, for example by delivering such information over the Internet.

Public health departments must provide the leadership in developing and using the tools for chronic disease care, because these departments' overriding core function involves improving the health of the population. They will also need to focus on more innovation in regard to finding and implementing the tools necessary to manage chronic diseases and improve health outcomes—innovation for which leadership is a very necessary prerequisite (Zenger, Folkman, and Edinger, 2009). In fact, the leader is capable of creating an environment in which new ideas develop and grow. This type of environment, in which followers trust and are inspired by the leader, is exactly what public health departments need to deal with the epidemic of chronic diseases. What is more, followers should have the freedom to be creative in their use of chronic disease data when developing educational prevention programs.

It has become abundantly clear that public health departments have to change the way they attempt to accomplish their most important goal, which is protecting the health of the population. Clawson (2009) argues that when we talk about providing leadership we are also discussing strategy development and change management. These important components of leadership actually overlap in the pursuit of successful outcomes. Public health leaders need to develop new strategies and manage change to unite this country in an effort to reduce chronic diseases, which in turn will reduce cost escalation in health care. This means moving beyond public health accomplishments of the past and toward fresh strategies for facilitating change in public health's responsibilities and direction.

The change that is required of public health departments will be monumental, and it demands public health leaders who are adaptable and capable of responding to the new challenges facing the health care system. Fairchild et al. (2010) believe that public health is well positioned to take its place as a part of the current reform movement in health care delivery. This will require empowered public health workers who can go far beyond their conventional roles in public health departments. New roles for public health workers will also entail greater collaboration with the medical community in order to improve the health of the entire population.

Balogun and Hailey (2008) argue that there are three parts to the change process: an assessment of the current organizational situation, a statement of the desired future state, and a plan to get to where the organization should go. The public health system in the United States has the skills necessary to reduce the incidence of chronic diseases and their complications. The problem has been the lack of appropriate funding and leadership to deal with such a large problem. Even when there are public health leaders with the vision of where public health departments need to go, inadequate funding for chronic disease interventions makes achieving success problematic.

The chronic disease challenge cannot be met by public health departments alone. It is also going to require leaders and followers in public health agencies to collaborate with members of the medical community to produce a medical home for managing chronic diseases and their complications. In addition to public health leadership, followership is critical. The public health leader must clear the roadblocks for his or her staff so that they can concentrate on health outcomes rather than on activities like counseling and testing infected individuals that may produce little value. Public health professionals have to move beyond reacting to population health problems and toward a proactive approach of preventing diseases before they occur.

Followership and team performance are also critical for the changing public health sector. Lighter (2009) argues that the delivery of quality medical care in America has become a matter of teamwork rather than the responsibility of individual leaders. This situation is also found in public health departments, which require leaders who appreciate the contributions of their followers and create an environment in which creativity can develop and grow. The opportunity for public health departments to lead the health care system out of chaos has arrived.

Value of Prevention Programs

Efforts to fight chronic diseases include health education programs to prevent the diseases and disease management programs to prevent the complications that may result from chronic diseases later in life. Public health departments then need to deliver the information necessary to prevent chronic diseases to younger audiences through health education programs. Further, disease management requires interventions for the community that facilitate patient self-care and involve rapid dissemination of health-related information. Public health departments have that information, and they must now become innovative in how they distribute this information to large community populations so that they can better manage their chronic diseases.

An article written by The Commonwealth Fund Commission on a High Performance Health System (2006) discusses the value of patient-centered primary care as a solution to many of the problems in health care delivery.

This article cites patients' engagement in their own care as one of the most important attributes of patient-centered primary care. For patients to be thus engaged, health professionals must supply them with information on disease prevention, self-care, and treatment plans—which seems like a natural function for public health practitioners.

There is a new concept evolving in medical care that is gaining traction as a potential solution to complex medical problems. This innovative approach to patient care involves the **medical home,** which Bernstein (2008) describes as a way to better treat patients with chronic diseases and comorbidities. This strategy is especially appropriate for individuals who have developed one or more chronic diseases and are now facing disability, pain, suffering, and death. The medical home offers a way for patients to receive accessible and comprehensive primary care whenever they need it. One of the most important aspects of the medical home concept is the availability of accurate medical information to allow each patient to take initiative in his or her own medical care.

The Centers for Disease Control and Prevention pointed out in a 2009 report that Americans ages fifty to sixty-four require a comprehensive set of preventive services to remain healthy as they grow older (CDC, AARP, and American Medical Association, 2009). This report, *Promoting Preventive Services for Adults 50–64: Community and Clinical Partnerships*, revealed that only 25 percent of American adults in this age group regularly take advantage of preventive services, which poses a major problem because this is the time when adults are already incubating their chronic diseases. The report calls for public health departments to respond to this challenge with innovative education initiatives to increase these adults' knowledge about chronic diseases and aging.

Fulfilling the mission of public health to assure the health of the population includes developing, implementing, and evaluating prevention programs for all Americans. Maciosek et al. (2010) argue that public health departments need to make better use of a package of evidence-based clinical preventive services that offer value for the dollar to the patient. A number of recent research reports question the value of preventive services as an investment. In the short run, there is very little evidence that medical costs are reduced through an emphasis on prevention programs. There is even disagreement among researchers concerning the value in the long term of health education programs, health promotion activities, and screening tests that are expensive to administer and may or may not result in reduced medical costs and ultimately improved health status.

According to an article in the *Nation's Health* (Currie, 2010), prevention programs save lives as well as money. A recent study conducted by the National Commission on Prevention Priorities found that preventive services such as promotion of daily aspirin use, tobacco cessation support and alcohol abuse screening, and colorectal cancer screening can potentially save two million lives and nearly $4 billion annually. The study concluded that not all preventive services are equal in impact but that in some cases the benefits in regard to population health can be profound. The secret is to use only proven, cost-effective prevention programs and find an innovative way to get health information to the population. If the vision for public health is to offer innovative health education and health promotion programs to large numbers of people, then public health departments need to look outside of public health for new ways to deliver the message to the population. This could be accomplished, for example, through greater use of such social networks as Facebook and Twitter.

A recent report, *Prevention for a Healthier California* (Levi, Cohen, and Segal, 2008), was completed through a partnership among Trust for America's Health, Prevention Institute, the New York Academy of Medicine, and the Urban Institute. This study involved a range of community-based programs in California. The purpose of this study was to focus on actions that California policymakers could take to make prevention a greater priority, with the goal of reducing health care costs and improving the health of the population. This groundbreaking study validated the idea that community-based prevention saves money and improves lives. It demonstrated that an investment in prevention programs following a relatively simple model that incorporates proven population-based preventive services can reduce health care costs by billions of dollars.

Figure 11.1 shows how the model works, and Figure 11.2 demonstrates the return on investment for California. Figure 11.3 expands the model used for California to the entire country.

Figure 11.4 demonstrates how the cumulative benefits of the use of primary prevention programs are measured. The underlying strategy here would include improved health from the reduction of the target condition along with the reduction in the prevalence of associated conditions. There would also be increases in the productivity and the work attendance of working individuals who have achieved better health status from the prevention effort. These increased

FIGURE 11.1 Community Intervention Logic Model

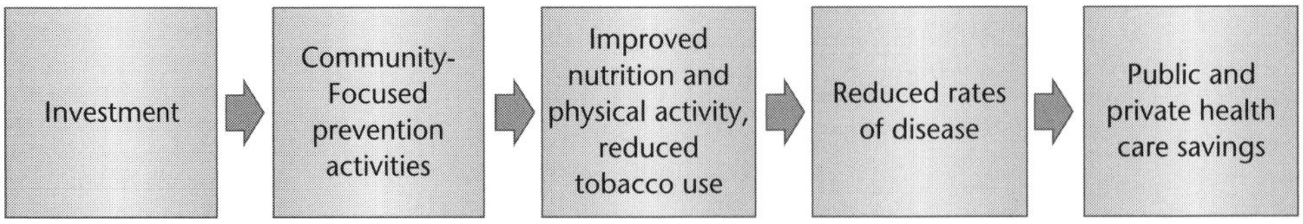

Investment → Community-Focused prevention activities → Improved nutrition and physical activity, reduced tobacco use → Reduced rates of disease → Public and private health care savings

Source: Levi et al., 2008, p. 2.

FIGURE 11.2   California Return on Investment of Ten Dollars per Person

	1–2 Years	5 Years	10–20 Years
Total State Savings	$621,400,000	$2,092,700,000	$2,297,700,000
State Net Savings (Net savings = Total savings minus intervention costs)	$262,900,000	$1,734,300,000	$1,939,300,000
ROI for State	0.73:1	4.84:1	5.41:1

Source: Levi et al., 2008, p. 2.

FIGURE 11.3   National Return on Investment of Ten Dollars per Person

	1–2 Years	5 Years	10–20 Years
U.S. Total	$2,848,000,000	$16,543,000,000	$18,451,000,000
ROI	0.96:1	5.6:1	6.2:1

Source: Levi et al., 2008, p. 2.

FIGURE 11.4   Return on Investment

In general, ROI compares the dollars invested in something to the benefits produced by that investment:

$$ROI = \frac{(\text{benefits of investment} - \text{amount invested})}{\text{amount invested}}$$

In the case of an investment in a prevention program, ROI compares the savings produced by the intervention, net of the cost of the program, to how much the program costs:

$$ROI = \frac{\text{net savings}}{\text{cost of intervention}}$$

When ROI equals 0, the program pays for itself. When ROI is greater than 0, then the program is producing savings that exceed the cost of the program.

Source: Levi et al., 2008, p. 2.

FIGURE 11.5   Multiplier Effects

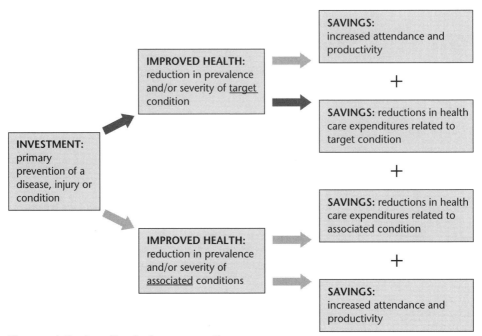

The cumulative benefits of primary prevention:

The arrows indicate the customarily studied savings pathway, but investments in primary prevention result in improved health in conditions other than the one targeted and savings accrue in three areas not captured by conventional models.

Source: Levi et al., 2008, p. 8.

side effects that go beyond addressing the targeted condition and associated conditions are the result of the multiplier effects of well-designed community prevention efforts (see Figure 11.5).

This study demonstrated that prevention programs can produce substantial health care savings if the right programs are offered to the population. Focusing prevention programs on the population can also produce such significant economic improvements as heightened productivity in the work process, reduced disability, and even increased school attendance. The problem is how to get prevention information to the entire population in an understandable format and at a reasonable cost.

One of the major problems with the American health care system is that the consumer (patient) has usually been a passive recipient of health services that the health care system provides. The consumer is not well educated in health care and, therefore, is not usually rational when it comes to purchasing health services. His or her demand for health care is a derived demand for good health, meaning that the consumer is not really demanding health services but rather an improvement in health status. The consumer delegates his or her demand when it comes to health care, placing it in the hands of the physician. This is because our health care system is structured with **information asymmetry,** which is present in decision transactions in which one party has more or better information than the other party—as is certainly the case when a patient deals with the physician who is making decisions concerning the patient's health. The consumer allows this imbalance or ignorance because medical knowledge costs a great deal to acquire and has small expected benefits for the individual patient. The average patient usually does not pay the full cost of medical care because of health insurance and trusts the better-educated physician to provide advice on what is required to remain healthy.

The patient does not know when to seek care and is not completely convinced that preventive health care is worth the time and investment necessary to avert future illness. The patient is also unable to evaluate physician recommendations for care, is unable to evaluate the quality of care, and is unaware of the price of medical care. In order to improve the population's situation in regard to their dearth of medical knowledge, especially that pertaining to the value of preventive services, there needs to be innovation in the distribution of this vital information to the population. This is the opportunity that is available to public health departments today.

Public health departments have the medical information that the patient requires to become a rational consumer of health care services. The problem for public health departments has been finding an effective and inexpensive way of distributing health information, especially data concerning the prevention of chronic diseases, to the entire population on a regular basis. This is where innovation, community collaboration, and public health leadership combine to become the catalyst necessary to accomplish the mission of public health in America.

The Process of Innovation

One of the more important qualities of the leader over years of research remains the ability to develop a vision and be able to get his or her followers to follow that vision. Strong leaders and the companies they work for have been successful in recent years in allowing creativity and innovation to flow in the workplace, and the ability to innovate has become a necessity for survival in the modern world of business. This innovation is also necessary for public health departments to meet their goals of assuring conditions that promote the health of the population.

This is going to require the public health leader to make bold moves toward changing the way public health departments function. The mission of public health is to assure conditions in which people can be healthy, but public health leaders have not done a great deal to reduce the challenge of the epidemic of chronic diseases in this country. The leader needs to build a culture among his or her followers that is dedicated to the vision of meeting the chronic disease challenge.

Thanks to technology, consumers are now able to find out a great deal about a product or service before they purchase it. This is true for all industries in the United States except the health care sector—and there lies the opportunity for public health departments to reinvent themselves through innovation. We began this chapter by asking two questions.

1. Do people really want to develop life-threatening and disability-producing chronic diseases as they grow older? (The answer, we believe, is no.)
2. How does a public health agency make preventing these diseases as easy as possible for the population? (The answer is innovation.)

The answer to both questions is found in the ultimate vision for innovation in public health departments. This vision entails assuring conditions that promote the health of the population through the provision of life-changing health education that is made possible through innovation in how information is delivered.

Summary

The delivery of health care in the United States is in a state of chaos, requiring immediate attention. The major culprits in the cost escalation in health care are the epidemic of chronic diseases and their complications. It has become very clear that our current system of medical care in this country is not capable of dealing with this very different type of epidemic. The current epidemic of chronic diseases along with the chaotic medical care system are producing the very real possibility of a bankrupt U.S. health care system.

The need to quell this epidemic is also producing a tremendous opportunity for public health leaders and their followers to offer their creativity and pursue innovation to restore the health of the population. This can only be accomplished, however, if the population has access to up-to-date information about chronic diseases and the prevention of complications that usually follow the development of chronic diseases.

Public health departments have to change how they seek to accomplish their most important goal—protecting the health of the population. Public health professionals need to receive extensive training in leadership, in the use of technology, and in developing communication and collaboration skills in order to fulfill their new challenges. They also need to move from a bureaucratic organizational structure to a more organic form of administration that encourages creativity and innovation in the delivery of services. Public health departments are quite capable of continuing and expanding on their past successes in improving the health of Americans, but in order to do so they must be given the necessary resources to win the war against chronic diseases.

Key Terms

Disruptive innovation

Information asymmetry

Medical home

Risk communication

Discussion Questions

1. Why is our system of health care delivery in chaos?
2. How can the tools of marketing help public health departments increase their budget for addressing the chronic disease epidemic?
3. Why are creativity, technology, and innovation so very necessary as public health departments develop health promotion programs to deal with the escalation of chronic diseases in the United States?
4. How can public health departments improve upon their creativity and innovation in addressing the major challenges faced by our current health care system?

CHAPTER 12

LOCAL SOLUTIONS TO REDUCE INEQUITIES IN HEALTH AND SAFETY

**Larry Cohen, Anthony Iton,
Rachel Davis, Sharon Murriguez**

LEARNING OBJECTIVES

- Understand the importance of addressing the underlying determinants of health inequities
- Articulate the necessity of employing both health care and community-focused strategies to prevent inequities in health and safety
- Identify how health inequities are systematically created and delineate elements of an effective strategy within health care and at the community level to reduce inequities in health and safety

Equitable Health: A Four-Pronged Solution

In Alameda County, California, where the authors live and work, an African American child born in Oakland's flatlands will live an average of fifteen years less than a white child born in the Oakland hills neighborhood (Alameda County Public Health Department, 2008). *Further, for every $12,500 in income difference between families, people in the lower-income family can expect to die a year sooner. Tragically, public health data confirms this same jarring reality all across American cities, suburbs, and rural areas.*

Good health is precious. It enables people to enjoy their lives and focus on what is important to them—their families, friends, and communities. It fosters productivity and learning, and it allows people to capitalize on opportunities. However, good health is not experienced evenly across society: heart disease, cancer, diabetes, stroke, injury, and violence occur in higher frequency, earlier, and with greater severity among low-income people and communities of color—especially African Americans, Native Americans, Native Hawaiians, certain Asian groups, and Latinos (Smedley, Stith, and Nelson, 2003). For example:

- Compared to whites, American Indians and Alaska Natives are 2.3 times more likely to have diagnosed diabetes, African Americans are 2.2 times more likely, and Latinos are 1.6 times more likely (CDC, 2007).
- Among African Americans between the ages of ten and twenty-four, homicide is the leading cause of death. In the same age range, homicide is the second leading cause of death for Hispanics, and the third leading cause of death for American Indians, Alaska Natives, and Asian/Pacific Islanders (Centers for Disease Control and Prevention [CDC], 2006). Homicide rates among non-Hispanic, African American males ten to twenty-four years of age (58.3 per 100,000) exceed those of Hispanic males (20.9 per 100,000) and non-Hispanic, white males in the same age group (3.3 per 100,000) (CDC, 2008e).
- Native Americans have a motor vehicle death rate that is more than 1.5 times greater than whites, Latinos, Asian/Pacific Islanders, and African Americans (CDC, 2006; U.S. Department of Transportation, 2006).
- Poverty is associated with risk factors for chronic health conditions, and low-income adults report multiple serious health conditions more often than those with higher incomes (National Center for Health Statistics, 2007).
- The average annual incidence of end-stage kidney disease in minority zip codes is nearly twice as high as in nonminority zip codes (National Minority Health Month Foundation [NMHMF], 2007).
- Premature death rates from cardiovascular disease (i.e., between the ages of 5 and 64) are substantially higher in minority zip codes than in nonminority zip codes (NMHMF, 2007).
- Education correlates strongly with health. Among adults over age twenty-five, 5.8 percent of college graduates, 11 percent of those with some college, 13.9 percent

of high school graduates, and 25.7 percent of those with less than a high school education report being in poor or fair health (CDC, 2005b).

Health inequity is related both to a legacy of overt discriminatory actions on the part of government and the larger society, as well as to present day practices and policies of public and private institutions that continue to perpetuate a system of diminished opportunity for certain populations. Poverty, racism, and lack of educational and economic opportunities are among the fundamental **determinants of health** or alternatively poor health, lack of safety, and health inequities, contributing to chronic stress and building upon one another to create a weathering effect, whereby health greatly reflects cumulative experience rather than chronological age (Geronimus, 2001). Further, continued exposure to racism and discrimination may in and of itself exert a great toll on both physical and mental health (U.S. Department of Health and Human Services, 1999). Inequities in the distribution of a core set of health-protective resources also perpetuate patterns of poor health.

Historically, African Americans, Native Americans, Alaska Natives, and Native Hawaiians, in particular, have to varying extents had their culture, traditions, and land forcibly taken from them. It is not a mere coincidence that these populations suffer from the most profound health disparities and shortened life expectancies. In many of the low-income and racially segregated places where health disparities abound, a collective sense of hopelessness is pervasive, and social isolation is rampant. This individual- and community-level despair fuels chronic stress, encourages short-term decision making, and increases the inclination toward immediate gratification, which may include tobacco use, substance abuse, poor diet, and physical inactivity.

To date, the collective national response has focused on what happens after people get sick or injured. Improving the health care system by increasing access and quality remains an integral component of addressing health inequities. At the same time, recent data indicates we must do more. Despite a decade-long investment in launching clinically focused initiatives to reduce health disparities, the United States has made virtually no significant progress in this domain (Voelker, 2008; House and Williams, 2000).

The National Institutes of Health defines **health disparities** as "diseases, disorders, and conditions that disproportionately afflict individuals who are members of racial and ethnic minority groups" (National Institutes of Health, 2002, p. 7). **Health inequities** are "differences in health which are not only unnecessary and avoidable but, in addition, are considered unfair and unjust" (Whitehead, 1990, p. 5). Thus, equity and inequity are based on core American values of fairness and justice whereas *disparity* is a narrow descriptive term that refers to measurable differences but does not imply whether this disparity arises from an unjust root cause. For the purposes of this chapter, the term *inequity* is used when the referenced differences in health outcomes have been produced by historic and systemic social injustices, or the unintended or indirect consequences of social policies.

Health equity is everyone's issue, and finding solutions will significantly benefit everyone. As the United States population becomes increasingly diverse, achieving a healthy, productive nation will depend even more on keeping all Americans healthy. An equitable system can drastically lower the cost of health care for all, increase productivity, and reduce the spread of infectious diseases, thus improving everyone's well-being. Last—and most importantly—the idea of equity is based on core American values of fairness and justice. Everyone deserves an equal opportunity to prosper and achieve his or her full potential, and it is our moral imperative to accomplish this.

We can remedy the problem of inequities in health and safety outcomes by creating a new paradigm addressing the needs that are critical to achieving health equity, and the specific challenges that affect integrating solutions into practice and policy. The first need is for a coherent, sustainable health care system that adequately meets the requirements of the entire U.S. population and of racial and ethnic minorities in particular. The second need is for adequate community prevention strategies that target the factors underpinning why people get sick and injured in the first place. These should be integrated to form a unified system for achieving health, safety, and health equity in the United States.

In this chapter, we propose a set of solutions that are achievable within the local arena. By local, we mean state, regional, and community levels. These solutions not only address the critical needs but also bridge traditional health promotion, disease management, and health care solutions with more upstream work that focuses on preventing illness and injury in the first place. We will outline a composite of community and health care factors that affect health, safety, and mental health and that—most importantly—provide the framework for accomplishing a four-pronged solution:

1. Strengthen communities where people live, work, play, socialize, and learn.
2. Enhance opportunities within underserved communities to access high-quality, culturally competent health care with an emphasis on community-oriented and preventive services.
3. Strengthen the infrastructure of our health system to reduce inequities and enhance the contributions from public health and health care systems.
4. Support local efforts through leadership, overarching policies, and through local, state, and national strategy.

Policy and **institutional practices** are the key levers for change. Institutional practices along with public and private policy helped create the inequitable conditions and outcomes confronting us today. Consequently, we need to focus on these areas—in community, business/labor, and government—in order to "unmake" inequitable neighborhood conditions and improve health and safety outcomes. Policies and institutional/organizational practices significantly influence the well-being of the community; they affect equitable distribution of its services; and they help shape norms, which, in turn, influence behavior.

The following policy principles, adapted from *Life and Death from Unnatural Causes: Health and Social Inequity in Alameda County* (Alameda County Public Health Department, 2008), provide guidance for taking on the challenge of addressing health inequities:

- Understanding and accounting for the historical forces that have left a legacy of racism and segregation is key to moving forward with the structural changes needed. A component of addressing these historical forces should consider policy and reform related to immigrant groups—notably Latinos, Asians, and Arab Americans.
- Acknowledging the cumulative impact of stressful experiences and environments is crucial. For some families, poverty lasts a lifetime and is perpetuated to next generations, leaving its family members with few opportunities to make healthful decisions.
- Meaningful public participation is needed with attention to outreach, follow-through, language, inclusion, and cultural understanding. Government and private funding agencies should actively support efforts to build resident capacity to engage.
- Because of the cumulative impact of multiple stressors, our overall approach should shift toward changing community conditions and away from blaming individuals or groups for their disadvantaged status.
- The social fabric of neighborhoods needs to be strengthened. Residents need to be connected and supported and feel that they hold power to improve the safety and well-being of their families. All residents need to have a sense of belonging, dignity, and hope.
- While low-income people and people of color face age-old survival issues, equity solutions can and should simultaneously respond to the global economy, climate change, and U.S. foreign policy.
- The developmental needs and transitions of all age groups should be addressed. While infants, children, youth, adults, and elderly require age-appropriate strategies, the largest investments should be in early life because important foundations of adult health are laid in early childhood.
- Working across multiple sectors of government and society is key to making the necessary structural changes. Such work should be in partnership with community advocacy groups that continue to pursue a more equitable society.
- Measuring and monitoring the impact of social policy on health to ensure gains in equity is essential. This will include instituting systems to track governmental spending by neighborhood, and tracking changes in measurements of health equity over time and place to help identify the impact of adverse policies and practices.
- Groups that are the most impacted by inequities must have a voice in identifying policies that will make a difference as well as in holding government accountable for implementing these policies.

- Eliminating inequities is a huge opportunity to invest in community. Inequity among us is not acceptable, and we all stand to gain by eliminating it.

Critical Needs for Achieving Equitable Health in the United States: A Health System

We need a coherent, sustainable health care system that adequately meets the health requirements of the entire U.S. population and of racial and ethnic minorities in particular. When we talk about fixing the health care system in the United States, we assume there is a system that can be improved. The underlying problem, however, is that we have no coherent system in the first place. The Affordable Care Act (ACA) does take some important steps including expanding access and funding that reflects an awareness of the value of a comprehensive approach to health. Notably, the ACA's establishment of the Prevention and Public Health Fund and the development of a surgeon-general-led National Prevention Strategy all point to an increased understanding of and commitment to prevention in the first place. However, additional steps and policies will be necessary in order to arrive at a fundamentally new approach to health that addresses inequities by bridging exemplary services available to all with a focus on the factors that have the greatest influence on health. The last time the World Health Organization published data on international health rankings in their *World Health Report 2000—Health Systems: Improving Performance,* the United States ranked number one in health expenditure per capita but only ranked thirty-seventh in overall health system performance (World Health Report, 2000). Among industrialized countries, the United States came in twenty-fifth out of thirty on infant mortality and twenty-third out of thirty on life expectancy (Organisation for Economic Co-operation and Development, 2007). Even for those with adequate access to health care, the system is flawed. For example, there are huge inconsistencies in the delivery of recommended care across a wide range of conditions and population groups (Davis, Taira, and Chung, 2006); medical errors are estimated to result in approximately ninety-eight thousand unnecessary deaths and over one million excess injuries each year (CDC, 2005a; Institute of Medicine [IOM], 2000a); medical practitioners' job dissatisfaction rates are growing; and major shortages in nursing and allied health professions are projected (American Association of Colleges of Nursing, 2009).

In a time of financial crisis, we may focus exclusively on reforming the areas of greatest expense in the economy, narrowing in on the cost of specific items as we try to reduce that cost or at least slow its increase. Studies have revealed that the dramatic rise in the prevalence of chronic disease is a major factor responsible for growth in U.S. health care spending (Thorpe, 2006). This is a cost that can be reduced through prevention (Trust for America's Health [TFAH], Prevention Institute [PI], The Urban Institute [UI], and New York Academy of Medicine [NYAM], 2008). An economic analysis revealed that investing even the modest amount of ten dollars per person in community-level initiatives aimed at reducing tobacco consumption, improving nutrition, and increasing physical activity results in a return on investment within two years and an estimated annual savings of over $15 billion nationally within five years (TFAH, PI, UI, and NYAM). Each year thereafter, the five-to-one return on investment is projected to increase. The savings from an investment in prevention in disenfranchised communities should be even greater because they experience the greatest burden of ill health. In addition to this chronic disease analysis, studies reveal that other health-related investments also yield a significant return. For instance, one dollar invested in breastfeeding support by employers results in three dollars in reduced absenteeism and health care costs for mothers and babies and improved productivity (United States Breastfeeding Committee, 2002); one dollar invested in lead abatement in public housing returns two dollars in reduced medical and special education costs and increased productivity (Brown, 2002); and one dollar invested in workplace safety measures returns four to six dollars in reduced illnesses, injuries, and fatalities (Occupational Safety and Health Administration, 2009).

The ACA provisions are one step forward in institutionalizing and catalyzing prevention. Even after current ACA provisions go into effect, the health care system and its reimbursement structure needs to do more to incentivize the necessary community-based prevention. Such community-based prevention efforts also aid in the *management* of existing chronic diseases and injuries and thus reduce costs and better meet the health needs of communities across our nation.

As we reform and redesign the health care system, we need to explicitly take the issue of equity into account, since anything done to reformulate how care is delivered can either mitigate or exacerbate the problem of inequity. Therefore, quality improvements to any health care component (e.g., prevention, access, and quality) have to embrace principles of cultural competency, diversity, and equity.

We need to create a coherent, comprehensive, and sustainable health care system that is culturally and linguistically appropriate, affordable, effective, and equally accessible to all people—especially disenfranchised populations. The overall health system should start with community strategies—reducing the likelihood that people will get sick or injured in the first place and helping to maintain the well-being of those who are already sick and injured. The overall system should also offer a full set of services (e.g., medical, dental, mental health, and vision), including screening, diagnostic, and disease management services, within the communities where people live.

We need adequate community prevention strategies that target the factors underpinning why people get sick and injured in the first place. Health care is vital but alone it is not enough. The health care system has great strength in its committed providers and in its ever-improving diagnosis, procedures, and medicines. Many formerly fatal diseases are now treatable and even curable. Yet, as important as it is to improve the quality of health care services, it is only part of the solution to improving health and reducing health inequities. Patterns of disease and injury that follow the socioeconomic status gradient would still remain (Adler and Newman, 2002). While health care is vital, there are three reasons why addressing access to and quality of health care services alone will not significantly reduce disparities:

1. Health care is not the primary determinant of health. Of the thirty-year increase in life expectancy since the turn of the century, only about five years of this increase are attributed to health care interventions (Pincus, Esther, DeWalt, and Callahan, 1998). Even in countries with universal access to care, people with lower socioeconomic status have poorer health outcomes (IOM, 2000a).
2. Health care treats one person at a time. By focusing on the individual and specific illnesses as they arise, medical treatment does not reduce the incidence or severity of disease among groups of people because others become afflicted even as others are cured (Smedley et al., 2003).
3. Health care intervention often comes late. Health care and intervention play important restorative or ameliorating roles after disease occurs. However, many of today's most common chronic health conditions, such as heart disease, diabetes, asthma, and HIV/AIDS, are never cured. It is extremely important to prevent them from occurring in the first place and, when they occur, their ongoing prognosis will depend on a number of factors in addition to health care.

In order to successfully address inequities in health and safety, we must pose the following questions: Why are people getting sick and injured in the first place? What impedes their ability to recuperate? Are their neighborhoods conducive to good health? What products are sold and promoted? Is it easy to get around safely? Is the air and water clean? Are there effective schools and work opportunities? Are there persistent stressors in the environment, and what is the long-term impact of this stress on health? The frequency and severity of injury and illness are not inevitable.

People's health is strongly influenced by the overall life odds of the neighborhood where they live. Indeed, place matters. In many low-income urban and rural communities, whole populations are consigned to shortened, sicker lives. While residential segregation has declined overall since 1960, people of color are increasingly likely to live in high-poverty communities (Poverty and Race Research and Action Council, 2005). Racially and economically segregated communities are more likely to have limited economic opportunities, a lack of healthy options for food and physical activity, increased presence of environmental hazards, substandard housing, lower-performing schools, higher rates of crime and incarceration, and higher costs for common goods and services (the so-called "poverty tax") (Smedley, Jeffries, Adelman, and Cheng, 2008).

Conversely, people are healthier when their environments are healthier. For example, in African American census tracts, fruit and vegetable consumption increases by 32 percent for each supermarket (Morland, Wing, Roux, and Poole, 2002). When states moved to require infant car seats, the impact of policy far exceeded that of education in changing norms and thus behavior: usage for infants went from 25 percent maximum to nearly universal, and death and injury from car crashes decreased (National Highway Traffic Safety Administration, 2004).

Taking a step from a specific disease or injury reveals the behavior (e.g., eating, physical activity, and violence) or exposure (e.g., stressors and air quality) that increases the likelihood of the injury or disease. Through an analysis of the factors contributing to medical conditions that cause people to seek care, researchers have identified a set of nine behaviors and exposures strongly linked to the major causes of death: tobacco, diet and activity patterns, alcohol, microbial agents, toxic agents, firearms, sexual behavior, motor vehicles, and inappropriate drug use (Mokdad, Marks, Stroup, and Gerberding, 2004). Limiting unhealthy exposures and behaviors enhances health and reduces the likelihood and severity of disease and injury. In fact, these exposures and behaviors are linked to multiple medical diagnoses, and addressing them can improve health broadly. If we take a second step, we see that specific elements of the environments in which people live are major determinants of our exposures and behaviors and thus of our illnesses and injuries.

This framework, *Take Two Steps to Prevention* (detailed further in the following sections and illustrated in Figure 12.1 below) was developed as a tool for analyzing the underlying causes of illness and injury and health inequities and identifying the key opportunities for intervention and prevention. *Take Two Steps to Prevention* presents a systematic way of looking at needed health care services and then traveling back to the exposures and behaviors that affect illness and injury and then back to the underlying community conditions that shape patterns of exposure and behavior.

FIGURE 12.1   Trajectory of Health Inequities

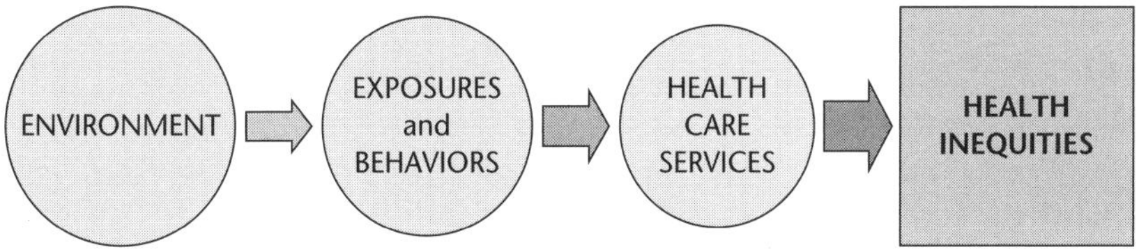

Source: Prevention Institute.

Take Two Steps to Prevention

Starting with Health Care Services. Health care services aim to improve health outcomes by focusing on identifying and treating specific medical conditions (e.g., heart disease, diabetes, and infections) with health care services. High-quality health care can prevent the onset of some medical conditions, diagnose problems early, reduce the severity of symptoms, and slow the progression of secondary conditions. The Institute of Medicine's *Unequal Treatment: Confronting Racial and Ethnic Disparities in Health Care* identified three primary ways to intervene to reduce health inequities through health care services (Smedley et al., 2003):

1. *Increase access to care:* Within our current system, lack of insurance and under-insurance, major barriers to accessing medical care, are not borne equally across racial and ethnic lines.

2. *Improve quality of care (diagnosis and treatment): Unequal Treatment* documents that "evidence of racial and ethnic disparities in healthcare is, with few exceptions, remarkably consistent across a range of illnesses and healthcare services" *Unequal Treatment* reveals that differences in diagnosis, quality of care, and treatment methods lead to consistently poorer health outcomes among people of color.

3. *Implement culturally and linguistically appropriate care:* A culturally competent system of care is measured both by achieving the desired health outcome and patient satisfaction with medical encounters.

The First Step: From Health Care Services to Exposures and Behaviors. Health care alone cannot eliminate health disparities. The first step is from health care to exposures and behaviors. Limiting unhealthy exposures and behaviors enhances health and reduces the likelihood and severity of disease. Through an analysis of the factors contributing to medical conditions that cause people to seek care, researchers have identified a set of nine behaviors and exposures strongly linked to the major causes of death: tobacco, diet and activity patterns, alcohol, microbial agents, toxic agents, firearms, sexual behavior, motor vehicles, and inappropriate drug use (Davis, Cook, and Cohen, 2005). These behaviors and exposures are linked to multiple medical diagnoses, and addressing them can improve health broadly. For example, tobacco is associated with a number of health problems including lung cancer, asthma, emphysema, and heart disease. Diet and activity patterns are associated with cardiovascular and heart disease, certain cancers, and diabetes, among other illnesses.

As a result, reducing exposures and unhealthy behaviors decreases the risk of multiple injuries and illnesses. It is also important to include analysis of exposure to the stressors of poverty, racism, lack of opportunity, etc. Exposure to these stressors affects low-income communities and people of color disproportionately, and similar to the nine listed above are contributing factors in multiple health conditions and opportunities for intervention.

The Second Step: From Exposures and Behaviors to the Environment. Exposures and behaviors are determined or shaped by the environments in which they are present, defined as anything external to individuals and shared by members of a community. Exposures, of course, are shaped by what in the environment one is exposed to, and behaviors are shaped (encouraged or discouraged) by what is available in communities and the norms that communities help shape. Taking the second step from exposures and behaviors to the environment, presents a tremendous opportunity to reduce health inequities by preventing illness and injury before their onset. The environment includes root factors (e.g., poverty, racism, and other forms of oppression), institutions, and community factors. THRIVE (Tool for Health and Resilience in Vulnerable Environments), a research-based framework created by Prevention Institute, offers a way to understand the community factors (Prevention Institute, 2004). THRIVE includes thirteen **community health factors** grouped into three clusters: people, place, and equitable opportunity. Similar work by other researchers confirms this overall approach. For example, in 2002 PolicyLink published very similar findings and factors in the report, *Reducing Health Disparities Through a Focus on Communities*.

The thirteen community THRIVE factors are organized into three interrelated clusters (see Figure 12.2): equitable opportunity, people, and place and either directly influence health and safety outcomes via exposures (e.g., air, water, soil quality; stressors) or indirectly via behaviors that in turn affect health and safety outcomes (e.g., the availability of healthy food affects nutrition). In addition, the environment also influences people's opportunity to access quality health care services, and these are included as a fourth cluster. The clusters are described here:

FIGURE 12.2   Community Clusters

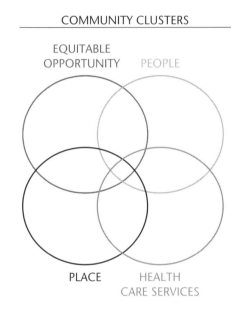

COMMUNITY CLUSTERS

EQUITABLE
OPPORTUNITY   PEOPLE

PLACE   HEALTH
CARE SERVICES

Equitable Opportunity This cluster refers to the level and equitable distribution of opportunity and resources. Root factors, including poverty, racism, and lack of educational and economic opportunities are among the fundamental determinants of poor health, lack of safety, and health inequities. They each contribute to chronic stress and can build upon one another to create a weathering effect, whereby health greatly reflects cumulative experience rather than chronological or developmental age (Geronimus, 2001). Chronic stress increases risk for coronary artery disease, stroke, cognitive impairment, substance abuse, anxiety, depression, mood disorders, and accelerated aging and cancer (Adler and Newman, 2002). Further, economic and racial segregation is one of the most powerful forces shaping health in the United States. The availability of jobs with living wages, absence of discrimination and racism, and quality education all affect health and safety (Lantz et al., 1998; Smedley et al., 2008). This segregation is not inevitable; it has been established and maintained through government policy and investment and the practices of institutions and organizations (Adler, 2002). Examples include redlining (wherein low-income neighborhoods and neighborhoods with primarily people of color are identified for discriminatory investment by banks and other lenders, historically by drawing a red line on a map); discriminatory application of GI Bill housing benefits; unequal investment in schools and transportation (leaving low-income communities at an educational and geographic disadvantage, which restricts social and economic mobility and development leading to further concentration of poverty); and judicial rulings such as the Supreme Court's recent ruling (*Parents Involved in Community Schools* v. *Seattle School District*) that reverses much of *Brown* v. *Board of Education,* which ruled that separate was not equal. Factors include:

- Racial justice, characterized by policies and organizational practices that foster equitable opportunities and services for all; positive relations among people of different races and ethnic backgrounds
- Jobs and local ownership, characterized by local ownership of assets, including homes and businesses; access to investment opportunities, job availability, and the ability to make a living wage
- Education, characterized by high-quality and available education and literacy development across the life span

   People This cluster refers to the relationships between people, the level of engagement, and norms, all of which influence health and safety outcomes. For instance, strong social networks and connections correspond with significant increases in physical and mental health, academic achievement, and local economic development, as well as lower rates of homicide, suicide, and alcohol and drug abuse (Buka, 1999; Wandersman and Nation, 1998); children have been found to be mentally and physically healthier in neighborhoods where adults talk to each other (Wilkenson, 1999). Social connections also contribute to a community's willingness to take action for the common good which is associated with lower rates of violence (Sampson, Raudenbush, and Earls, 1997), and improved food access (Pothukuchi, 2005). Factors include:

- Social networks and trust, characterized by strong social ties among persons and positions, built upon mutual obligations; opportunities to exchange information; the ability to enforce standards and administer sanctions
- Community engagement and efficacy, characterized by local/indigenous leadership; involvement in community or social organizations; participation in the political process; willingness to intervene on behalf of the common good
- Norms/accepted behaviors and attitudes, characterized by regularities in behavior with which people generally conform; standards of behavior that foster disapproval of deviance; the way in which the environment tells people what is okay and not okay

Place This cluster refers to the physical environment in which people live, work, play, and go to school. Decisions about place have multiple direct and indirect effects on health and safety. For example, physical activity levels are influenced by conditions such as enjoyable scenery (Jackson, Kochtitzky, 2009), the proximity of recreational facilities, street and neighborhood design (CDC, Active Community Environments Factsheet), and transportation design (Hancock, 2000); and the presence of alcohol distributors in a community is correlated with per capita consumption (Schmid, 1995). Factors include:

- What's sold and how it's promoted, characterized by the availability and promotion of safe, healthy, affordable, culturally appropriate products and services (e.g., food, books and school supplies, sports equipment, arts and crafts supplies, and other recreational items); limited promotion and availability, or lack, of potentially harmful products and services (e.g., tobacco, firearms, alcohol, and other drugs)
- Look, feel, and safety, characterized by a well-maintained, appealing, clean, and culturally relevant visual and auditory environment; actual and perceived safety
- Parks and open space, characterized by safe, clean, accessible parks; parks that appeal to interests and activities across the life span; green space; outdoor space that is accessible to the community; natural/open space that is preserved through the planning process
- Getting around, characterized by availability of safe, reliable, accessible, and affordable methods for moving people around, including public transit, walking, and biking
- Housing, characterized by availability of safe, affordable, and available housing
- Air, water, and soil, characterized by safe and nontoxic water, soil, indoor and outdoor air, and building materials
- Arts and culture, characterized by abundant opportunities within the community for cultural and artistic expression and participation and for cultural values to be expressed through the arts

Health Care Services Over the course of our lives we also all want and need health care, including good medical, mental health, and dental services. As a starting point, people need to be able to obtain quality health and dental care, which means people need adequate and affordable health insurance. To help maintain health, people need preventive care and chronic disease management. In crisis situations, we need reliable, immediate, and qualified emergency responses. When we suffer from acute or chronic conditions, we hope for quality health care to treat or cure our conditions, or help us manage them. For all of these services, culturally and linguistically appropriate patient care is critical for communicating with patients and addressing health concerns within the cultural context of the patient. Factors include:

- Preventive services, characterized by a strong system of primary, preventive health services that are responsive to community needs

- Cultural competence, characterized by patient-centered care that is understanding of and sensitive to different cultures, languages, and needs
- Access, characterized by a comprehensive system of health coverage that is simple, affordable, and available
- Treatment quality, disease management, in-patient services, and alternative medicine, characterized by effective, timely, and appropriate in-patient and out-patient care including for dental, mental health, and vision
- Emergency response, characterized by timely and appropriate responses in crisis situations that stabilize the situation and link those in need with appropriate follow-up care

Clearly, local solutions to health and safety inequities are central to success. Local work complements broader national change, and local solutions often help shape profound, long-lasting federal changes. Altering community conditions, particularly in low-income communities of color where the memory and legacy of dispossession remains, requires the consent and participation of a critical mass of community residents. Thus strategies that reconnect people to their culture, decrease racism, reduce chronic stress, and offer meaningful opportunities are ultimately health policies. Effective change is highly dependent upon relationships of trust between community members and local institutions. The process of inclusion and engaging communities in decision making is as important as the outcomes, which should directly meet the needs of the local population. Strategies such as democratizing health institutions, as was envisioned with the creation of community health centers, foster increased civic participation and serve as a health improvement strategy.

A quality health care system and community prevention are mutually supportive and constitute a health system. While health care and community prevention are often thought of as separate domains and operate independently, they actually are synergistic. Health care institutions have critical roles to play in ensuring an emphasis on health within communities as a key part of the solution. Health services must recognize that the community locale is an essential place for service provision, for example, by expanding community clinics, providing school health services, and giving immunizations in supermarkets. An effective health care institution will also provide broad preventive services, such as screening and disease management that address populations at risk and those that already have illnesses.

Health care also has a role to play in improving community environments. It is one of the nation's largest industries and is often the largest employer in a low-income community. As such, health care institutions can support pipeline development to recruit, train, and hire people from the community, especially from underserved sectors. They can also advocate for community changes that will positively impact disease management, such as healthier eating and increased activity; improve the local economy by purchasing local products; create a farm-to-institution program to incorporate fresh, local produce and other foods into cafeteria or patient meals; reduce waste and close incinerators to reduce local pollution; and enhance staff and community access to fresh produce by establishing accessible farmers' markets or farm-stand programs. For example, Kaiser Permanente, the nation's largest HMO, has instituted farmers' markets in some of the communities it serves, providing healthy options for the residents, offering a needed place to purchase quality food, and strengthening the nearby local farms.

Equally, community prevention efforts should be a part of the strategy to foster health and reduce health disparities by improving the success of treatment and injury/disease management even after people get sick or injured. Illnesses such as diabetes, cardiovascular disease, HIV/AIDS, and cancer require patients to do what the medical practitioner requests, such as eat healthy foods and be more active. It is important for health care institutions to recognize the ways in which poverty and other social structures impede a patient's ability to follow a doctor's recommendations. Disenfranchised people usually don't have safe places to walk or healthful food to eat. Overwhelmed with the requirements of work and daily life and coping with transportation and child-care issues, poor people can have more obstacles to keeping medical appointments as well. With community prevention efforts bolstering neighborhood environments and support structures, disease management strategies will be more effective.

Challenges and Opportunities to Achieving Health Equity Through Practice and Policy

Achieving equitable outcomes is challenging and will take concerted attention, leadership, and investment. The following challenges and opportunities are based on interviews with local health officers that informed the development of *Health Equity and Prevention Primer* (Prevention Institute, 2008) funded by the Robert Wood Johnson Foundation as part of the project Advancing Public Health Advocacy to Eliminate Health Disparities. Pinpointing specific challenges and opportunities is key to shaping responsive solutions.

Challenges

1. We haven't embraced the problem of health inequities at its roots.
We need to recognize that health inequities are rooted in historical policies and practices and are entrenched in social structures that create barriers to opportunity. This legacy remains invisible to many health care practitioners, policymakers, and the public. Practitioners and community spokespersons need to talk about race and social justice in new ways and often need guidance to do so effectively.

2. We don't have a good playbook for how to do this.
The people and institutions working for reform need more guidance and information in order to identify and realize the most effective, sustainable changes. They often lack standardized, comparative data; documented examples of success; protocols for adaptation, with attention to fidelity of core elements; a set of best practices; a framework to measure outcomes and successes; and clear goals for the community.

The roles of different players are not well defined. Many health issues can be traced to determinants that cross over into other public sectors, such as housing. Public health practitioners have indicated a need for guidance on strategies where public health can take the lead (Prevention Institute, 2008). Further, they don't always know how to coordinate with leadership in other sectors such as housing. In most cases, the charge to address health equity will require public health practitioners to step outside of the contemporary bounds of public health, but this will mean establishing effective communication channels, navigating turf issues, and clarifying shared goals and objectives.

Also, the role of other institutions needs clarification as part of a coherent effort. Banks, businesses, multiple government sectors, schools, and community groups all have a major influence on health equity outcomes, even though they may not realize it or consider it in their decision-making processes. While these players may not see themselves as having an active role, none should be taking actions that are detrimental to health outcomes.

3. A siloed system leads to a fragmented approach at best.

Even if there were a shared understanding of the root of health inequities, sectors are siloed without a mechanism to work collaboratively to provide a coherent, effective set of solutions. By and large, there is a lack of coordination and cross-fertilization across sectors, efforts, and disciplines (Prevention Institute, 2008). This is critical to address, because reducing health inequities cannot be achieved by any one organization or sector, let alone any single department or division within public health.

Not only are sectors siloed, but the health system itself is siloed. Even within public health departments, opportunities to create meaningful collaboration across divisions, sections, or departments are limited. Categorical funding—important because it provides dedicated resources to deliver essential programs and services—can reinforce siloed approaches. There is even a divide between public health and health care; the two don't work together systematically and strategically to catalyze, advocate for, and launch the kinds of solutions that can make a fundamental difference. Finally, community members are not consistently included in prioritizing problems or in shaping solutions.

4. Community-based, family-centered primary care is not a medical emphasis.

Medical reimbursement, prestige, and medical education norms can all favor specialization over community-based, family-centered primary care. Furthermore, there is a lack of value and incentive placed on allied health professionals, promotoras (i.e., community health workers), and patient navigators. We also need to incentivize preventive services and better train medical providers in prevention.

5. Disparities in health care are not an organizational priority for many U.S. hospitals.

Many hospitals consider disparities in care as a function of conditions beyond their control. They may be reluctant to openly address "disparities" collaboratively, because this might be viewed as an admission of inequitable care (Siegel et al., 2007). Often providers assume they administer equal care since it is their mission. Stratifying their publicly reported quality measures by patient race and ethnicity would be one way to confirm their assumption or identify areas for quality improvement work.

6. Health equity isn't embedded in most people's job descriptions; there are many competing demands.
Research and practice in equitable outcomes tend to occur either as a small part of one's job or as a specialty focus of a small group of experts within an organization. The challenge here is how to embed health equity into research and practice across and within organizations, bringing these efforts to scale, infusing them into the broader organizational culture, and propelling them to center stage.

Opportunities

1. Health reform can be leveraged.
The Affordable Care Act includes a number of provisions that support a focus on underlying determinants of health and health equity, including the creation of a Community Transformation Grant program and the development of a National Prevention and Health Promotion Strategy. As health reform moves into implementation, it is critical that we highlight opportunities in all parts of the bill to connect clinical and community efforts and to focus on underlying determinants of health. The economic case for community-oriented prevention is solid (TFAH, PI, UI, and NYAM, 2008). With a growing awareness of community conditions for health, of tools that help make the case for addressing the underlying causes of health inequities (e.g., the PBS documentary series, *Unnatural Causes: Is Inequality Making Us Sick?*), and of the role of culturally appropriate, family-centered primary care, the pieces are in place to inform a more equitable, health-producing health system that is sustainable for all. To reduce inequities in health and safety, health reform implementation will need to maintain or increase investment in community-level prevention to decrease the number of people getting sick and injured; shift the emphasis from delivery of services (quantity) to improved health and safety (quality), particularly for vulnerable populations; reimburse for health care services, including preventive health care services that are delivered in communities; and ensure that system redesign enables the delivery of high-quality, culturally appropriate health care services for all.

2. It makes a lot of sense to focus at the state and local levels to address inequities.
Over the past several decades, there has been a general shift toward moving social programs from federal to state governments—a "devolution of authority." Although federal initiatives provided the catalyst for health disparities to emerge as a public health issue, states are now poised to build on this opportunity and take the lead in sponsoring social programs that help reduce inequities. States are seen as a key place for health reform (Prevention Institute, 2008). Numerous health departments

are engaging in efforts to advance health equity in communities large and small, urban and rural (Prevention Institute, 2008). In some cases, departments are deeply engaged in equity-focused work and are creating organizational structures and processes to focus specifically on health equity. In other cases, departments are engaged in supportive ways, sharing resources and information with community-based organizations that are providing more of the leadership and energy behind equity efforts. Many health departments are in an exploratory phase, examining internal interest and opportunities for addressing health equity.

Focusing equity efforts at the state and local levels is promising because many of the social and economic health determinants can be acted upon at these levels. For example, a local health department seeking to ensure quality affordable housing can work with the local community development and housing agency to discuss proposed projects, provide data about their potential health impacts, and work with local residents to explore their needs and concerns. Commitment and optimism about health equity becoming a centerpiece of the public health agenda remains high within health departments as they strive to make the internal and external changes necessary to take on an equity-related focus. There remains a need to further coalesce and project a stronger community voice, though partnerships with community organizations and policymakers have proven successful (Prevention Institute, 2008).

3. Our ability to map, measure, and track is improving significantly.

Emerging technologies, coupled with new and expanding sources of data, are providing significant support in reducing health inequities. For instance, community-based organizations and public agencies are increasingly using maps to support social and economic change on a community level. Mapping is a powerful tool in two ways: (1) it makes patterns based on place much easier to identify and analyze and (2) it provides a visual way of communicating those patterns to a broad audience, quickly and dramatically (PolicyLink, 2001). Projects such as Healthy City in Los Angeles allow users with minimal technical skill to create a variety of maps that highlight patterns of community resources, community conditions (e.g., income level or air quality), and health and social outcomes (e.g., disease rates or high school graduation rates). These maps provide stark illustration of community issues and can be used as the focus of community decision making and organizing and as important evidence during advocacy campaigns.

There is a strong national trend toward using community-level health indicators and indicator data to monitor change over time, increase accountability among poli-cymakers, and engage communities in a dialog about local priorities. This movement is being supported by national institutions and resources, such as the Community Health Status Indicators Project, and implemented at regional and local levels. Well-selected community health indicators provide comparative data over time and are a step toward ensuring that actions are aligned with health interests, that the social determinants of health are monitored and acted upon, and that there is account-ability for improving community conditions. The process of selecting indicators and collecting data—in essence selecting what will be measured—is in itself valuable as a venue for developing community capacity, building partnerships, and engaging community members, along with representatives from the public and private sectors, in identifying, prioritizing, and setting benchmarks related to health and well-being. Prevention Institute conducted a review of more than ninety indicator reports and report cards for the study *Good Health Counts: A 21st Century Approach to Health and Community for California* (2007). This review revealed that success was achieved through both a carefully developed set of indicators that reflect the determinants of health within the community and a well-orchestrated, transparent process.

Movement toward the use of electronic medical records and shared data among hospitals also holds promise for examining differences in access and equity in hospitals and clinics. As hospitals and clinics move toward electronic systems, the capacity to analyze differences by race and ethnicity increases as does the potential to address issues of high rates of missing race/ethnicity data—a key parameter for establishing the presence of disparities. Taking appropriate steps to protect privacy, we can link this data to GIS mapping to yield powerful information about the impact of community environment on health.

4. What's good for our natural environment is good for our health.

The mounting concern over environmental degradation and the increased focus on prioritizing solutions have introduced an opportunity to align issues of health and health equity with those of the environment and improve both simultaneously. For instance, greenhouse gas emissions are bad for the environment generally, accelerate climate change, and also have direct repercussion on health (e.g., asthma rates). In our efforts to solve these challenges, we can build powerful partnerships and address health issues that might otherwise be diminished. Strategically improving the physical environment could reduce the number of people getting sick and injured in the first place as well as the severity of those diseases. In effect this could reduce the demand for health care services and the burden on the health care system, which has the potential to increase the accessibility and affordability of quality health care and reduce the ecological footprint of our health care institutions.

Shifting toward a more sustainable food system and altering our transportation systems to support public transportation, walking, and biking, are among the initiatives that hold multiple environmental and health benefits by virtue of reducing greenhouse gases and our dependence on fossil fuels while improving air quality and increasing physical activity. There is potential to engage in strategies that simultaneously improve environmental conditions and support the health of vulnerable populations. Policies and practices are needed to improve the environmental and health conditions of communities—including ensuring clean air and water; preserving agricultural lands; reducing exposure to toxins; and providing economic opportunity, quality housing, and safe streets. However, such work must be done cautiously. For instance, rises in gas prices without simultaneous expansion of public transportation may have a positive impact in terms of greenhouse gases but can have disastrous effects on low-income people who live in communities that have been designed around automobile travel and where access to employment and resources such as healthy food are contingent on driving. As another example, popular "cap and trade" policies need to be implemented with safeguards against high polluters moving into communities with limited political capital to oppose such moves.

5. Internal organizational diversity helps to move along an equity-focused health agenda.

Achieving greater diversity within the health professions has been identified as a key strategy for ensuring a culturally competent workforce. Greater diversity across all levels of an organization can seed new and creative strategies for tackling health inequities. A number of health organizations are currently at the forefront of efforts to address health equity, and all these organizations—including health departments, health care organizations, and community-based organizations—have the opportunity to increase the diversity of their staffs. Diversity goes beyond racial and ethnic diversity to include factors such as age, gender, socioeconomic status, sexual preference, and professional skills. Ways to build and sustain diverse leadership include proactive efforts to recruit, hire, train, and retain staff that will contribute to diversity (Prevention Institute, 2008). Many organizations explicitly looking to address health equity have found that workforce development strategies can build the capacities of current staff and attract skilled and committed individuals to partake in the mission to achieve health equity. Organizations, as a result, seed new and creative ideas for tackling health inequities.

Local Solutions for Advancing Equity in Health and Safety

Community Solutions

Strengthen communities where people live, work, play, socialize, and learn.

C1 Build the capacity of community members and organizations. Capacity building enables the residents and grassroots groups affected by poor health outcomes to better solve the community problems undermining health and safety. Strategies include:

- Train public sector staff to encourage local capacity building and to empower residents to take action in partnership with city and county governments and community-based organizations to improve their neighborhood conditions.
- Invest in both established and developing community organizations. Encourage and strengthen the capacity of these and other institutions and of individuals via financial support, technical assistance, and sharing best practices.
- Foster structured community planning and prioritization efforts to implement neighborhood-level strategies to address unfavorable social conditions.

C2 Instill health and safety considerations into land use and planning decisions. Land use, transportation, and community design (the built environment) influence health, including physical activity, nutrition, substance abuse, injuries, mental health, violence, and environmental quality. Strategies include:

- Ensure that health, safety, and health equity are accounted for in General Plans, Master Plans, or Specific Plans; zoning codes; development projects; and land-use policies.
- Engage community residents in developing zoning laws and general plans to integrate health and equity goals and criteria into community design efforts.
- Train public health and health care practitioners to understand land use and planning and to advocate for policies that support health and safety.

C3 Improve safety and accessibility of public transportation, walking, and bicycling. Transportation is the means to accessing key destinations such as schools, workplaces, hospitals, and retail venues. Shifting the dominant mode of transportation from driving to greater public transportation use, walking, and/or bicycling is a key step to increasing physical activity, reducing traffic injuries, and reducing developmental and respiratory illnesses from poor air quality. Strategies include:

- Implement land-use strategies such as high-density, mixed-use zoning, transit-oriented development, and interconnected streets that promote walking and bicycling as a means of transportation.
- Adopt complete streets policies in state and local transportation departments to ensure that roads are designed for the safety of all travelers including pedestrians, bicyclists, wheelchairs, and motor vehicles.
- Ensure that public transportation options are safe, easily accessible, reliable, and affordable.
- Design public transit routes to connect community residents to grocery stores, health care, and other essential services.
- Prioritize federal transit funding toward biking, walking, and public transportation.

C4 Enhance opportunities for physical activity. Home, school, and community environments can either promote or inhibit physical activity. Physical activity is essential to preventing chronic illnesses and promoting physical and mental health. It is imperative to establish a foundation of activity behaviors from an early age and to provide environments with access to parks, open space, and recreational facilities that support people in attaining the daily recommended levels of physical activity (Active Living Research, 2005). Strategies include:

- Develop and promote safe venues and programming for active recreation. Ensure parks, playgrounds, and playing fields are equitably distributed throughout the community.
- Facilitate after-hour (joint) use of school grounds and gyms to improve community access to physical activity facilities.

- Require recess and adopt physical education policies to ensure all students engage in developmentally appropriate moderate-to-vigorous physical activity on a daily basis.
- Establish state licensing and accreditation requirements/health codes and support implementation of minimum daily minutes of physical activity in after-school programs and child-care settings.

C5 Enhance availability of healthy products and reduce exposure to unhealthy products in underserved communities. The food retail environment of a neighborhood—the presence of grocery stores, small markets, street vendors, local restaurants, and farmers' markets—plays a key role in determining access to healthy foods. Communities of color and low-wealth neighborhoods are most often affected by poor access to healthful foods (Larson, Story, and Nelson, 2009). Research suggests that the scarcity of healthy foods makes it more difficult for residents of low-income neighborhoods to follow a good diet compared with people in wealthier communities (Sloane et al., 2003). Strategies include:

- Invest in Fresh Food Financing Initiatives to provide grants, low-interest loans, training, and technical assistance to improve or establish grocery stores, small stores, and farmers' markets in underserved areas.
- Encourage neighborhood stores to carry healthy products and reduce shelf space for unhealthy foods through local tax incentives, streamlined permitting, and zoning variances.
- Ensure grocery stores, small stores, and farmers' markets are equipped to accept Supplemental Nutrition Assistance Program (SNAP) (formally known as the Food Stamp Program) and Special Supplemental Nutrition Program for Women, Infants, and Children (WIC) benefits.
- Establish and enforce regulations to restrict the number of liquor stores and their hours of operation.

C6 Support healthy food systems and the health and well-being of farmers and farmworkers. What farms grow, how they grow it, and how it gets to the consumer have a profound impact on what we eat, on our health, and on our environment. U.S. farm policy and agricultural research and education have contributed to the proliferation of industrial farms that grow grains, oil seeds, corn, meat, and poultry that serve as raw ingredients for cheap soda, fast food burgers, and other highly processed products. These industrial farms pollute the air, water, and soil while harming our nutritional health. Small- and mid-size farmers are struggling to make a living under the current system. Farmers of color face discrimination in access to loans. Farmworkers are exposed to hazardous levels of pesticides (Reeves, Katten, and Guzman, 2002), dangerous working conditions, and poor wages and living conditions. Strategies include:

- Support small- and mid-sized farmers, particularly farmers of color, immigrants, and women through grants, technical assistance, and help with land acquisition, marketing, and distribution.
- Establish incentives and resources for growers to produce healthy products, including fruits, vegetables, and foods produced without pesticides, hormones, or nontherapeutic antibiotics.
- Establish policies that support the health and well-being of farmworkers, including enforcing occupational safety and health laws and regulations as well as banning pesticides that may pose health risks. Government entities can also facilitate wage increases for farmworkers by providing grants and incentives for growers to engage in labor-sharing strategies with other growers.

C7 Increase housing quality, affordability, stability, and proximity to resources. High-quality, affordable, stable housing located close to resources leads to reduced exposure to toxins and stress, stronger relationships and willingness to act collectively among neighbors, greater economic security for families, and increased access to services (including health care) and resources (such as parks and supermarkets) that influence health. Strategies include:

- Support transit-oriented development and other policies and zoning practices that incentivize density, mixed-use, and mixed-income development.
- Ensure that housing standards; building permits for new buildings and rehabilitation; and housing inspections include safety and health considerations regarding design, the use of materials, and construction requirements.
- Protect affordable housing stock via rent control laws and condominium conversion policies, increase funding for emergency housing assistance, and maintain single-room-occupancy hotels.
- Support home ownership by creating community land trusts, increasing funds for and utilization of first-time home buyer programs, and establishing inclusionary zoning ordinances.

C8 Improve air, water, and soil quality. Environmental toxins present in air, water, soil, and building materials, including lead in soil and buildings, air pollution from motor vehicle traffic, and water pollutants, such as oil and human waste, have a substantial effect on health. Strategies include:

- Minimize diesel trucks in residential neighborhoods to reduce exposure to diesel particulates.
- Expand monitoring of air and water quality for impact on low-income and vulnerable populations.
- Enforce national water quality standards.
- Strengthen penalties for industrial and agricultural polluters.

- Replicate effective local lead abatement programs.
- Require public health input on air and water pollution impacts in local land use planning and development decisions.

C9 Prevent violence using a public health framework. Violence contributes to premature morbidity and mortality and is a barrier to health-promoting activities, such as physical activity, and to economic development. Strategies include:

- Invest in citywide, cross-sector planning and implementation with an emphasis on coordinating services (Weiss, 2008), programming, and capacity building in the most highly impacted neighborhoods, drawing on such tools as the UNITY RoadMap (Prevention Institute, 2008).
- Support local intervention models to reduce the immediate threat of violence, such as the Chicago CeaseFire model (Skogan, Hartnett, Bump, and Dubois, 2008).
- Institute changes in clinical and organizational practices in health care settings to support and reinforce community efforts to prevent intimate partner violence, which results in injury and trauma from abuse, contributes to a number of chronic health problems (Family Violence Prevention Fund, n.d., *The Facts on Health Care and Domestic Violence*) and disproportionately impacts immigrant women ("The Facts on Immigrant Women and Domestic Violence," Family Violence Prevention Fund, n.d., *The Facts on Immigrant Women and Domestic Violence*; Salber and Taliaferro, 2006).

C10 Provide arts and culture opportunities in the community. Artistic and cultural institutions have been linked with lower delinquency and truancy rates in several urban communities (Stern and Seifert, 2000), and participation in the arts has been associated with academic achievement, election to class office, school attendance (Heath et al., 1998), appropriate expression of anger, effective communication, increased ability to work on tasks, less engagement in delinquent behavior, fewer court referrals, improved attitudes and self-esteem, greater self-efficacy, and greater resistance to peer pressure (Catterall, 1997). Strategies include:

- Support community art centers and other opportunities for creativity in the community.
- Integrate art and creative opportunities into existing programs and businesses.
- House art commissions within state or city government.
- Work with large art institutions, local policymakers, and residents to bring "Big Art" (e.g., museums and orchestras) to low- and middle-income communities.
- Implement a policy to receive a portion of every ticket sold in the community for movies, sporting events, etc. as an alternate source of funding for arts and culture. Another funding mechanism involves redirecting a portion of hotel and car rental taxes, since art contributes to enhancing the community.

Health Care Service Solutions

Enhance opportunities within underserved communities to access high-quality, culturally competent health care with an emphasis on community-oriented and preventive services.

HC1 Implement and extend health reform efforts in order to provide high-quality, affordable health coverage for all. Everyone, including the most vulnerable populations, should have equal access to health care, including health care, dental, vision, and mental health services. There currently are a disproportionate number of racial and ethnic minorities who either do not have any health insurance or are enrolled in "lower-end" health plans (Smedley et al., 2003) and this could persist after ACA implementation. Strategies include:

- Equalize access to high-quality health plans to limit fragmentation of health care services. For example, Medicaid beneficiaries should be able to access the same health services as privately insured patients (Smedley et al., 2003).
- Ensure that all eligible children and families enroll in and access the State Children's Health Insurance Program (SCHIP).
- Support safety net hospitals through state insurance coverage and state and local subsidies (Smedley, 2008).
- Ensure equitable support for dental and mental health services.
- Improve access through equitable and fair sharing of health care costs; streamline public health insurance enrollment and increase affordability of services within existing public programs, such as Medicaid; evaluate outreach to and enrollment of underserved populations; and support state and local legislative proposals for universal access to quality health care.

HC2 Institute culturally and linguistically appropriate screening, counseling, and health care treatment. Culture shapes beliefs, behavior, and expectations surrounding health and health care. Physicians and other health care providers should deliver quality services in a culturally competent and sensitive manner. This approach can increase patient satisfaction, patient adherence to treatment plans, and the probability of improved health outcomes. Strategies include:

- Adopt standards of practice that are sensitive to the language and cultural needs of all patients.
- Provide training for providers to conduct screening, counseling, and treatment in both a culturally appropriate and sensitive manner.
- Promote culturally and linguistically appropriate screening programs for specific populations, such as Asian women for cervical cancer and other targeted groups for breast and cervical cancer.
- Ensure an effective communication strategy that takes into account the patient's health literacy and preferred language.
- Ensure patient-system concordance (i.e., a setting of care delivery that optimizes patient adherence and a sense of security and safety).

HC3 Monitor health care models/procedures that are effective in reducing inequities in health and data documenting racial and ethnic differences in care outcomes. Detailed documentation of health care models/procedures will delineate the key elements of success. Currently, hospital practices for data collection vary widely as do the racial and ethnic classifications used. Strategies include:

- Standardize data: collect race and ethnicity data in all health institutions. Coordinate state standards for data collection on race and ethnicity with federal standards to track the health of minorities (Trivedi et al., 2005). Although it may be difficult to use data to compare institution-to-institution, hospitals can use it to identify existing disparities in care and track trends for different patient populations within a hospital.
- Coordinate data collection and data systems beyond individual institutions and the health care system: multiple partners from various sectors should be involved in outreach to different populations. For example, when addressing asthma management, school systems would be able to reach out to a broad range of school-aged children. Public health can play a key role in coordinating data collection at the community level and comparing it across systems.
- Disaggregate the data: ensure that data reflects differences within the broad categories of race and ethnicity (particularly among Latino and Asian/Pacific Islander populations), as well as income levels, and duration of residence in the United States. Adopt uniform patient classifications in health information technology to make quality analysis easier and quicker. Analysis should be included in quality improvement initiatives.
- Incorporate new accreditation standards and mandates that account for equitable health care.
- Apply emerging data practices to better determine what medical procedures are most effective for different populations. (One size does not necessarily fit all.) Explore the Expecting Success disparities collaborative as one such example. Upon submission of their LOI, although the majority (97 percent) of the 122 hospitals were collecting patient race and ethnicity data, almost none reported using the data for quality improvement purposes at that time. Currently, they are among the most likely to have begun using quality data to reduce inequities in care (Siegel et al., 2007).

HC4 Take advantage of emerging technology to support patient care. Recent advances in health care technology can strengthen medical treatment. To the extent that technology is used as an element of quality health care, it's important to ensure that these advances fully benefit everyone. Cell phones are one area where there is a high degree of market penetration among all groups and so we should capture their potential to support medical treatment so as not to exacerbate disparities. When technology is not equally available (e.g., computers in every home), alternatives should be provided that are efficacious. Strategies include:

- Institute electronic health records that protect privacy but ensure caregivers have all needed information.
- Use telephone and e-mail reminders to increase frequency of appointments and testing compliance, reduce failure to take pills, and encourage following procedures.
- Make tailored health information easily accessible and responsive.

HC5 Provide health care resources in the heart of the community. Strengthening the presence of health care services located in communities of high need reinforces the connection between health care and community and can remove pervasive access barriers such as inadequate transportation options or not being able to seek health care during traditional working hours. Strategies include:

- Support community-based clinics. Clinics have an essential role in improving community health and providing services for uninsured and underserved populations. Clinics should establish organizational practices to increase access to equitable health care. Health reform funds designated for community-based clinics should be used both to expand services and also to expand the role of the clinic as a hub for community health (e.g., development of intersectoral partnerships to work on issues affecting health such as housing and transportation).
- Expand availability of school-based health clinics.
- Provide support groups that enhance self-efficacy in engaging in healthy behaviors.
- Provide culturally appropriate care such as translation services, disease prevention counseling, advocacy for quality health care, and other services to patients directly in the community, not just in health care settings.
- Expand the use of community health workers. Reforming reimbursement is essential, including state grants and seed funding as resources (Smedley, 2008).
- Change the available work hours and locations to meet the needs of patients.

HC6 Promote a medical home model. Having a designated health provider for every patient and, ideally, every family has enormous benefits. Primary care becomes more accessible, continuous, comprehensive, family-centered, coordinated, compassionate, and culturally effective. Patient-centered care is given within a community and cultural context. In 2007, the American Academy of Family Physicians, American Academy of Pediatrics, American College of Physicians, and American Osteopathic Association released the Joint Principles of the Patient-Centered Medical Home. Far fewer people of color have a medical home, which is strongly associated with prevention, screening, and specialty care referral (Beal et al., 2007). Strategies include:

- Design interventions to incorporate detection, prevention, and management of chronic disease with full deployment of multidisciplinary teams that are family- and patient-centered.

HC7 Strengthen the diversity of the health care workforce to ensure that it is reflective and inclusive of the communities it is serving. The diversity of health care professionals is associated with increased access to and satisfaction of care among patients of color. States can adopt strategies such as loan repayment programs and service grants, health profession pipeline programs, and other incentives for service (Smedley, 2008). Strategies include:

- Train clinic providers to conduct culturally appropriate outreach and services.
- Address the imbalance of health care providers by offering incentives to work in underserved communities (Smedley, 2008). States could provide incentives that include funding graduate medical programs focusing on underserved populations, tuition reimbursement, and loan forgiveness programs that require service in Health Professional Shortage Areas (HPSAs).
- Expand use of Community Health Workers (CHWs) as a means of diversification. By acting as health connectors for populations that have traditionally lacked access to adequate health care, CHWs meet the ever-changing health needs of a growing and diverse population. Their unique ties to the communities where they work allow CHWs to understand cultural and linguistic needs and provide a resource for populations that are not necessarily connected or trusting of the health care system.

HC8 Ensure participation by patients and the community in health care–related decisions. Research suggests that the consistency and stability of the relationship between patient and doctor is an important determinant of patient satisfaction and access to care. However, people of color are less likely to have a consistent relationship with a provider, even when insured at the same levels as white patients (Smedley et al., 2003). Strategies include:

- Develop and strengthen patient education programs to help patients navigate the health care system (Smedley, 2008).
- Promote community health planning, which actively involves community residents in planning, evaluation, and implementation of health care efforts (Smedley, 2008).

HC9 Enhance quality of care by improving availability and affordability of critical prevention services. Access to culturally competent, accessible clinical preventative services is a key ingredient to keeping people healthy. Examples include:

- Immunizations of children, adults, and seniors
- Regular monitoring of children's growth
- Assessment of prevention and safety behaviors (e.g., alcohol, tobacco, gun use; vehicle safety devices; family violence; risks including guns, STDs)
- Medical testing and screening
- Patient education, counseling, and referrals (e.g., smoking cessation, dietary counseling, and physical activity programs)
- Oral health, a key element of health care that is too often overlooked

HC10 Provide outspoken support for environmental policy change and resources for prevention. In order to reduce racial and ethnic disparities, public policies and practices must address factors beyond health care services that impact health outcomes and disparities, specifically the community recommendations in this document. Strategies include:

- Advocate for community changes that will improve health outcomes and support disease management by speaking up in the media, community, and political environments and within health care institutions and associations and the broader health care community.
- Support pipeline development to recruit, train, and hire people from the community, especially from underserved sectors.
- Reduce waste and close incinerators to reduce local pollution.
- Purchase products and services from local businesses and organizations, such as food from nearby farms.
- Be attentive to community impact (e.g., reducing noise and emphasizing public transportation).

Systems Solutions

Strengthen the health system infrastructure to reduce inequities and enhance the contributions from public health and health care systems.

S1 Enhance leadership and strategy development to reduce inequities in health and safety outcomes. High-level leadership at state and local levels and clear strategic direction are essential to achieving equitable health outcomes. Strategies include:

- Engage civic leadership at the highest levels (e.g., mayors and governors) to coalesce influential partners, establish the priority of reducing inequities, ensure accountability, and use the bully pulpit to elevate the problem and solutions.
- Develop local and state plans that clarify what prioritized actions will be taken in order to achieve health equity.

S2 Enhance information about the problem and solutions at the state and local levels. A central challenge of twenty-first-century American health policy is to characterize the powerful relationship between social inequities and health inequities and to identify comprehensive multidisciplinary community-level interventions that systematically reduce social inequity. Strategies include:

- Develop, test, and disseminate new tools such as Connecticut's Health Equity Index, BARHII's social gradient analyses, San Francisco's Healthy Development Measurement Tool, and other innovative tools that integrate information from varied domains to illuminate relationships between social measures and health status.

- Invest in better communicating the problem so that the general public and potential partners understand the underlying contributors to disparities and can evaluate the broader elements and potential solutions (e.g., the PBS documentary series, *Unnatural Causes: Is Inequality Making Us Sick?*).

S3 Establish sustainable funding mechanisms to support community health and prevention. Prevention rarely rises to the level of urgency that would support adequate funding, because public budgets remain in crisis mode and the payoff from prevention comes two or five or ten years down the road. Strategies include:

- Educate the broad public about the cost savings of health care and government investments in prevention.
- Create a wellness trust to collect, manage, and expend prevention funding, including indexing prevention to health care costs.
- Reinvest prevention savings in further prevention efforts.

S4 Build the capacity of state and local health agencies to understand and lead population-based health equity work. Having a public health workforce that is equipped to address issues of health equity and to convene key partners is a critical component of success. Public health practitioners have expressed an eagerness to address health equity and social justice along with awareness that organizational support and staff capacity are crucial to moving this forward (Prevention Institute, 2008). Strategies include:

- Build the capacity of health departments to address issues of equity, including retraining and repooling of all staff working in public health and health service to have a solid grounding in the social determinants of health, health equity, and how to work with diverse sectors.
- Recruit and build a diverse health workforce reflective of underserved communities: institute health equity studies in public health graduate programs; emphasize community-based equity work as a core public health competency and hiring criteria; build a diverse leadership team that includes people most affected; and develop pathways and pipelines for public health professionals to move from community-based equity work into leadership positions.
- Bolster Offices of Minority Health to support multiple sectors/efforts by serving as convener and coordinator of work that spans multiple departments and agencies; providing data sets that help inform and track progress; providing information on most effective practices and solutions; developing policy solutions to be implemented by multiple sectors; and providing training and capacity building to support communities, public health, and other sectors to reduce inequities in health.

S5 Collaborate with multiple fields to ensure that health, safety, and health equity are considered in every relevant decision, action, and policy. Ensuring health in every policy will be essential in significantly improving health and safety outcomes and achieving health equity. Strategies include:

- Engage and coordinate the efforts of multiple sectors and diverse government agencies (e.g., business, labor, educators, public health, housing, transportation, environmental protection, and planning) to establish policies and efforts in support of health equity, including reducing barriers and improving incentives.
- Establish health and health equity impact/analyses: evaluate proposed policies and funding streams with a "health lens" to determine impact on health, safety, and equity and ensure that consideration of health equity runs through all practices and policies within health institutions and beyond.

S6 Expand community mapping and indicators. Community mapping and indicators are emerging techniques that provide the opportunity to have collective community dialogues, to define the elements that comprise a healthy community, to translate community priorities into data that can be monitored over time, and to aggregate inexpensive, compelling, easy-to-use evidence for community advocacy. Strategies include:

- Develop and provide necessary data sets.
- Provide technical assistance on the technology and advocacy potential of maps and in support of local indicator projects.
- Establish standards and guidance for indicators and indicator reports to track improvements in inequities (i.e., the community characteristics and the health outcomes).
- Enhance state and local public health departments' ability to access electronic health records and data to facilitate timely public health surveillance, trend and outbreak detection, and geographical analysis to link environmental determinants to patterns of disease distribution.
- Link the mapping of medical conditions and community conditions to better assess their interplay and develop effective environmental solutions that reduce the incidence of these conditions (e.g., compare traffic injury data to neighborhoods or diabetes rates to supermarket locations).

S7 Provide technical assistance and tools to support community-level efforts to address determinants of health and reduce inequities.

- Provide access to tools and resources to assess and address the elements that can maximize health (e.g., indicators and report cards, maps, and community assessment tools).
- Provide access to high-quality, culturally appropriate technical assistance and training in planning, implementing, and evaluating.

Overarching Solutions

Support local efforts through leadership, overarching policies, and through local, state, and national strategy.

01 Develop a national strategy to promote health equity across racial, ethnic, and socioeconomic lines, with specific attention to preventing injury and illness in the first place. A national strategy could provide an overall framework and direction and set a clear expectation that reducing health inequities is a national priority. Although this chapter is about local efforts, there is a critical interplay of the local, state, and national, and thus we identify some of the national steps that must be taken in support of local approaches. Components of a national strategy should include:

- Establishing high-level leadership at the White House and the department level to serve as a focal point for strategy on health equity and to ensure collaboration among government agencies
- Building the capacity of federal, state, and local health agencies to lead health equity work
- Expanding funding for community-based initiatives
- Providing technical assistance and tools to support community-level efforts to address determinants of health, improve health care outcomes, and reduce disparities
- Supporting the development of national, state, and local data systems to inform community efforts, foster accountability, and build a stronger understanding of what it takes to achieve health equity
- Furthering research on and significantly expanding the amount and proportion of federal research dollars for population-based prevention and health equity, with an emphasis on translating the findings into targeted, community-specific strategies
- Fostering new leadership to advance health equity work and ensure that attention to achieving health equity is embedded into the priorities, practices, and policies of government entities, private organizations, the health care system, and communities

02 Provide federal resources to support state and local community-based prevention strategies. Strategies for federal health agencies (such as Health and Human Services, the Centers for Disease Control and Prevention, Health Resources Services Administration, and the National Institutes of Health) include:

- Build upon recently passed legislation to fund local public health agencies to craft local, flexibly designed community prevention strategies that are relevant to local conditions.
- Align existing strategies and policies with those of other federal agencies such as the Department of Education, Environmental Protection Agency, United States Department of Agriculture, Housing and Urban Development, and Department of

Transportation so that states and local communities can leverage resources and efforts.

• Grant regulatory waivers to states seeking to create financial incentives for community-based prevention efforts that reduce health care costs.

• Reimburse such strategies as fall prevention for seniors, nursing home visitation for high-risk infants, asthma environmental risk reduction initiatives, diabetes peer counseling, promotoras programs, and other proven and promising community-based prevention efforts.

O3 Tackle the inequitable distribution of power, money, and resources—the structural drivers of the conditions of daily life that contribute to inequitable health and safety outcomes—and especially address race, racism, and discrimination in institutions and polices; racial and socioeconomic segregation; and socioeconomic conditions. Poverty, racism, and lack of educational and economic opportunities are among the fundamental determinants of poor health, lack of safety, and health inequities. Strategies include:

• Assess institutional policies and practices for race, racism, and discrimination—including holding discussions about race and racism within institutions—and modify practices and policies accordingly.

• Conduct a comprehensive review of policies and practices that contribute to racial and socioeconomic segregation, delineate recommended policies to reverse segregation, and include attention to demonstrated promising strategies to reverse residential segregation.

• Improve socioeconomic conditions by (1) raising incomes of the poor, especially those with children (increase enrollment in income support programs; raise the state minimum wage; implement local living wage ordinances); (2) assisting poor people in accumulating assets (provide education and financial counseling to increase access to savings accounts and investment programs; expand home ownership and microenterprise opportunities); and (3) supporting job creation and workforce development (negotiate community benefits agreements; preserve industrial land for well-paid jobs; expand local green-collar jobs; increase access to education, training, and career ladders; fund job readiness and skill-building programs).

• Reform criminal justice laws to address disproportionate incarceration rates for African Americans, Latinos, and low-income people such as by decriminalizing addiction and implementing community programs for drug offenders in lieu of prison; supporting mental health treatment for those in need, including those with post-traumatic stress disorder; and supporting effective reentry programs.

O4 Improve access to quality education and improve educational outcomes. Educational attainment is one of the strongest predictors of income, and there is a strong relationship between income and health (Freudenberg and Ruglis, 2007; Ross and Mirowsky, 1999). Even independent from income, education is associated with improved health outcomes: each additional year in school correlates to increased life expectancy and better health (Lleras-Muney, 2005). Strategies include:

- Reform school funding to equalize access to quality education in K–12, including providing equal access to technology to develop job readiness for twenty-first-century jobs.
- Invest in recruiting, training, and retaining teachers, particularly to work in disadvantaged schools, and create incentives for teachers to remain in these schools.
- Provide need-based supports to schools, students, and parents—including positive interventions for at-risk middle and high school students and creating greater support for low-income parents of color to participate in their child's education.

05 Invest in early childhood. During the first five years of life, every encounter a child has or lacks is formative. For healthy development, young children need a range of supports, social and emotional care, and nurturing (Consultative Group on Early Childhood Care and Development, n.d.). Strategies include:

- Provide high-quality and affordable child care and preschools; ensure equitable distribution of and access to preschools and provide subsidies.
- Invest in home visiting initiatives such as the Nurse-Family Partnership.
- Invest in recruiting, training, and retaining child-care providers.

Conclusion: A Time of Opportunity

As interviews with public health leaders confirm, this is a time of opportunity. Nationally, health and health care have emerged as major economic issues and top priorities. There is growing understanding of the importance of healthy communities, the influence of their underlying health determinants, and of the role of culturally appropriate, family-centered primary care in accomplishing health equity.

Over the past several decades, there has been a general shift toward moving social programs from federal to state governments—a "devolution of authority." Although federal initiatives provided the catalyst for health disparities to emerge as a public health issue, states are now poised to build on this opportunity and take the lead in sponsoring policies and social programs that help reduce inequities. States are seen as a key place for health reform (Smedley, 2008) and have significant roles and responsibilities in implementing the Affordable Care Act. Numerous health departments are engaging in efforts to advance health equity in communities large and small, urban and rural (Prevention Institute, 2008).

Focusing equity efforts at the state and local levels is promising because many of the social and economic health determinants can be acted upon at these levels. There is a strong national trend toward using community-level health indicators and indicator data to monitor change over time, increase accountability among policymakers, and engage communities in a dialogue about local priorities.

What's good for our health is good for our overall well-being. For example, the mounting concern over environmental degradation and the increased focus on prioritizing solutions have introduced an opportunity to align issues of health and health equity with those of the environment and improve both simultaneously. Health is not only a major issue in and of itself, but it aligns with many of the other major concerns of our society.

In real estate, there are only three things that matter—location, location, location. Our conclusion as authors is that policy is vital and changing our organizational practices is critical; and it all must be done in service of people, where they live, work, play, socialize, and learn. In other words—community, community, community.

Key Terms

Community health factors

Determinants of health

Health disparities

Health equity

Health inequities

Institutional practices

Discussion Questions

1. How are a quality health care system and community prevention mutually supportive?
2. Why is a multisectoral approach to health critical for addressing health inequities?
3. How have organizational practices and policies contributed to inequities in health and safety?
4. What are some local strategies and solutions for reducing inequities in health and safety?

CHAPTER 13

CHALLENGES IN THE NEW WORLD OF PUBLIC HEALTH PRACTICE

LEARNING OBJECTIVES

- Describe the complex problems challenging public health organizations
- Discuss the value of evidence-based public health practice
- List examples of global initiatives to improve public health
- Identify some goals for the future of public health practice

The status quo of poor health outcomes and social inequities is reinforced by beliefs that individuals are solely responsible for making unhealthy choices, that life is not fair and health and wealth disparities are just part of life, and that nothing short of a revolution can be done to change these conditions (Rogow, Adelman, Poulain, and Cheng, 2008). Moving beyond these limiting concepts is our common challenge and one that we can meet by reframing the health dialogue into questions about how we put an end to dangerous conditions, create healthy places and spaces, and help communities organize and build partnerships that create and sustain policies protecting the public good in regard to health (Rogow et al., 2008). Reducing community populations' vulnerability to significant threats to health by planning and implementing evidence-based global and local public health strategies will require a redesign of current public health services to ensure a primary focus on population-centered prevention policies, programs, and actions. Evidence-based public health strategies are interventions that have been evaluated and determined to improve health outcomes. The increasing rates of chronic diseases, the effect of climate change on human health and the world ecosystem, and the long-term repercussions of human violence on countries and their populations are just some of the complex threats affecting the health of many communities and nations. Such complex health problems are best addressed by a public health system skilled at providing population-based health services based on the best available knowledge.

Determinants of Health

As the costs of health care in the United States continue to rise with little change in national health status and quality of health, questions have surfaced about what actions, programs, or policies create good health and how much is too much to pay for health care. Awareness is growing that health is about more than access to health care and that those at the bottom of the socioeconomic scale get sicker and die younger than those who are well employed and prospering. Studies of the increasing rates of health disparities point to racism as an added health burden, in part due to the stress of discrimination and the relegation of many people of color to lower socioeconomic status (SES), resulting in exclusion, feelings of hopelessness, and reduced access to health care (Rogow et al., 2008). Under these conditions the stress in people's lives is intensified along with levels of cortisol, a stress hormone. As observed by Stanford biologist Robert Sapolsky, living with a stress response for thirty years, even at a low level, will increase your risk for *every* chronic disease (California Newsreel, 2008).

Changing individual health behaviors by marketing healthier choices, such as eating more nutritious foods, has been the focus of many prevention programs in the field of public health. Within the local public health agency, government-funded programs emphasize health education as part of a medical visit. For instance, women seeking family planning services are counseled and educated about safe sex, folic acid, healthy diets, and the effects of tobacco use on health. However, an increasing number of public health practitioners are recognizing that choices people make are often shaped by the choices they have. New evidence demonstrates that the places where we live and work clearly affect our health (Wilson et al., 1998). People living in poorer communities often have limited choices, exemplified by the abundance of fast food chains, convenience marts, and liquor stores compared to the limited presence of grocery stores filled with fresh produce, fish, meat, and whole grain foods.

The status of economic, social, and built environments is a result of the decisions that a society has made in the form of government policies, and these decisions shape health. The characteristics of walkable and mixed-use neighborhoods (that is, neighborhoods with parks, businesses, homes, and stores or restaurants with healthy food choices) are related to an improved sense of community and social capital (Dearry, 2004). Unsafe neighborhoods with vacant buildings, limited space for recreation, damaged or nonexistent sidewalks, crime, fumes from motor vehicles, and other similar hazards are less walkable and have fewer possibilities for mixed use. The increased presence of hazards in poorer communities creates health inequities and reduces overall health status. Reducing inequality and implementing policies that protect all people from threats to their health, regardless of their economic status, skin color, or geographical location, are changes that we can make to ensure healthier outcomes and promote the public good (Rogow et al., 2008).

For many developing countries, the situation is much grimmer as people struggle to survive in the midst of civil war, as occurred in Rwanda in 1994 and El Salvador during the 1980s, or armed conflict with another nation—exemplified by the United States' war with Iraq starting in 2003 and the conflict between Pakistan and India from 1990 to 1992. People living in countries involved directly in armed conflict face the complete devastation of their infrastructure, a frequent consequence of war.

Modern-day health is also seriously affected by the economic interdependence and interconnectedness of today's world, which are transforming the spread of diseases and risk factors for poor health into much larger menaces for global communities. Countless opportunities exist for the rapid spread of communicable diseases, including the potential for outbreaks associated with the accidental or intentional release of infectious agents (World Health Organization [WHO], 2007). Worldwide export and import of consumer goods exposed to contaminants create an easy environment for the immediate disbursement of illness across the planet. The same can be said for humans exposed to microbial contamination or toxic agents who travel from country to country, potentially exposing thousands and more to new viruses, such as severe acute respiratory syndrome (SARS), or reemerging diseases, including multi-drug-resistant tuberculosis (MDR-TB) and extensively drug-resistant tuberculosis (XDR-TB). Over 120 different diseases, most including multiple cases, occur daily around the world and are tracked by HealthMap (http://healthmap.org/en). A sudden health crisis in China, for example, can easily spread to other parts of the world, as we witnessed with the deadly SARS outbreak in 2003 that sparked an international alert.

In 2009 an influenza pandemic was declared, and by 2010, 214 countries reported confirmed cases of H1N1, resulting in over eighteen thousand deaths. The particular H1N1 strain had never been seen in humans before, and, although it was not the fearsome event expected by many public health practitioners, its occurrence uncovered the lack of readiness for dealing with a potentially more deadly pathogen. In the presence of monumental medical advances over the past century, a new and highly contagious disease still has the potential to destroy populations and wreak havoc on social, economic, political, and legal structures around the world (Harmon, 2010). A new, virulent virus could kill millions, resulting in countries' closing their borders, which would affect global commerce and trade, and potentially abridging basic human rights to prevent the spread of the disease. This situation could last years as each changing season brings new surges of the disease (Harmon).

The World Health Organization (WHO, 2007, p. 5) has issued a call for action, proactive and reactive, "to minimize vulnerability to acute public health events that endanger the collective health of populations living across geographical regions and international borders." This effort is known as the *Global Public Health Security in the 21st Century*. WHO's call for worldwide health security recognizes that a sudden health crisis in one region of the world is now just hours away from threatening another part of the world. Chronic diseases have surfaced as a serious global health threat in the past few decades, attributed primarily to the exportation of the U.S. lifestyle to developing countries and other world economies. Armed conflicts around the world also contribute to the spread of disease, increased rates of violence both during and after wars, and economic disparities across countries. The rest of this chapter presents more detail on the major causes of disease and injury in the world today and calls upon public health practitioners to respond with population-centered public health approaches.

Obesity Epidemic

The **obesity epidemic** stems from the 1.1 billion overweight adults and 312 million obese people in the world (James, Rigby, Leach, International Obesity Task Force, 2004). The rates of obesity have doubled, possibly tripled, in less than two decades. When we consider children as a population, the rates are rising much more quickly in parts of Europe. The burden of disease from obesity is great—obesity is considered to be among the top five risk factors for poor health (James et al., 2004). In the United States about 68 percent of the population over the age of twenty is either overweight or obese (IOM, 2010a). Annual medical expenditures related to obesity have doubled in the last decade, estimated to be almost $147 billion per year (RTI International, 2009). More than 80 percent of people with type 2 diabetes are either overweight or obese. Being overweight increases the risk of heart disease. People who are overweight or obese are also at higher risk for hypertension or high blood pressure, greatly raising their risk of heart attack, stroke, and kidney failure. Obesity adversely affects metabolic or endocrine disorders, one of the fastest-growing obesity-related health concerns in the United States, creating current and future health problems for almost a quarter of the U.S. population—forty-seven million people. Childhood obesity rates continue to increase in the adolescent young population. Some experts predict that one-third of the children born in 2000 will develop obesity-related diabetes, and half of these cases will occur in Latino or African American communities (The Endocrine Society, 2009). Obese children suffer from lung, liver, heart, and musculoskeletal afflictions and also experience psychological problems.

Chronic, noncommunicable diseases are also increasing at disturbing rates in other countries (Hossain, Kawar, and El Nahas, 2007). Around the world, diabetes and hypertension are the major causes of eighteen million deaths each year from cardiovascular disease. The growing prevalence of overweightness and obesity over the past decade is the major contributor to the increases observed in diabetes and hypertension in developing countries that are already suffering from underweightness, malnutrition, and infectious diseases. Being poor in a very poor developing country where the annual income is less than eight hundred dollars a year per capita increases the likelihood of being underweight or malnourished, whereas being poor in a middle-income developing country, where the annual income is estimated at three thousand dollars per year, is associated with increased risk of obesity. In some developing countries parents are obese while children are underweight (Hossain et al.).

The tripling of obesity rates in developing counties is attributed to the adoption of a Western lifestyle, which results in decreased physical activity and overconsumption of inexpensive, energy-dense foods made available through fast food chains and processed foods suppliers. The biggest threats are to the Middle East, the Pacific Islands, Southeast Asia, and China. From 2 to 7 percent of total health care costs in developing countries are due to obesity (WHO, 2009).

The increased rates of diabetes will reach pandemic levels by 2030, affecting more than 220 million people (Hossain et al., 2007). The economies of developing countries can easily become overwhelmed by the increase in serious forms of cardiovascular disease and other health complications associated with obesity and diabetes at a time when they are still struggling to contain communicable diseases. In China alone, 92.4 million people are estimated to be diabetic, with another 148.2 million in the prediabetic state, a risk factor for developing type 2 diabetes and cardiovascular disease (Yang et al., 2010). Given its large population, China will most likely experience the greatest burden of diabetes compared to all other countries. An alarming factor for public health experts is the large proportion of Chinese who remain undiagnosed and, hence, untreated. China is expected to lose over $558 billion in income due to the presence of this illness in its population during the ten-year period from 2005 to 2015 (WHO, 2009).

Diabetes has become a major global health problem. Diabetes is preventable, but action is required to produce fundamental social and policy change, making healthy foods more affordable and available and expanding community-wide educational and informational campaigns coupled with increased opportunities for physical activity. WHO recently issued objectives for developing countries to improve the nutritional content of school meals and promote healthy living (Hossain et al., 2007). Some countries are now monitoring policies and programs that target obesity and poor nutrition. However, given the newness of such programs, few data are available on their costs and outcomes. Such initiatives are also expected to generate fierce opposition from food manufacturers and consumer groups that are opposed to any restrictions that affect civil liberties (Hossain et al.).

In the United States, the Centers for Disease Control and Prevention publishes evidence-based practices for increasing rates of physical activity and reducing obesity in the Guide to Community Preventive Services (Community Guide Branch, n.d.). Recommended practices for behavioral interventions to reduce screen time (TV, computers, and so on); multicomponent counseling or coaching to effect and maintain weight loss; and workplace wellness programs to prevent or control obesity and overweightness can be found in the Community Guide. In 2009 the Institute of Medicine reviewed what it believed to be the relevant information for community, environmental, and policy-based obesity prevention programs. The group found a clear evidence gap and developed the LEAD framework (**L**ocate evidence, **E**valuate it, **A**ssemble it, and inform **D**ecisions) to support innovative approaches to identify, evaluate, and build the evidence base using a broad, transdisciplinary approach—one that takes a systems perspective (IOM, 2010a).

WHO reports that simple lifestyle measures are known to effectively prevent or delay the onset of type 2 diabetes, such as achieving and maintaining healthy body weight; being physically active, getting at least thirty minutes of regular, moderate-intensity activity on most days; eating a healthy diet of between three and five servings of fruit and vegetables a day and reducing sugar and saturated fat intake; and avoiding tobacco use, which increases the risk of cardiovascular disease (WHO, 2009). However, as stated earlier, the choices people make are based on the choices they have, and policies are needed to ensure that all communities have access to healthy foods, safe areas for recreation, and community-wide efforts to promote and support healthier lifestyles.

Obesity is a complex, population-centered health problem. The IOM's goal in creating the LEAD framework is to provide guidance for gathering and compiling evidence in a transparent manner and in a real-world context. The process is an alternative to randomized experiments and focuses on learning from ongoing policies and practices that can be evaluated for effectiveness and then generalized to address the obesity epidemic on a county, state, national, or global scale (IOM, 2010a). The use of the LEAD framework by public health practitioners with decision-making responsibilities and their key partners, along with researchers working on obesity prevention and other complex public health issues, is an important initiative for understanding and disseminating information about which programs and policies effectively reduce obesity rates. Public health practitioners and decision makers will have the most relevant and accurate knowledge as they work to reverse the rates of obesity by applying the best available evidence and by planning interventions with a keen eye on the importance of measuring their progress and the effect of the planned changes on obesity outcomes. Examples of evidence-based public health interventions developed using the LEAD framework can be reviewed in the CDC's Guide to Community Preventive Services (Community Guide Branch, n.d.).

Climate Change

Climate change is any significant shift in climate, as measured by temperature, precipitation, wind, and storms, lasting decades or longer. According to the Centers for Disease Control and Prevention (CDC, 2011a), the world's climate is becoming warmer, and extremes in weather are more common. Climate change has the potential to create intense heat waves, heavy rain, severe and numerous droughts, air pollution, rising sea levels, and such extreme weather events as flooding, hurricanes, and tornadoes.

Climate and health are inextricably linked. The presence of some diseases and conditions that threaten our health are attributed to the climate in which we live. Heat causes hyperthermia, cold causes hypothermia, and droughts cause famine. Hurricanes, tornadoes, floods, and forest fires cause injuries, deaths, disruption, and relocation. Climate and weather affect the distribution and risk of vector-borne diseases, such as malaria or dengue fever (Frumkin et al., 2008). The effect on human health from global warming will be great; injuries and fatalities are expected to increase due to severe weather events, extremes of temperature and rainfall, the spread of vector-borne infectious diseases, respiratory problems related to pollution and poor air quality, and famine. Increased temperatures can result in a range of health effects, from mild heat rashes to deadly heat strokes. Heat increases ground-level ozone concentrations that cause lung injury and exacerbate such respiratory diseases as asthma and chronic obstructive pulmonary disease (COPD). Longer bouts of higher temperatures lead to drought and ecosystem changes, such as shifting migratory patterns of disease vectors that can be very deleterious to health. Agricultural products are significantly affected by drought conditions, creating food insecurity and increasing hunger.

Seas are expected to rise as a result of the warming atmosphere, and this will affect coastal communities, particularly in developing countries where resources are inadequate for protection from changes in sea levels. Climate change will also affect biodiversity and the goods and services from the ecosystem on which humans rely (Haines, Kovats, Campbell-Lendrum, Corvalan, 2006).

Global warming has become possibly the most complex issue facing the world today. Scientific evidence continues to mount concerning the increasing dangers from the buildup of greenhouse gasses. The world's climate has been warming primarily due to the buildup of greenhouse gasses in the atmosphere, which is attributed in great part to the burning of fossil fuels and deforestation. Evidence of warming is found in increased global average temperatures and ocean temperatures, extensive melting of snow and ice, and rising average global sea levels. Climate warming is expected to continue and accelerate—end-of-the-century projections for the overall increase in temperature approach 1.4°C to 5.8°C (2.5°F to 10.4°F) (Haines et al., 2006). Although the lower estimate of warming could be tolerated, increased temperatures of 10°F or more would result in disastrous long-term effects on ecosystems and economies.

Global warming has been linked to increased incidences of extreme weather, including more floods and more frequent and intense storms. Increases in natural disasters are expected to produce widespread psychological distress and increases in social disruption, physical problems, and psychological disorders, particularly among those who are most vulnerable, such as young children, older adults, impoverished communities, and those suffering from chronic conditions (Jenkins and Phillips, 2009). Mental health problems are expected to grow as more and more communities experience devastating storms and floods. Table 13.1, produced by the CDC, highlights the effects of climate on health.

Reducing global warming and reversing, or at least mitigating, its effects calls for a worldwide effort that addresses technological, economic, political, and social issues—a systems approach. The challenges of reaching a global treaty on global warming have proven to be overwhelming during the early part of the twenty-first century. The best we can achieve for the foreseeable future is a reduction in emissions and increased aid for developing countries to help them adapt to the effects of global warming and climate change. The concern for developing countries is centered on their lack of resources to defend against the effects of climate change, including rising sea levels, increased incidence and intensity of tropical storms, and the expansion of tropical diseases. In 2009 the world's leaders agreed upon a dangerous climate threshold, 1.3°F above the current average global temperature of 57°F, or no more than a 3.6°F–increase in temperature from the time of the Industrial Revolution (Baker, 2009). The

Table 13.1   Weather Events and Health Effects

Weather Event	Health Effects	Populations Most Affected
Heat waves	Heat stress	Extremes of age, athletes, people with respiratory disease
Extreme weather events (rain, hurricane, tornado, flooding)	Injuries, drowning	Coastal, low-lying land dwellers, low SES
Droughts, floods, increased mean temperature	Vector-, food-, and water-borne diseases	Multiple populations at risk
Sea-level rise	Injuries, drowning, water and soil salinization, ecosystem and economic disruption	Coastal, low SES
Drought, ecosystem migration	Food and water shortages, malnutrition	Low SES, elderly, children
Extreme weather events, drought	Mass population movement, international conflict	General population
Increases in ground-level ozone, airborne allergens, and other pollutants	Respiratory disease exacerbations (COPD, asthma, allergic rhinitis, bronchitis)	Elderly, children, those with respiratory disease
Climate change generally; extreme events	Mental health	Young, displaced, agricultural sector, low SES

Source: CDC, 2009c.

eight industrial powers also agreed to a 50-percent reduction in global emissions by 2050 that would require the richest countries to lower their emissions by 80 percent. China and India, the two fastest developing nations in the world, did not join the other eight industrial powers in agreeing to lower emissions.

Public health professionals, including their community partners and stakeholders, have recognized the need to respond to climate change for practical as well as ethical reasons (Frumkin et al., 2008). Quality public health services are characterized as being population-centered, proactive, equitable, risk reducing, and effective (U.S. Department of Health and Human Services, 2008). Preventing the effects of climate change requires public health practitioners to work with others to slow, stabilize, or reverse climate change. We must also anticipate and prepare for the harmful effects of climate change by reducing risks and the health burden on populations, paying particular attention to those most vulnerable. Identifying such groups in advance—being proactive—will provide crucial information for planning and preparedness and prevent avoidable loss of lives.

The Centers for Disease Control and Prevention (2009c) has identified the following priority health actions for climate change for public health organizations:

1. Serve as a credible source of information on the health consequences of climate change for the U.S. population and globally.
2. Track data on environmental conditions, disease risks, and disease occurrence related to climate change.
3. Expand capacity for modeling and forecasting health effects that may be climate-related.
4. Enhance the science base to better understand the relationship between climate change and health outcomes.
5. Identify locations and population groups at greatest risk for specific health threats, such as heat waves.
6. Communicate the health-related aspects of climate change, including risks and ways to reduce them, to the public, decision makers, and healthcare providers.
7. Develop partnerships with other government agencies, the private sector, nongovernmental organizations, universities, and international organizations to more effectively address U.S. and global health aspects of climate change.
8. Provide leadership to state and local governments, community leaders, healthcare professionals, nongovernmental organizations, the faith-based communities, the private sector and the public, domestically and internationally, regarding health protection from climate change effects.
9. Develop and implement preparedness and response plans for health threats such as heat waves, severe weather events, and infectious diseases.
10. Provide technical advice and support to state and local health departments, the private sector, and others in implementing national and global preparedness measures related to the health effects of climate change.
11. Promote workforce development by helping to ensure the training of a new generation of competent, experienced public health staff to respond to the health threats posed by climate change.

The World Health Organization's work plan on climate change is aimed at supporting health systems in all countries, particularly in low- and middle-income nations and small island states; building capacity for assessing and monitoring risks to and impacts on populations due to global warming and climate change; developing strategies and actions to protect human health, with a focus on the most vulnerable; and sharing knowledge and good practices (WHO, 2010). Some of the strategies WHO is promoting to reduce the impact of warming are (1) advocating to raise awareness about the threats to human health; (2) partnering with agencies to ensure representation of health on the climate change agenda; (3) building the scientific evidence on the links between climate change and health, pursuing a global research agenda; and (4) strengthening the health system to work with countries on assessing their vulnerability to the effects of climate change and building capacity to reduce health consequences (WHO, 2010).

War and Armed Conflicts

Wars and their aftermath produce arguably as much mortality and morbidity as many major diseases combined. More than 191 million people died as a result of war, over half of whom were civilians, during the twentieth century (Levy and Sidel, 2008). Many civilian casualties occurred when innocent people were caught in the cross fire between combatants. Wars are devastating to individuals, families, communities, and, at times, entire states or nations by the killing, maiming, and displacement of people. Millions have died as a result of starvation and disease brought about by the destruction of infrastructure and agricultural systems, and by being forced, along with entire communities, to flee their homes (Taipale, 2002). A large proportion of soldiers and civilians are disabled because of injuries suffered during war. Survivors of war suffer long-term health consequences, including physical, psychological, and emotional problems from their exposure to the brutalities of war that include torture, rape, the violent death of loved ones, and the destruction of entire communities. People who spend much of their lives in armed conflict or exposed to war will think of violence as the solution for many problems, and in this environment criminal acts and domestic violence rates will rise in communities. Women are particularly vulnerable during wars in which rape is used as a weapon to humiliate and assault female family members of enemies (Levy and Sidel). Children are also vulnerable, suffering or dying from malnutrition, disease, or violence during a war, and experiencing extreme psychological trauma in its aftermath.

The loss of human lives is the most significant cost of war. War also has economic consequences that affect both industrialized and developing nations because major resources are devoted to war and the preparation for war. Almost all wars since 1948 have been fought in developing countries (Taipale, 2002). The resources spent on arms pose a great burden to developing countries, draining already scarce resources that could be used for development. Regions at war experience the destruction of their infrastructure, including health systems, and their resources are redirected toward efforts that damage, rather than promote, the health of populations. Medical care facilities, energy generating plants, food supply, water systems, sanitation facilities, transportation, and communication are routinely destroyed as a result of war (Levy and Sidel, 2008). Developing countries are most severely affected by the economic costs of militarism, which create delay or reversal of economic development and produce huge gaps in essential nutrition, housing, education, and health services for populations (Taipale). Many industrialized countries have spent enormous financial and human resources on armed conflicts they could not afford, leaving their children with huge debts to repay (Taipale). The diversion decreases the amount of money available for health and human services. In the United States, individuals from minority communities form a disproportionate number of those on active military duty, exposing a greater percent of minority groups to the very real risks of early mortality and disabling injuries. War veterans suffering from mental and physical health problems due to their tour of duty during wartime often find inadequate support to address the many areas of life affecting their well-being, including economic, social, physical, community, and policy factors.

War and its effects are preventable. Public health practitioners can work to prevent war and its repercussions by conducting surveillance and reporting on the short- and long-term effects of war on the health of soldiers and civilians. Public health professionals can use this information to raise awareness and educate communities on the human and economic costs of war, including the ability or inability of the health care system to care for the casualties of war. Supporting policies to prevent war and its health consequences are also areas for public health professionals to develop in partnership with others concerned about the impact of war on community health.

Summary

The obesity epidemic, climate change, and war are major, complex public health problems facing twenty-first-century public health practitioners around the world. Public health policies and actions directed at preventing or mitigating the effects of these important health problems for populations would prevent human and economic costs. Devising strategies for addressing these problems requires skilled public health professionals capable of planning and implementing interventions across multiple levels of the system based on the best available evidence and knowledge. The skills of surveillance and communication are also needed to monitor improvements; evaluate the effect of interventions in addressing multiple, complex health problems; and build advocacy for policy changes that prevent disease or injury and reduce the impact on people and communities adversely affected by these complex problems.

Key Terms

Climate change

Global warming

Obesity epidemic

Wars

Discussion Questions

1. Explain the phrase "The choices people make are often shaped by the choices they have." How is public health practice informed by this perspective?
2. What are the advantages of considering global health issues for public health practitioners in the United States?
3. Obesity has been called an epidemic. Explain what factors contribute to identifying this health risk as a worldwide epidemic.
4. What can local public health practitioners do to help their communities prepare for as well as reduce the effects of climate change?
5. Do you concur that war is a public health issue? Why or why not? What role can public health practitioners play in addressing the health problems arising from armed conflict?

CASE STUDIES

INNOVATION IN HEALTH EDUCATION PROGRAMS

HEALTH EDUCATION and health promotion programs are capable of reducing the incidence of chronic diseases. One way in which nonprofit health care organizations can benefit communities is by providing resources for community health projects. Nonprofit health care organizations must produce some community benefit in order to maintain tax-exempt status. Nonprofit organizations' concern in regard to this Internal Revenue Service (IRS) regulation was used to acquire money from a third-party health insurer to complete a health assessment of a county in order to develop a Web site for giving information to county residents about the health problems uncovered by the survey.

Emanuel (2008) points out that our country loses a larger percentage of individuals to diabetes than other industrialized countries because fewer Americans have a primary care physician. Therefore, they are not as well-versed in the value of avoiding high-risk health behaviors. Our system devotes precious few resources to public health and health education programs.

The irony in our attempt to find a solution to the health care crisis is that we have had that solution ever since public health departments in this country began to realize the value of prevention programs. Moving past the mission of public health—to prevent disease and improve the health of the population—it is very clear that public health departments have the tools to keep people healthy. These tools of prevention should be utilized by the entire health care system to keep people healthy rather than allowing them to become ill.

Public health departments in the United States have been unable to capitalize on their accomplishments in improving the life expectancy of most Americans. Their funding is reduced every year, they are losing many of their most experienced workers to retirement, and they have been unable to move past their previous success. Herbold (2007) introduced the legacy concept, whereby an organization becomes convinced that because it has achieved past success with a certain approach it is entitled to future success using the same approach. This attitude makes businesses and agencies resistant to new approaches for solving current problems.

An example of the legacy concept in public health is found in the strategy public health departments have embraced in dealing with human immunodeficiency virus (HIV), which has plagued this country since 1981. This approach calls for using the counseling and testing approach to HIV even though it has not worked and will not work. HIV has become a chronic disease and will never be eliminated or even controlled unless health education becomes the new strategy to deal with this deadly infection.

Financing Health Promotion Programs

Missed workdays and lower employee productivity due to illness as well as expenses associated with the treatment of chronic diseases cost the U.S. economy $1.3 trillion annually, and it is estimated that this figure will grow to $4.2 trillion by 2023 (DeVol and Armen, 2007). However, with modest improvements in prevention and early treatment of chronic diseases forty million cases of chronic diseases (with an annual economic impact of $1.1 trillion) could be avoided by 2023 (DeVol and Armen). One key to achieving this outcome lies with local health departments (LHDs), which use health education programs to reduce the incidence of chronic diseases among community residents. Although these departments have had great success in reducing the high-risk health behaviors that result in the development of chronic diseases later in life, their programs' sustainability is intrinsically tied to the availability of appropriate funding.

LHDs are financed through a complex, fragmented, and often confusing combination of federal and state grants, appropriations, and fees. One major source of funding for LHDs is the CDC's Preventive Health and Health Services (PHHS) Block Grants. These grants, established by Congress in 1981, give LHDs the flexibility to tailor health promotion programs to the specific needs of their respective communities. Examples of chronic disease prevention activities to which many LHDs devote PHHS funds include screening programs and programs that promote healthy eating and physical activity. However, cuts in the 2009 CDC budget would eliminate these PHHS funds (CDC, 2008a). The CDC raises the need to improve efficiency and effectiveness as the rationale for the elimination of funding, stating that "other existing resources will continue to be available for programs which have traditionally addressed similar public health issues" (CDC, 2008a, p. 13). However, the National Association of County and City Health Officials (NACCHO, 2008) estimates that the elimination of the PHHS funds would cause a loss of $40.8 million for chronic disease programs and $11.2 million for infectious disease programs. This is just one example of how LHDs are faced with a continuing pattern of declining funding and as a result are forced to explore alternative methods of funding to improve chronic disease prevention. One alternative financing mechanism LHDs have employed has been to use the IRS community benefit standard to form a community partnership with a third-party health insurer to acquire funding for health promotion initiatives at the local level.

Internal Revenue Service—Community Benefit Standard

The IRS grants tax-exempt status to health care and related service organizations under section 501(c)(3) of the Internal Revenue Code. Under this section, an organization must not only operate on a nonprofit basis but also qualify as a charitable organization by serving the public interest through what is called the "community benefit standard." The community benefit standard was first established in 1969 under Revenue Ruling 69-545, in which the IRS recognized that programs promoting health are considered to have a charitable purpose under the common law of charity. Promotion of health is deemed beneficial to the community as a whole even though the class of individuals eligible to receive a direct benefit from activities does not include all community members, provided that the class is not so small that its relief is not of benefit to the community.

For nonprofit health care organizations, providing community benefit is the principal standard for maintaining tax-exempt status. However, it is becoming increasingly difficult to differentiate for-profit health care organizations from the nonprofit ones, and as a result, both the IRS and Congress have begun to challenge the appropriateness of the community benefit standard. The IRS wants to make tax-exempt entities more accountable for their activities and to quantify the supply of community benefit provided. One way in which nonprofit health care organizations can demonstrate benefit to their communities is to engage in community partnerships, providing resources for the development, implementation, and evaluation of educational efforts geared toward prevention of high-risk health behaviors.

The health care consultant who was trying to start the Luzerne County Health Department in Pennsylvania used the community benefit standard to request seed money. Hospitals and insurance providers contributed the money.

This seems like a logical way for a health care organization to maintain its nonprofit status and improve the health of its community.

In January 2008 the program director for a graduate program in health care administration met with the CEO from a large health insurance provider in regard to the development of an innovative health education program. The program director mentioned the community benefit standard as the reason why the CEO should consider providing funds for this new education program. The CEO accepted the request, and the health insurance provider supplied funding to conduct a community health assessment that was to be the catalyst in the development of a Web-based education program designed to provide free health information to residents concerning the health problems the assessment uncovered.

The major cause of the continuing escalation in the costs of health care in the United States is the epidemic of chronic diseases. These diseases are expected to cost the U.S. economy more than $1 trillion a year, and this figure could rise to $6 trillion by 2050. These diseases are the result of practicing poor health behaviors like using tobacco, maintaining a poor diet, and being physically inactive over the years. Today's public health system needs to position itself to capitalize on the many opportunities available as the focus and goals of the health care system are being reorganized. These opportunities for improving the health of the population are also available to such other nonprofit agencies as insurance providers, health care organizations, and colleges.

Health education and health promotion programs are capable of reducing the incidence of chronic diseases and have also been effective in reducing the costly complications that result from these diseases over time. Such educational efforts have had great success in reducing the high-risk health behaviors that result in the development of chronic diseases. However, the success of these programs is dependent on community partnerships that increase the amount of resources available to support the expansion of programs with proven best practices.

LHDs can use the community benefit standard to pressure nonprofit health facilities to provide resources for the development, implementation, and evaluation of educational efforts geared toward the prevention of high-risk health behaviors. One way in which a nonprofit health care organization can act to benefit its community is to provide resources for community health projects. LHDs need to use this IRS regulation to acquire money from third-party health insurers and nonprofit hospitals to develop and implement population-based health education programs for reducing high-risk health behaviors that lead to chronic diseases.

Discussion Questions

1. How have the problems facing public health departments changed since the early 1900s?
2. Explain how the Internal Revenue Service community benefit standard can be used to expand local health department programs in the United States.
3. Why has the public health system been unable to capitalize on its past accomplishments?

DISABILITIES

Jill D. Morrow-Gorton

S TATE GOVERNMENTS face many issues related to assessing the safety and efficacy of the programs that they provide and fund. Also, different constituent groups outside of government monitor events occurring in these programs and advocate for change where they see problems. These groups communicate their concerns to their government in many ways including formal letters as well as verbal contact. The state government must evaluate these claims in regard to their accuracy and develop a plan to approach addressing the findings. This case study provides the opportunity to apply principles of public health to this scenario.

Case Study (Student Version)

You are the director of the Division of Epidemiology for a large state. In your state the Division of Epidemiology provides statistical support to all of the program offices in the Department of Health and Welfare. This includes the Office of Programs for People with Disabilities (OPPD), which provides services and supports for people with developmental disabilities, including intellectual disabilities (formerly called mental retardation), cerebral palsy and other physical disabilities, and autism spectrum disorders.

The director of the OPPD comes to you with the information that the advocates for the OPPD are concerned that people living in residential settings, which are licensed by the state and run by private provider entities, use emergency departments and are admitted to the hospital more than people without disabilities living in the same geographical areas. These residential settings generally consist of three or four individuals with disabilities living in the same home with paid staff members who work in the home and provide their care. These homes are houses or apartments located in communities. The advocates maintain that this is because the staff members working with these individuals have little knowledge about health and medical conditions, and they have asked that the director of the OPPD address these concerns. The director is asking you for help in analyzing and addressing them. Outline your recommendations for analyzing the accuracy of these concerns, using the following questions to guide your response:

1. What types of data would you look at in order to evaluate this concern?
2. What demographic characteristics of this population might be different from those of the general population and require adjusting the data?
3. What health characteristics and medical conditions might need to be considered when analyzing this information?

Your analysis of the data reveals that indeed this population has a higher rate of use of both emergency departments and hospital care. In addition, this care is related to conditions common to the general population like congestive heart failure, diabetes, and respiratory illnesses as well as those more common to the population of people with developmental disabilities, such as seizures and problems requiring orthopedic surgery. The literature shows that people with greater health knowledge about particular medical conditions are more likely to get better health care and have better control of their disease condition. You present this information to the director of the OPPD and suggest that increasing the health knowledge of the people responsible for the day-to-day support of these individuals with disabilities might result in better care and control of their chronic diseases. Describe some ways to provide health education to this population.

The director of the OPPD took your suggestions and created a group of units across the state to provide health education to the staff working with people with disabilities in residential settings. These units assess the health and medical conditions of the population of people living in their area and then develop educational activities to teach the staff members how to better manage common diseases like congestive heart failure, diabetes, and chronic lung disease. Some of the classes include specific information about a disease, whereas others address some of the barriers to better management and provide training in how to give medication consistently. The units have nurses that gather health data from a random sample of people living in residential settings. They have identified that of the people in residential settings with a diagnosis of high blood pressure who are on medication, about 84 percent of them have a normal blood pressure compared with 28 percent of the general population who are not in residential settings (Centers for Disease Control and Prevention, 1999a; Morrow and Breen, 2001).

One of the reasons for this difference is probably individuals' level of compliance with taking prescribed medication, given that staff members giving medication in the licensed residential settings document each dose of medication administered as taught to them in a course about medication administration. Thus, health knowledge can have a significant impact on chronic disease management.

Case Study (Teacher Version)

You are the director of the Division of Epidemiology for a large state. In your state the Division of Epidemiology provides statistical support to all of the program offices in the Department of Health and Welfare. This includes the Office of Programs for People with Disabilities (OPPD), which provides services and supports for people with developmental disabilities, including intellectual disabilities (formerly called mental retardation), cerebral palsy and other physical disabilities, and autism spectrum disorders.

The director of the OPPD comes to you with the information that the advocates for the OPPD are concerned that people living in residential settings, which are licensed by the state and run by private provider entities, use emergency departments and are admitted to the hospital more than people without disabilities living in the same geographical areas. These residential settings generally consist of three or four individuals with disabilities living in the same home with paid staff members who work in the home and provide their care. These homes are houses or apartments located in communities. The advocates maintain that this is because the staff members working with these individuals have little knowledge about health and medical conditions, and they have asked that the director of the OPPD address these concerns. The director is asking you for help in analyzing and addressing them. Outline your recommendations for analyzing the accuracy of these concerns, using the following questions to guide your response:

1. What types of data would you look at in order to evaluate this concern?
   - Discussion should include evaluation of hospitalization and emergency department use for both this population and the general population in order to make a comparison between the two. Possible sources of information include Behavioral Risk Factor Surveillance System (RFSS) data, data from the National Center for Health Statistics, such state-specific sources as unusual incident reporting systems common to many state developmental disability offices, hospitalization data reported to the state, claims data from Medical Assistance or Medicare, and so on.

2. What demographic characteristics of this population might be different from those of the general population and require adjusting the data?
   - Demographic issues include age differences in sample populations, as many developmental disability agencies only serve adults in residential settings, and also because a number of individuals with genetic conditions die as infants or young children as a consequence of their disability. Gender is important because many developmental disorders including intellectual disabilities and autism spectrum disorders are more prevalent in males than females. Race or ethnicity may be important if those characteristics differ between the residential and general populations (for example, there may be cultural factors that would predict that the racial makeup of the residential population would not be representative of that of the state as a whole if a particular racial or ethnic group tended not to use residential settings). Urban versus rural populations could also be considered.

3. What health characteristics and medical conditions might need to be considered when analyzing this information?
   - Some medical conditions are more prevalent in a population of people with developmental disabilities. These include hypothyroidism, seizure disorders, congenital heart disease with congestive heart failure, and chronic respiratory disease.
   - People with motor disorders like cerebral palsy or spina bifida tend to have more surgical procedures related to their developmental disability. For example, individuals with spina bifida often have hydrocephalus and require shunts. These shunts may fail, thus necessitating replacement. People with cerebral palsy develop contractures of the muscles and need to have surgery to release them.
   - People with disabilities also have the same chronic medical conditions that are present in the general population—including diabetes, heart disease, and so on.

Your analysis of the data reveals that indeed this population has a higher rate of use of both emergency departments and hospital care. In addition, this care is related to conditions common to the general population like congestive heart failure, diabetes, and respiratory illnesses as well as those more common to the population of people with developmental disabilities, such as seizures and problems requiring orthopedic surgery. The literature shows that people with greater health knowledge about particular medical conditions are more likely to get better health care and have better control of their disease condition. You present this information to the director of the OPPD and suggest that increasing the health knowledge of the people responsible for the day-to-day support of these individuals with disabilities might result in better care and control of their chronic diseases. Describe some ways to provide health education to this population.

- Students should provide some thoughts about how to effectively identify the appropriate topics and develop education materials, and describe how to get this type of knowledge to this population. Ideas might address the following:
  - Strategies to identify appropriate topics based on the information gathered about health conditions
  - Strategies to develop training materials, including such issues as who will develop the materials (internal departmental staff members or a contractor), what separate groups will be created, who will prepare materials for use, and what formats would be most effective for those materials
  - Methods of providing the information, including face-to-face training, electronic training, train-the-trainer modules, and so on
  - The use of focus groups and other similar entities to best identify how to get the information to people in this group
  - Ways to assess the impact of the provision of this information
  - Ways to make the educational materials available to people, taking into account appropriate reading level and so on

The director of the OPPD took your suggestions and created a group of units across the state to provide health education to the staff working with people with disabilities in residential settings. These units assess the health and medical conditions of the population of people living in their area and then develop educational activities to teach the staff members how to better manage common diseases like congestive heart failure, diabetes, and chronic lung disease. Some of the classes include specific information about a disease, whereas others address some of the barriers to better management and provide training in how to give medication consistently. The units have nurses that gather health data from a random sample of people living in residential settings. They have identified that of the people in residential settings with a diagnosis of high blood pressure who are on medication, about 84 percent of them have a normal blood pressure compared with 28 percent of the general population who are not in residential settings (Centers for Disease Control and Prevention, 1999a; Morrow and Breen, 2001). One of the reasons for this difference is probably individuals' level of compliance with taking prescribed medication, given that staff members giving medication in the licensed residential settings document each dose of medication administered as taught to them in a course about medication administration. Thus, health knowledge can have a significant impact on chronic disease management.

Discussion Questions

1. What types of data would you look at in order to evaluate this concern?
2. What demographic characteristics of this population might be different from those of the general population and require adjusting the data?
3. What health characteristics and medical conditions might need to be considered when analyzing this information?

FORMATION OF COMMUNITY PARTNERSHIPS TO PREPARE FOR H1N1

Marc C. Marchese

D URING INFLUENZA PANDEMICS the medical community and the general public need up-to-date information. This information must be easy to understand and readily available for large numbers of people if the pandemic occurs. The time to prepare the information is long before the outbreak of disease so that individuals will know what to do if and when public health authorities begin to report the disease. This type of information development and distribution works best if several agencies work together on the project because collaboration often yields more ideas and available resources.

The IOM (2002) has argued that the use of information technology in the improvement of the health of communities presents great opportunities and challenges. This prestigious group recommends that public health agencies should use information technology to collect and disseminate information more efficiently in order to help the public and public officials better understand what health services should be offered. This would include conveying to a large number of people the advantages of using preventive services for circumventing or postponing the development of chronic diseases and their complications. According to Novick et al. (2008), information management systems have evolved as some of the most important tools available to public health departments because of the sheer volume of health data available and the emergence of technology to swiftly disseminate these data.

According to Herzlinger (2007), approximately ninety-five million Americans use the Internet to retrieve health care information, and six million use the Web on a daily basis to learn about health problems. Employing this type of technology is definitely one way to better educate the consumer about the dangers of high-risk health behaviors. The nice part about this kind of intervention is that it is an inexpensive way to make accurate health information available to many.

Due to the availability of computing technology, public health departments are now able to rapidly gather health-related data, analyze these data, and share them with those responsible for the improvement of the health of the population (Novick et al., 2008). The future holds great promise for the further development of information technology to be used in delivering public health information to larger audiences. Information delivered by public health departments, especially at the local level, should include notices pertaining to education programs to prevent diseases and their complications, notifications about other preventive services, and data concerning quality of care issues. Also necessary to improve health outcomes is a partnership with patients, which should involve sharing medical information with them and helping each patient to understand the relevance of that information to the quality of his or her life and the lives of family members. Information sharing can help patients implement their own prevention strategies in order to avoid chronic diseases and their complications.

Health education and health promotion programs are capable of reducing the incidence of epidemics of communicable diseases like influenza. According to the Centers for Disease Control and Prevention (CDC, 2009g), health risk communication strategies are very important in the protection of the population in the event of an influenza pandemic. Community partnerships can be used to develop health communication programs for rapidly sharing vital information to large segments of the population. Vaughan and Tinker (2009) point out that health communication programs can help the public become an effective partner by encouraging them to instigate prevention activities and enabling them to respond to the changing nature of a communicable disease pandemic.

The attempt to develop a proactive approach for dealing with the almost certain epidemic of H1N1 influenza began in August 2009 at King's College in Wilkes-Barre, Pennsylvania. The director of the Health Care Administration Program was an epidemiologist for the Pennsylvania Department of Health for twenty-five years before assuming his current position at the college. The director recognized the need for collaboration in rapidly developing an education initiative designed to answer the public's questions about the potential epidemic of influenza throughout the country in fall 2009. A second purpose of the program was to help employers in the community prepare for the H1N1 pandemic. This included educating employers on how the disease is contracted and how long an employee can be contagious, offering recommendations for sick leave policies, suggesting proactive measures to reduce the spread of infection, and so on.

As already mentioned, one way in which information can be shared quickly with large segments of the population is through the use of the Internet. Community agencies, especially at the local level, can deliver online information that includes virtual preventive services and education programs to prevent diseases and their complications. One such program was developed through a partnership that involved the American Red Cross, a city health department, and a graduate program in health care administration at King's College. This program was in the form of a voice-narrated PowerPoint presentation about how to prevent infection with H1N1. This presentation also included a short pretest and was followed by a posttest to determine the effectiveness of this program. The program was launched on the Health Care Administration Program's Web site and was made available to all partner agencies.

Community partnerships can be used to obtain additional human and material resources necessary to combat population-based health problems, as was the case with efforts to prepare for H1N1. Rashid et al. (2009) argue that when agencies collaborate in their work on health problems there is a greater chance for the development of improved solutions and effective interventions that can then be shared with other agencies.

Discussion Questions

1. Explain how community partnerships can be used to share information about chronic diseases with large segments of the population.
2. Can you think of other forms of technology that will be useful in the education of large segments of the population about the prevention of disease?
3. How can virtual health education programs be marketed to the general public?

MUNICIPAL HEALTH DEPARTMENT LEADERSHIP INSIDE OUT

Ted Kross

EXPERIENCE, EDUCATION, and training in one's personal life as well as professional career can bridge many gaps in one's quest through a life span. I entered into my nursing life in 1979 at the age of eighteen when I began school at Pittston School of Nursing in Pittston, Pennsylvania. The three-year diploma program had an emphasis on hands-on training in a hospital or other clinical environment enriched with classroom education. My grandmother and parents persuaded me in this direction due to my inherent ability to communicate with and help people. I was told, "No one could ever take your education away from you." Uncertain if I would succeed, I forged through many uncomfortable and difficult times as a nurse and a human being. I can remember my initial encounters with patients when I had no prior professional training or experience. The first person I cared for could not speak as a result of a stroke. I can picture him almost perfectly today, thirty-two years later, and can visualize his appreciation when I had to help him with breakfast because his dominate side was paralyzed. I fed him scrambled eggs, and was amazed how much he swallowed—at least, so I thought. I had not been told that his swallowing reflex was also affected; he began to choke, but fortunately he expelled the eggs all over his beside table and food tray before any further complication. Training, education, and experience might have led me to a different approach to feeding him that morning.

I have worked in the private sector of health care in a hospital setting for most of my career to date as an emergency department registered nurse. I gained insurmountable personal satisfaction by challenging myself daily with critically ill persons. I took the next step and worked as a prehospital nurse and flight nurse to satisfy my ambition to help people and save lives. I returned to school and attended King's College in Wilkes-Barre, Pennsylvania, to attain both an undergraduate and graduate degree in health care administration. I wanted to teach people how to not only care for individuals but also take health care in a direction of both professional and ethical excellence. I managed in emergency nursing for nearly fourteen years in Pennsylvania and nearby Maryland. Change is critical to success in family life and one's career; therefore, I sought a new direction in health care!

Approximately two years ago I entered into a much different health care environment, public health (or community health). Personal satisfaction remains high on my radar, along with the pursuit of helping people. Community health deals with different challenges to a much larger and more diverse population with unique diseases ranging from influenza to tuberculosis. Managing a municipal health department is exciting and has offered me opportunities in the form of new challenges, experience, and education. As director of this health department I am responsible for the health care of Wilkes-Barre residents, in addition to my financial responsibilities of grant writing and balancing a budget. Pennsylvania has three other municipal health departments (York, Allentown, and Bethlehem) along with six county departments. Philadelphia's local health department is responsible for many lives and acts almost independently of the entire state.

The city of Wilkes-Barre has a population of more than forty-one thousand individuals in a geographic area of approximately nine square miles. The Wilkes-Barre City Health Department comprises several different divisions and types of personnel. The health department is located in the Kirby Health Center near the city's center. The Kirby family built this facility in the early 1930s and currently operates the health center, which houses various public entities to meet the needs of Wilkes-Barre residents and the surrounding communities. A board of health directs our activities and is made up of several local physicians, a school nurse, community members, and a medical director. The health department comprises four nurses—an associate director of nursing, two community health nurses (a registered nurse and a licensed practical nurse), and a director chosen and supported by not only the city of Wilkes-Barre but also the state health department's leadership. Two health educators promote several programs under three separate state and federal grants: Maternal and Child Health, Injury Prevention, and chronic disease funding (osteoporosis, diabetes, and heart and lung diseases). An animal enforcement officer is part of the department, which controls many aspects of animal surveillance in the city including licensing animals, monitoring animal bites (rabies prevention), and ensuring animal control and behavior as outlined by the ordinances set forth through its local government (Mayor Thomas Leighton and an elected city council). Three health inspectors are responsible for inspecting and licensing over three hundred restaurants and caterers on both an annual basis and throughout the year. The health inspectors and department ensure all aspects of any health-related issue in the geographic confines of the city of Wilkes-Barre. A public health preparedness coordinator actively ensures readiness of the city of Wilkes-Barre to react to any natural or bioterrorist public health threat. Many of the city's employees and community volunteers are educated and trained to prepare and practice for these events. Federal and state funding allows for this training and ability to practice planning and procedures in preparation for a bioterrorism event. The events of September 11, 2001, prompted department members to devise a plan to better prepare for and react to acts of terrorism through improved communication. Although the events surrounding this tragedy in New York that affected the world were courageously conquered by many employed and volunteer emergency medical services (EMS), police, fire department, and health care workers, a few fundamental issues were uncovered. Number one was the need for a common communication network to allow all personnel involved to communicate with each other and with leaders. Police, fire, EMS, and command personnel were on different radio frequencies and communication devices, and the health and welfare of many of these heroes were in jeopardy. The state and federal government subsequently introduced an 800 MHz radio tool that all personnel can use for emergency communications. E-mail messages and emergency personnel radio discussions can take place with field and hospital personnel. The country has pushed all kinds of emergency response personnel to train, educate, and exercise many community groups to prepare for continued threats to our homeland security.

Most recently, in spring 2009 the world was confronted with an apparent epidemic of a new strain of influenza virus termed *novel influenza A (H1N1)*. With H1N1 positioned to be one of the biggest threats and challenges in today's world, our country began vigorously preparing to battle this respiratory disease and engage four pharmaceutical companies worldwide to begin careful research in and development of a vaccine. Concurrently, the Wilkes-Barre City Health Department began to plan for vaccine distribution to large numbers of individuals through Points of Distribution (POD) and patient care delivery disaster plans. Weekly planning meetings with leadership of the various departments (EMS, police, fire, health, and administration) in the city of Wilkes-Barre began in late spring 2009 and continued throughout the summer.

The health department was challenged in October 2009 by being one of the region's first public health entities to receive the H1N1 vaccine and distribute it to residents and nearby communities for high-risk individuals (children six months to twenty-four years, pregnant women, persons twenty-five to sixty-four with certain chronic health conditions, health care workers, and caregivers of children under six months). The philosophy of this health department, expressed through its leaders and nursing personnel, was to receive and distribute this scarce vaccine in the early availability era to the residents of Wilkes-Barre. We scheduled several clinics in cooperation with the Kirby Health Center leadership at our building on North Franklin Street. Three nurses and various health department and city personnel organized one of the country's first vaccine distribution efforts from 1:00 A.M. to 6:00 P.M. We were immediately challenged with many issues ranging from nonresidents seeking the vaccine to people outside the risk groups identified nationally pursuing our services. Great communication and organization allowed the handful of personnel to distribute over six hundred doses of the vaccine in mid-October. The media had been anticipating these events and promoted the vaccine and distribution over the next several weeks. Shortages of the vaccine quickly became an issue, and cooperation from nearby Allentown to share five hundred additional doses of the vaccine with Wilkes-Barre allowed continued distribution. In early January 2010 the state health department partnered with the Wilkes-Barre City Health Department to implement a state-organized mass immunization clinic at the Kingston Armory just outside of Wilkes-Barre. Thousands of nasal and injectable vaccine doses were distributed to all citizens from the region through a well-organized pre-event registration and this mass immunization clinic.

Cooperation, knowledge, leadership, training, and education led our health department to a very successful program that saved many lives and decreased morbidity caused by this new strain of influenza. The personnel involved were left with a huge sense of accomplishment both personal and professional, having contributed to a humanitarian effort not experienced in community health in the recent past.

Leadership has been my passion for the last fifteen years and has led to my personal satisfaction as a public service provider and humanitarian. Experience in the many facets of my professional career has been crucial to the achievement of my goals.

Discussion Questions

1. What is the fundamental difference between public health (community health) departments and the traditional acute health care system accessed today?
2. Life experience is essential to health care practice. How can an individual gain life experience and survive the many challenges faced as a new health care provider?
3. How does strong leadership in public health contribute to improved health and quality of life?

THE POWER OF DATA: OSCEOLA COUNTY SECURES A FEDERALLY QUALIFIED HEALTH CENTER

Julia Joh Elligers

OSCEOLA COUNTY (Florida) has the power of data and knows how to use it to connect residents to services. With a growing population, large percentage of underserved minorities, and high rate of uninsured, Osceola County faced serious health challenges. Assessment data, strategic planning, and cooperative action have allowed Osceola County to improve access to public health services by developing a health center system and obtaining federally qualified health center (FQHC) status.

Located in central Florida, Osceola County includes Poinciana, Kissimmee, and St. Cloud, making it a popular vacation destination. While the county attracts tourists, much of the region is undeveloped. Ninety percent of the population lives on the borders of Polk and Orange Counties near Orlando, while the remainder of the area is rural.

The county has a diverse and growing population. The population grew more than 60 percent since 2000 from approximately 174,000 to over 280,000

Funding for this story was provided by the Centers for Disease Control and Prevention under Cooperative Agreement Numbers 5U38HM000449-02 and HM08-80502CONT09. The contents of this document are solely the responsibility of the National Association of County and City Health Officials (NACCHO) and do not necessarily represent the official views of the sponsor.

in 2010 (Florida Charts, n.d.). Forty-two percent of the county's population is Hispanic or Latino, 40 percent of which is uninsured. Many other residents are uninsured because they do not receive health benefits as part-time employees of the tourist industry.

MAPP as the Catalyst

In an effort to meet the unique public health needs of the county's growing population, Osceola County implemented the Mobilizing for Action through Planning and Partnerships (MAPP) process. MAPP provides a framework for creating, implementing, and evaluating a community health improvement plan. Using MAPP, communities build partnerships, develop a shared community vision, and conduct a series of assessments. MAPP assessment data provide a comprehensive picture of the community's health and are used to identify strategic issues that must be addressed in order for the community to achieve its vision. Communities then formulate goals, strategies, and activities that are implemented and evaluated in an iterative MAPP action cycle. Karen van Caulil, executive director of the Health Council of East Central Florida, made the following comment in regard to MAPP:

> The MAPP process is easy to understand. It has been the catalyst for moving things along and looking at them in a comprehensive way. It has been a wonderful process for being able to convene stakeholders in an organized fashion; to get information out to the community on issues and trends; and to do something about the information. Too often we do needs assessment, we present data, and then everybody stands there and says now what? The MAPP process really tells you what to do with that data. It has allowed us to really have great success in identifying initiatives that have made a difference.

Community Vision, a nonprofit organization, facilitated the MAPP process and convened representatives from different entities such as the local health department, hospitals, advocacy groups, school system, and faith-based institutions. Together, these community partners completed three iterations of the MAPP process and developed and implemented three community strategic plans over the course of ten years.

Improving Access to Care

In all three iterations of the MAPP process, access to care was identified as a major strategic issue. While assessment data consistently identified barriers to care, the assessment phase also revealed solutions. In the first iteration of the

MAPP process, the county developed a specialty care network and a medical home program and decreased the number of patients using emergency rooms for primary care and ambulatory care visits. In the second and third iterations, the county built the capacity to address access to care through mobile units, a volunteer specialty network, cultural competence training and awareness, and federally qualified health centers.

The county used MAPP assessment data to increase its capacity to improve access to care. "We needed the data to describe the magnitude of the problem so that grant funding could be secured to implement these initiatives," says van Caulil. "We certainly had compelling statistics, and we had folks who have expertise in writing grants. Now, every organization uses the data from the MAPP process for writing grants, developing initiatives, and targeting their initiatives."

Osceola County's ability to secure federally qualified health centers was a particularly proud achievement. "Our health issue taskforce initiated a mobile medical express to increase access to remote areas. At the same time, a health center was being created in a modular building. Then, Belinda Johnson-Cornett [Osceola County Health Department director] was able to grab hold of FQHC designation and turn other health centers into FQHCs. It was a rapid fire turnover to FQHC," recalls van Caulil.

Johnson-Cornett adds, "FQHCs are strategically placed throughout the county. The primary site was in a community that was contained. No one would go there unless they lived there. It is a forty-five-minute drive from there to our other two sites. Transportation is an issue here. Being able to expand it and move it to the other two larger communities was great."

Furthermore, "I really don't think that the FQHC idea would have necessarily floated to the top had it not been for the MAPP process and people getting together to figure out that we need to increase access to care," says Johnson-Cornett.

Measuring Outcomes

Osceola County is now monitoring how its hard work is improving health outcomes. Karen van Caulil shares, "Our theory is if you're offering comprehensive and high-quality care in the community and there is ample access, you won't find high rates of admission for chronic conditions in the emergency rooms and hospitals." The county is monitoring patient health improvements over time in programs associated with conditions like diabetes and cardiovascular disease. The county has also started an emergency room diversion program and is measuring the type of patients referred, costs, retention, and how many patients get into case management programs.

Another example of how the county monitors outcomes is related to infant mortality. The county's Fetal and Infant Mortality Review (FIMR) committee, which is led by the Osceola County Health Department and includes representatives from law enforcement, social services, clinical staff, and community providers, addresses the issue of infant mortality as it relates to access to care. "We track indicators associated with infant mortality and access to care to see if we have programs to address those issues, and if we do not, we decide what we need to put into place as a community to be able to address those issues," says Johnson-Cornett.

The Way to Get Things Done

While MAPP implementation requires resources, the process also uncovers and secures resources for health improvement. Johnson-Cornett advises:

> In this particular environment, with the economy the way it is, [MAPP] is going to be the only way to get things done in your community. You're going to need to get people together, on the same page, willing to share resources and ideas. It's the shared resources that are going to get you there. Individually, it's not financially feasible for any one organization to do all these things. MAPP brings together different levels of expertise to identify where the resources are [and] the best people to provide those resources, and really pulls your community together so you are providing comprehensive care to the population you serve.

For those apprehensive about undertaking the MAPP process, van Caulil says, "There is nothing to be afraid of because the NACCHO Web site lays it out for you very easily. There are so many good case studies and tools that the process can be easily started."

Discussion Questions

1. What are some characteristics of Osceola County that would make a community health improvement initiative like MAPP challenging?
2. How did Osceola County use MAPP assessment data?
3. How did Osceola County benefit from the MAPP process?

USING MAPP TO *GET UP &
GO!* IN ST. CLAIR COUNTY

Lisa Jacobs

A New Way of Doing Business

S T. CLAIR COUNTY Health Department (Illinois), as a county health department in Illinois subject to the state's Illinois Project for Local Assessment of
Needs requirements, was well versed in strategic planning when staff first
learned of Mobilizing for Action through Planning and Partnerships (MAPP).
While partnerships and collaboration were not new to St. Clair, with more
than sixty health and human services organizations rooted in the county, MAPP
presented a unique opportunity to engage community members and partners
in collective assessment, planning, and action. Now, six years since the first
MAPP meeting, the process is continuing to generate excitement as community
members and local leaders collectively confront some of the most challenging
public health issues.

Over the course of nine months, the St. Clair Health Care Commission,
an appointed body that serves as the MAPP Steering Committee, facilitated a
community visioning process, assessment design, and data collection and analysis.
Findings from the four MAPP assessments were then used to identify six strategic
issues that, when addressed, will help St. Clair County achieve its shared vision
of a healthy community. Data points from the county's Community Themes and

Funding for this story was provided by the Centers for Disease Control and Prevention under Cooperative
Agreement Numbers 5U38HM000449-02 and HM08-80502CONT09. The contents of this document
are solely the responsibility of the National Association of County and City Health Officials (NACCHO)
and do not necessarily represent the official views of the sponsor.

Strengths Assessment revealed perceived disparities in quality of life, safety risks, and a need to more effectively engage young people (Arras and Peters, 2009). Based on these data points and data from the other three MAPP assessments, a need for greater community connectedness emerged as the first strategic issue on the county's to-do list.

St. Clair County is part of the St. Louis Metropolitan Area and is composed of comingling urban, suburban, and rural landscapes. St. Clair encompasses more than 650 square miles and is home to 260,000 residents. Socioeconomic and environmental diversity define the region. Brownfields from former heavy industry, impoverished communities experiencing significant health inequities, and St. Louis "bedroom communities" all exist within the same county lines. Community leaders knew that cultivating a cohesive sense of community might be difficult in this varied landscape.

From Planning to Action

MAPP stakeholders began by developing an asset map to identify attributes that contribute to community connectedness in pockets of the county. Once equipped with a more acute understanding of the components that contribute to a shared sense of community in St. Clair, stakeholders began generating ideas for how to actualize community connectedness throughout the county. With assessment data in hand, stakeholders crafted a plan to improve community connectedness by collectively addressing two of the county's priority health issues: troubling rates of cardiovascular and respiratory diseases.

The *Get Up & Go!* campaign was conceived to answer the question "How can the county's health care community create a broader sense of community connectedness?" MAPP stakeholders developed a blueprint for a thirty-day fitness challenge designed to catalyze new investments in personal and community health and well-being. Within several months, the *Get Up & Go!* committee garnered two grants to promote the campaign, and a local Web designer was enlisted to develop the campaign's Web site, which now features announcements about local fitness events and resources, accounts of participant activities, local officials' endorsements, links to Internet resources, and more (Arras and Peters, 2009).

Getting Active and Getting Healthy *Together*

With thousands of Web site hits, a growing cadre of volunteers, and the pledged support of thirteen of nineteen mayors throughout the county, the campaign held its official kickoff event the following spring. The event included blood pressure and weight screenings and a group walk to dedicate a new walking trail. In less than a year, the campaign galvanized 110 teams—as small as a single family and as large as an entire town—representing twenty-three thousand individuals to join the effort to *Get Up & Go!* (Arras and Peters, 2009).

Two years after the official launch, the campaign was selected to join the YMCA's national Pioneering Healthy Communities initiative. As a result, community leaders were funded to participate in a policy training in Washington DC, and the campaign received a grant to develop policy-level strategies to nurture healthy lifestyles and promote community connectedness in St. Clair. The *Get Up & Go!* campaign has since expanded from a thirty-day challenge to an entire season of community events driven by growing partnerships between local government, community-based organizations, and residents. In addition, the campaign, now a freestanding coalition, has expanded to include a "policy arm" that recently hosted a community-wide health policy summit and has developed work groups to begin assessing and implementing policy-level healthy eating and active living strategies.

Beyond the anticipated outcomes, health department leaders argue that the MAPP process and associated campaign have nurtured goodwill between local mayors and county leadership and improved the county's ability to respond to public health emergencies. According to St. Clair County Health Department Executive Director Kevin Hutchison:

> Relationships we developed through MAPP partnerships were extremely helpful during actual public health emergencies such as major power outages resulting from ice storms and the H1N1 pandemic. These relationships add distinct value to a local health department's ability to rapidly engage community partners and provide a unified foundation for the local public health system response to a public health emergency. MAPP is not something else we have to do. It is what we do in public health. It's not an extra step or another task; it's the essence of good public health practice.

Moving Forward

Stakeholders in St. Clair County are preparing to launch into a second iteration of MAPP and are anxious to build stronger evaluation components into their process and more rigorously measure the impact of their work on health outcomes and community connectedness. When asked about the greatest outcomes of the process to date, Mark Peters, St. Clair County Health Department director of community health, replied that "we are much more community minded, and I think the community is much more public health minded."

Discussion Questions

1. What was a major theme that emerged from St. Clair County's MAPP process?
2. What was the purpose of St. Clair County's *Get Up & Go!* campaign?
3. How did St. Clair County benefit from the relationships built through the MAPP process?

PARTNERING FOR IMPROVED INFANT HEALTH IN STANISLAUS COUNTY

Lisa Jacobs

Trendsetting in Central California

I N THE HEART of central California, Stanislaus County stretches more than 1,500 square miles and is divided by the north-flowing San Joaquin River. With a rich agricultural tradition rooted in California's wine, nut, and dairy industries, the county includes everything from small farming towns to "bedroom communities" for San Francisco commuters. While the communities that make up Stanislaus may not be as well known for trendsetting as their Bay Area neighbors, members of the Stanislaus County public health system were among the first in the nation to set the tone for community-driven health improvement, and they're beginning to see the fruits of their labor.

Stanislaus County is home to just over half a million people, primarily of European and Latino origin. Stanislaus County, like others in the Central Valley, has chronically higher rates of poverty and unemployment and lower educational attainment than the state as a whole. As a rapidly urbanizing county, Stanislaus County's health challenges don't always reflect those seen in other

Funding for this fact sheet was provided by the Centers for Disease Control and Prevention under Cooperative Agreement Numbers 5U38HM000449-02 and HM08-80502CONT09. The contents of this document are solely the responsibility of the National Association of County and City Health Officials (NACCHO) and do not necessarily represent the official views of the sponsor.

parts of the golden state. For example, a recent California County Health Status Profiles report revealed that Stanislaus County bears a disproportionate burden of chronic disease and poor infant health outcomes as compared to other counties in the state (Health Services Agency/Public Health Community Assessment, Planning and Evaluation Unit, 2010). Further, the county's infant mortality, low birth weight, and premature birth rates are all higher than state averages. According to one of the county's epidemiologists, in many ways, health outcomes in the Central Valley have more in common with Appalachia than with other counties in California.

Since 2002, the Stanislaus County Health Services Agency has used the Mobilizing for Action through Planning and Partnerships (MAPP) process to engage public health partners and county residents in community health assessment and improvement. Now in their second iteration, partnerships between local governmental agencies and grassroots, community-based organizations have grown, and Stanislaus County is continuing to make inroads toward improving priority health outcomes.

A New Community Anchor

During Stanislaus's first iteration of MAPP, data from the 2003 comprehensive health assessment—especially concerns about troubling infant health outcomes—inspired community leaders to develop what soon became known as Family Resource Centers. This new community resource, first piloted in 2005, began with three locations and has since grown to include ten sites distributed throughout the county. Family Resource Centers are funded largely through Proposition 10—the California Children and Families Act—with contracts managed by the Stanislaus County Health Services Agency. Family Resource Centers are embedded in the communities they serve and act as independent nonprofit organizations.

Members of the Stanislaus Health Services Agency cite the creation and development of Family Resource Centers among the proudest and most profound outcomes of MAPP. The centers grew out of a combination of initiatives, namely MAPP and asset-based community development and partnership efforts that occurred throughout the county in the first part of the millennium. Data and partnerships generated by the MAPP process created the foundation for Family Resource Centers.

Family Resource Centers represent a new anchor in the communities that make up Stanislaus County and provide opportunities for community residents to access everything from mental health services to the Healthy Birth Outcomes program, an education and support service for pregnant and parenting women and teens. Further, according to a local health educator, the Family Resource Centers have become a trusted venue for residents to exchange information about community-based activities and initiatives occurring throughout Stanislaus.

Improving Birth Outcomes

Community-wide concern about the health of Stanislaus's youngest residents initiated the design and promotion of the Healthy Birth Outcomes program, which now serves as one of the Family Resource Centers' foundational programs in cooperation with the Health Services Agency and the Children and Families Commission. The Healthy Birth Outcomes program focuses on improving birth and child health outcomes by increasing the number of babies born at term and at adequate weights and by improving family functioning and maternal/child support systems. The program consists of three components: intensive case management services (for women with medical problems such as diabetes, substance abuse, and behavioral health issues), community-based services, and provider/county outreach. Services include assessment, service plan development, prenatal care referral, medical/preventive health services, social services, infant care/parenting education, and support services (Stanislaus County, n.d.). Annual enrollment has grown from 306 women in 2005 to 554 women in 2009.

In a county where prematurity, infant mortality, and low birth weight are chronic challenges, local epidemiologists are thrilled to finally report progress. According to one of the county's epidemiologists, the percentage of premature births among women enrolled in the Healthy Birth Outcomes program (5 percent) is lower than the rest of the county (11.1 percent) as a whole, despite the fact that some of the women enrolled are experiencing "high-risk" pregnancies.

Looking Back and Moving Forward

Looking back on a decade's worth of partnerships, planning, and action, Stanislaus County Health Services Agency's MAPP mastermind, Cleopathia Moore, notes that "if you spend the time up front, the results will pay off. Not the short term, but the long-term gain." Public health staff members in Stanislaus are eager to share the range of new programs and relationships that have formed as a result of MAPP—from policy initiatives to reduced obesity rates to the establishment of a Certified Farmers' Market and a new walking trail. As a local health educator put it, "The process takes on a life of its own and starts developing like in a web.

Everybody took something and developed it further." Looking toward the decade ahead, there's no doubt that the growing sense of community, new partnerships, and focus on system change will aid public health stakeholders as they continue to tackle chronic and emerging health challenges in Stanislaus.

Discussion Questions

1. What were the major health issues affecting Stanislaus County?
2. What is the purpose of Stanislaus Family Resource Centers?
3. How has the MAPP process benefited Stanislaus County?

INNOVATION IN COLORECTAL CANCER EDUCATION PROGRAMS

C OLORECTAL CANCER (CRC), the second most common cause of cancer death in the United States, is preventable if detected at an early stage. A readily available screening test can prevent many cases of this cancer by identifying precancerous polyps, which are then removed. Unfortunately, the majority of eligible Americans are not screened.

The rate of colorectal cancer in Luzerne County, Pennsylvania, is alarming, approximately 20 percent higher than the state average and nearly 40 percent higher than the national average. This case study demonstrates a way to increase the screening rate and reduce the incidence of this disease through the use of marketing strategies. These strategies include developing a target market; using a marketing mix, which involves the product, price, place, and promotion; conducting a SWOT analysis, which includes looking at the strengths, weaknesses, opportunities, and threats; and promoting and disseminating information concerning the return on investment (ROI) to other employers in the county in order to enroll more businesses in this project.

This colorectal cancer education program was developed and implemented by members of the Luzerne County Colorectal Cancer Task Force and initially involved two businesses in Luzerne County that agreed to aggressively market a colorectal cancer screening program to their employees over age fifty. A marketing plan was designed to increase awareness of the need for the screening beginning at age fifty and the dangers of ignoring this very preventable cancer. Information about the screening test was made available to all employees on each company's Web site for a two-week period before the online education program was conducted.

This online education program was developed on a local college's SharePoint site, which is a dedicated virtual site where data can be entered. It began with a pretest, which consisted of a series of questions about the epidemiology of colorectal cancer, the testing procedure, those at high risk of developing the disease, and a testimonial from a colorectal cancer survivor. The pretest was followed by an eleven-minute colorectal cancer education program, which comprised a series of voice-narrated PowerPoint slides discussing the risk factors for developing colorectal cancer, the various tests available for this disease, and recommendations for those at high risk for developing this disease. The program concluded with a posttest, incorporating all of the questions from the pretest, which was designed to assess the knowledge participants gained from the education program.

Program 1

The first colorectal cancer education program was completed during May 2009. There were 504 employees eligible to take advantage of the program, and the employer offered incentives to encourage employees to complete it. There were 184 employees who participated in the program, representing 36.5 percent of those eligible to attend.

Information concerning the availability of the program was sent by e-mail and in letters to all employees on two separate occasions. An incentive was offered to program participants for attendance (a ten-dollar Barnes & Noble gift card or two free movie tickets). There were twenty-eight employees who indicated a willingness to receive a follow-up phone call from the American Cancer Society six months after program completion.

The first three items in Table CS1 were used to assess the subjects' knowledge in regard to CRC. For all three items the subjects' knowledge of CRC significantly improved in the posttest compared to the pretest. Item 4 was inserted in both the pretest and the posttest to make sure the subjects were carefully reading the items. Because the pre- and posttests were administered over a short time period, as expected, there was not a significant difference in scores on this item. Item 5 was used to see if the program may influence subjects' behavioral intentions in relation to CRC. As indicated in Table CS1, a significantly higher percentage of subjects intend to get screened for CRC as a result of the program. Moreover, item 6 pertains to another aspect of the subjects' behavior: the vast majority of the subjects clearly intend to share what they have learned with their family and friends. Only 1.6 percent of the subjects responded "no" to this item. Overall, these subjects learned key information on CRC and are likely to take action to help prevent or at least detect CRC in themselves and others they care about.

Table CS1   Pre- and Posttest Results for Program 1 (n = 184)

Item	Pretest Score	Posttest Score	Significant Change ($p<.05$)
1. You are at risk for CRC if . . . (% indicated "all of the above" for the following: age fifty or older, have had a colon/rectal polyp, family history of CRC)	76.6%	84.2%	Yes
2. Signs and/or symptoms of CRC include . . . (% indicated "all of the above" for the following: change in bowel habits, rectal bleeding, unexplained weight loss)	85.3%	95.7%	Yes
3. An effective screening method for CRC is . . . (% indicated "fecal occult blood test")	58.0%	88.6%	Yes
4. Have you ever been tested for CRC? (% indicated "yes")— control question	41.8%	43.5%	No
5. I plan to ask my doctor to be screened for CRC (% indicated "very likely" or "definitely")	29.4%	39.1%	Yes
6. I plan to share what I learned about CRC with friends and family (% indicated "very likely" or "definitely")—posttest only	n/a	66.8%	n/a

Note: Statistically significant change was determined by a pairwise t-test (df = 183).

Program 2

The second colorectal cancer education program was completed during June and July 2009. There were 298 employees who were eligible to take advantage of this program, and the City of Wilkes-Barre offered incentives to encourage them to complete it. There were 51 employees who participated in the program, representing 17.1 percent of those eligible to attend.

Information concerning the availability of the program was sent by e-mail and in letters to all employees on two separate occasions. An incentive was offered to program participants for attendance (a ten-dollar gas card). There were thirteen employees who indicated a willingness to receive a follow-up phone call from the American Cancer Society six months after program completion.

Table CS2   Pre- and Posttest Results for Program 2 (n = 51)

Item	Pretest Score	Posttest Score	Significant Change (p<.05)
1. You are at risk for CRC if... (% indicated "all of the above" for the following: age fifty or older, have had a colon/rectal polyp, family history of CRC)	78.4%	82.4%	No
2. Signs and/or symptoms of CRC include... (% indicated "all of the above" for the following: change in bowel habits, rectal bleeding, unexplained weight loss)	94.1%	98.0%	No
3. An effective screening method for CRC is... (% indicated "fecal occult blood test")	76.0%	92.2%	Yes
4. Have you ever been tested for CRC? (% indicated "yes")— control question	37.3%	39.2%	No
5. I plan to ask my doctor to be screened for CRC (% indicated "very likely" or "definitely")	35.3%	51.0%	Yes
6. I plan to share what I learned about CRC with friends and family (% indicated "very likely" or "definitely")—posttest only	n/a	72.6%	n/a

Note: Statistically significant change was determined by a pairwise t-test (df = 50).

The results from this program were somewhat comparable to the findings from program 1. As shown in Table CS2, for all three knowledge questions, scores improved from the pretest to the posttest. However, in only one item (item 3) was this change statistically significant. One reason why significant changes were not found in the first two knowledge questions is the smaller sample size in program 2 compared to program 1. Further, the subjects in program 2 had a much stronger knowledge of the signs and symptoms of CRC prior to the education program. Thus, there was very little room for improvement. Similar to subjects in program 1, as expected, subjects in program 2 did not indicate a significant change in prior testing for CRC. Moreover, these subjects are also more willing to be screened for CRC after the program as compared to before the program. Finally, a very large percentage of subjects plan to share this CRC information with their loved ones.

Conclusion

Both groups gained valuable knowledge from this education program on CRC. In addition, both groups appear to have intentions to help prevent or detect CRC in themselves and their loved ones. Thus, the program had value in meeting this important health promotion objective.

Colorectal cancer screening is a cost-effective preventive program that is being used by far too few individuals despite its being readily available and paid for by most health insurance programs. Recent research clearly indicates that colorectal cancer screening is often a missed opportunity that will save many lives and result in a reduction in the costs associated with this expensive and deadly form of cancer.

The results from this colorectal cancer education program offer strong support for the accomplishment of the goals put forth in the Luzerne County Colorectal Task Force's original mission statement. For example, on the posttest, as compared to the pretest, a significantly higher percentage of the employees in program 1 and program 2 indicated that they are likely to ask their doctor to be screened for colorectal cancer—a desired outcome of the program. Almost all of the participants in both programs indicated that they are likely to share what they learned from the program with friends and family members, which represents another intended outcome of the program.

Discussion Questions

1. Can this approach of developing online health education programs work with other chronic diseases?
2. Can employers use marketing skills to increase the participation rates in online education programs?
3. What is the best way to share the results of the program discussed in this case study with other communities?

REFERENCES

Active Living Research. (2005). *Investigating Policies and Environments to Support Active Communities*. Robert Wood Johnson Foundation. www.activelivingresearch.org/files/briefing0305.pdf.

Adler, N. E., and Newman, K. (2002). Socioeconomic Disparities in Health: Pathways and Policies. *Health Affairs*, *21*(2), 60–76.

Agency for Healthcare Research and Quality. (2002). Expanding Patient-Centered Care to Empower Patients and Assist Providers. *Research in Action*, no. 5. www.ahrq.gov/qual/ptcareria.htm.

Alameda County Public Health Department. (2008). *Life and Death from Unnatural Causes: Health and Social Inequity in Alameda County*. Oakland, CA: Alameda County Public Health Department.

American Academy of Family Physicians, American Academy of Pediatrics, American College of Physicians, and American Osteopathic Association. (2007). Joint Principles of the Patient Centered Medical Home. www.pcpcc.net/content/joint-principles-patient-centered-medical-home.

American Association of Colleges of Nursing. (2009). Nursing Shortage Fact Sheet. www.aacn.nche.edu/Media/FactSheets/NursingShortage.htm.

American Medical Association. (2010). Humana Bolstering Chronic Disease Management Service. www.ama-assn.org/amednews/2010/09/27/bise0929.htm.

Arras, R., and Peters, M. (2009). Health Education in Practice: Using MAPP to Connect Communities: One County's Story. *Health Educator*, *41*(2), 77–84.

Aschengrau, A., and Seage, G. (2003). *Essentials of Epidemiology in Public Health*. Sudbury, MA: Jones & Bartlett Learning.

Association for Community Health Improvement. (2006). Advancing the State of the Art in Community Benefit. www.communityhlth.org/communityhlth/resources/communitybenefit.html.

Association of American Medical Colleges. (1998, June). *AAMC Contemporary Issues in Medicine: Medical Informatics and Population Health: Medical School Objectives Project Report 11*. Washington DC: Association of Medical Colleges.

Baicker, K., Cutler, D., and Song, Z. (2010). Workplace Wellness Programs Can Generate Savings. *Health Affairs*, *29*(2), 1–8.

Bailey, S.B.C. (2010). Focusing on Solid Partnerships Across Multiple Sectors for Population Health Improvement. *Preventing Chronic Disease*, *7*(6). http://www.cdc.gov/pcd/issues/2010/nov/10_0126.htm.

Baker, P. (2009, July 9). Poorer Nations Reject a Target on Emissions Cut. *The New York Times*, p. A–1.

Balogun, J., and Hailey, V. H. (2008). *Exploring Strategic Change* (Third Edition). New York: Prentice Hall.

Barnett, K. (2009). Beyond the Numerical Tally: Quality and Stewardship in Community Benefit. Oakland, CA: Public Health Institute.

Barton, P. (2010). *Understanding the U.S. Health Services System* (Fourth Edition). Chicago: Health Administration Press.

Batalden, P., and Davidoff, F. (2008). What Is Quality Improvement and How Can It Transform Health Care? *Quality & Safe Health Care, 16*(1), 2–3.

Beal A. C., Doty, M. M., Hernandez, S. E., Shea, K. K., and Davis, K. (2007). *Closing the Divide: How Medical Homes Promote Equity in Health Care: Results from the Commonwealth Fund 2006 Health Care Quality Survey.* The Commonwealth Fund.

Beerel, A. (2009). *Leadership and Change Management.* Thousand Oaks, CA: Sage.

Beltsch, L. M., Brooks, R. G., Menachemi, N., and Libbey, P. M. (2007). Public Health at Center Stage: New Roles, Old Props. *Health Affairs, 25*(4), 911–922.

Berkowitz. E. N. (2006). *Essentials of Health Care Marketing* (Second Edition). Sudbury, MA: Jones & Bartlett Learning.

Bernstein, S. J. (2008). A New Model for Chronic-Care Delivery. *Frontiers of Health Services Management, 25*(2), 31–38.

Berwick, D. (1996). A Primer on Leading the Improvement of Systems. *British Medical Journal, 312*(7031), 619–622.

Berwick, D., James, B., and Coye, M. (2003). Connections Between Quality Measurement and Improvement. *Medical Care, 41*(1[Supplement]), I-30–I-38

Bodenheimer, T., Chen, E., and Bennett, H. D. (2009). Confronting the Growing Burden of Chronic Disease: Can the U.S. Health Care Workforce Do the Job? *Health Affairs 28*(1), 64–74.

Bodenheimer, T., Wagner, E. H., and Grumbach, K. (2002). Improving Primary Care for Patients with Chronic Illness: The Chronic Care Model, Part 2. *Journal of the American Medical Association, 288*(15), 1909–1914.

Bossidy, L., and Charan, R. (2002). *Execution: The Discipline of Getting Things Done.* New York: Crown Business.

Brinkerhoff, J. (2002). Assessing and Improving Partnership Relationships and Outcomes: A Proposed Framework. *Evaluation and Programming, 25*(3), 215–231.

Brooks, R. G., Beitsch, L. M., Street, P., and Chukmaitov, A. (2009). Aligning Public Health Financing with Essential Public Health Service Functions and National Public Health Performance Standards. *Journal of Public Health Management and Practice, 15*(4), 299–306.

Brown M. J. (2002). Costs and Benefits of Enforcing Housing Policies to Prevent Childhood Lead Poisoning. *Medical Decision Making, 22*(6), 482–492.

Brown, R. (1997). Leadership to Meet the Challenges to the Public's Health. *American Journal of Public Health, 87*(4), 554–557.

Brownlee, S. (2007). *Overtreated: Why Too Much Medicine Is Making Us Sicker and Poorer.* New York: Bloomsbury USA.

Brownson, R. C., Fielding, J. E., and Maylahn, C. M. (2009). Evidence-Based Public Health: A Fundamental Concept for Public Health Practice. *Annual Review of Public Health, 30,* 175–201.

Brownson, R. C., Remington, P. L., and Davis, J. R. (1998). *Chronic Disease Epidemiology and Control* (Second Edition). Washington DC: American Public Health Association.

Buka, S. (1999). *Results from the Project on Human Development in Chicago Neighborhoods.* Proceedings from the 13th annual California Conference on Childhood Injury Control, San Diego, CA.

California Newsreel. (2008). Unnatural Causes. www.unnaturalcauses.org/resources.php?
topic_id=2.

Catterall, J. S. (1997). Involvement in the Arts and Success in Secondary School. *Americans for the Arts MONOGRAPHS, 1*(9). www.americansforthearts.org/NAPD/files/9393/Involvement
%20in%20the%20Arts%20and%20Success%20in%20Secondary%20School%20%28
%2798%29.pdf.

Centers for Disease Control and Prevention (CDC). (1991). Assessment Protocol for Excellence
in Public Health. http://wonder.cdc.gov/wonder/prevguid/p0000089/p0000089.asp
#head002000000000000.

Centers for Disease Control and Prevention (CDC). (1995). Framework for Program Evaluation
in Public Health. *Morbidity and Mortality Weekly Report, 48*(11), 1–40.

Centers for Disease Control and Prevention. (1997). *Principles of Community Engagement.* Public
Health Practice Program Office. www.cdc.gov/phppo/pce/.

Centers for Disease Control and Prevention (CDC). (1999a). *Healthy People 2010: A Systematic Approach to Health Improvement.* www.healthypeople.gov/2010/Document/html/
uih/uih_2.

Centers for Disease Control and Prevention (CDC). (1999b). Ten Great Public Health
Achievements—United States, 1900–1999. *Morbidity and Mortality Weekly Report, 48*(12),
241–243.

Centers for Disease Control and Prevention (CDC). (2005a). *National Health Interview Survey
2001–2005.* National Center for Health Statistics. www.cdc.gov/nchs/nhis.htm.

Centers for Disease Control and Prevention (CDC). (2005b). Deaths and Mortality. National
Center for Health Statistics. www.cdc.gov/nchs/fastats/deaths.htm.

Centers for Disease Control and Prevention (CDC). (2006a, December 22). Preface: Sixty Years
of Public Health Science at CDC. *Morbidity and Mortality Weekly Report, 55*(Supplement), 1.

Centers for Disease Control and Prevention (CDC). (2006b). Web-Based Injury Statistics
Query and Reporting System (WISQARS). National Center for Injury Prevention and
Control. www.cdc.gov/injury/wisqars/index.html.

Centers for Disease Control and Prevention (CDC). (2007). Chronic Disease Publications.
www.cdc.gov/nccdphp/publications/index.htm.

Centers for Disease Control and Prevention (CDC). (2008a, July 8). *Budget Request Summary:
Fiscal Year 2009.* www.cdc.gov/fmo/PDFs/FY09budgetreqsummary.pdf.

Centers for Disease Control and Prevention (CDC). (2008b). *Key Findings from Public Health
Preparedness: Mobilizing State by State.* www.bt.cdc.gov/publications/feb08phprep/pdf/
feb08phpkeyfindings.pdf.

Centers for Disease Control and Prevention (CDC). (2008c). National Public Health Performance Standards Program (NPHPSP). www.cdc.gov/od/ocphp/nphpsp/
PresentationLinks.htm.

Centers for Disease Control and Prevention (CDC). (2008d). Preventing Tobacco Use.
www.cdc.gov/NCCphp/publications/factsheets/Prevention/tobacco.htm.

Centers for Disease Control and Prevention (CDC). (2008e). *Youth Violence Data Sheet.* National
Center for Injury Prevention and Control. www.cdc.gov/ncipc/dvp/YV_DataSheet.pdf.

Centers for Disease Control and Prevention (CDC). (2009a). Chronic Disease Prevention and
Health Promotion. www.cdc.gov/nccdphp/.

Centers for Disease Control and Prevention (CDC). (2009b). Chronic Diseases: The Power to
Prevent at a Glance. www.cdc.gov/nccdphp/publications/AAG/chronic.htm.

Centers for Disease Control and Prevention (CDC). (2009c). Climate Change and Public
Health: CDC Policy. http://cdc.gov/climatechange/policy.htm.

Centers for Disease Control and Prevention (CDC). (2009d). Healthy People 2020. *Proposed Healthy People 2020 Objectives*. www.healthypeople.gov/hp2020/default.asp.

Centers for Disease Control and Prevention (CDC). (2009e). Leading Causes of Death. www.cdc.gov/nchs/fastats/lcod.htm.

Centers for Disease Control and Prevention (CDC). (2009f). National Nosocomial Infections Surveillance System. www.cdc.gov/ncidod/dhqp/nnis_pubs.html.

Centers for Disease Control and Prevention (CDC). (2009g). Outbreak of Swine-Origin Influenza A (H1N1) Virus Infection—Mexico, March–April, 2009. *Morbidity and Mortality Weekly Report*, *58*(17), 467–470.

Centers for Disease Control and Prevention (CDC). (2010a). Garnering Partnerships to Bridge Gaps Among Mental Health, Health Care, and Public Health. www.cdc.gov/pcd/issues/2010/jan/09_0127.htm.

Centers for Disease Control and Prevention (CDC). (2010b). Healthy People 2010 Leading Health Indicators at a Glance. www.cdc.gov/nchs/healthy_people/hp2010/hp2010_indicators.htm.

Centers for Disease Control and Prevention (CDC). (2011a). Climate Change and Public Health. www.cdc.gov/ClimateChange/default.htm.

Centers for Disease Control and Prevention. (2011b). Epi-X: The Epidemic Information Exchange. www.cdc.gov/epix/#1.

Centers for Disease Control and Prevention (CDC). (n.d.). *Active Community Environments Factsheet*. http://www.sprawlwatch.org.

Centers for Disease Control and Prevention (CDC). (n.d.). *National Public Health Performance Standards Program* (Brochure). www.cdc.gov/od/ocphp/nphpsp/PDF/Brochure.pdf.

Centers for Disease Control and Prevention (CDC), AARP, and American Medical Association. (2009). *Promoting Preventive Services for Adults 50–64: Community and Clinical Partnerships*. Atlanta, GA: National Association of Chronic Disease Directors. www.cdc.gov/aging2010.

Centers for Medicare and Medicaid Services. (n.d.). National Health Expenditure Data. U.S. Department of Health and Human Services. www.cms.gov/NationalHealthExpendData/02_NationalHealthAccountsHistorical.asp#TopOfPage.

Christensen. C. M., Bohmer. R., and Kenagy, J. (2000). Will Disruptive Innovations Cure Health Care? *Harvard Business Review*, *78*(5), 103–111.

Christensen, C. M., Grossman, J. H., and Hwang, J. (2009). *The Innovator's Prescription: A Disruptive Solution for Health Care*. New York: McGraw-Hill.

Christoffel, T., and Gallagher, S. S. (2006). *Injury Prevention and Public Health* (Second Edition). Sudbury, MA: Jones & Bartlett Learning.

Clark, N. M., and Weist, E. (2000). Mastering the New Public Health. *American Journal of Public Health*, *90*(8), 1208–1211.

Clawson, J. G. (2009). *Level Three Leadership: Getting Below the Surface* (Fourth Edition). Upper Saddle River, NJ: Prentice Hall.

Coker, A. (2005). Opportunities for Prevention: Addressing IPV in the Health Care Setting. *Family Violence Prevention and Health Practice, 1*.

Collins. J. (2009). *How the Mighty Fall and Why Some Companies Never Give In*. New York: HarperCollins.

Committee on Public Health Strategies to Improve Health. (2010). *For the Public's Health: The Role of Measurement in Action and Accountability*. Institute of Medicine. www.nap.edu/catalog/13005.html.

The Commonwealth Fund. (1999). *Medicaid Managed Care and Cultural Diversity in California.* www.commonwealthfund.org/usr_doc/Coye_Medicaid_managed_311.pdf.

The Commonwealth Fund Commission on a High Performance Health System. (2006, September). *Why Not the Best? Results from a National Scorecard on U.S. Health System Performance.* www.commonwealthfund.org/usr_doc/Commission_whynotthebest_951.pdf? section=4039>.

The Commonwealth Fund Commission on a High Performance Health System. (2009). *The Path to a High Performance Health System: A 2020 Vision and the Policies to Pave the Way.* www.commonwealthfund.org/Content/Publications/Fund-Reports/2009/Feb/ The-Path-to-a-High-Performance-US-Health-System.aspx.

Community Guide Branch. (n.d.). Guide to Community Preventive Services. Centers for Disease Control and Prevention. http://www.thecommunityguide.org/index.html.

Consultative Group on Early Childhood Care and Development. (n.d.). What is ECCD? www.ecdgroup.com/what_is_ECCD.asp.

Corso, L. C., Wiesner P. J., Halverson, P.K., and Brown, C.K. (2000). Using the Essential Services as a Foundation for Performance Measurement and Assessment of Local Public Health Systems. *Journal of Public Health Management and Practice*, *6*(5), 1–18.

Currie, D. (2009). Nation's Health Not Improving: Obesity, Tobacco Use to Blame. *Nation's Health*, *39*(1). http://thenationshealth.aphapublications.org/content/39/1/4.1.full?sid= ecacb72e-ce0a-4c6e-8d5c-60b72f6d994d.

Currie, D. (2010). Prevention Saves Lives as Well as Money, New Research Confirms. *Nation's Health*, *40*(9), p. 5.

Curtis V. A., Garbrah-Aidoo, N., and Scott, B. (2007). Ethics in Public Health Research: Masters of Marketing: Bringing Private Sector Skills to Public Health Partnerships. *American Journal of Public Health*, *97*, 634–641.

Davis, J. W., Taira, D., and Chung R. S. (2006). Health Disparities in Thirty Indicators of Recommended Clinical Care. *Journal of Healthcare Quality*, *28*(3), 32–41.

Davis, R., Cook, D., and Cohen, L. (2005). A Community Resilience Approach to Reducing Ethnic and Racial Disparities in Health. *American Journal of Public Health*, *95*(12), 2168–2173.

Dearry, A. (2004). Impacts of Our Built Environment on Public Health. *Environmental Health Perspectives*, *112*(11), A600–A601.

DeVol, R., and Armen, B. (2007, October). *An Unhealthy America: The Economic Burden of Chronic Disease.* Milken Institute. www.milkeninstitute.org/publications/publications.taf?function =detail&ID=38801018&cat=ResRep.

DioData, C., Likosky, D., DeFoe, G., Groom, R., Shann, K., Krumholz, C., Warren, C., Pieroni, J., Benak, A., McCusker, K., Olmstead, E., Ross, C., O'Connor, G. (2008). Cardiopulmonary Bypass Recommendations in Adults: The Northern New England Experience. *Journal of Extracorporeal Technology*, *40*(1), 16–20.

Dlugacz, Y. (2010). *Value-Based Health Care: Linking Finance and Quality.* San Francisco: Jossey-Bass.

Dodder, R. (2000). *Complex Adaptive Systems and Complexity Theory: Inter-Related Knowledge Domains.* http://web.mit.edu/esd.83/www/notebook/ComplexityKD.PDF.

Doll. R., and Hill, A. B. (1950). Smoking and Carcinoma of the Lungs: Preliminary Report. *British Medical Journal*, *2*(4682), 739–748.

Dubrin, A. J. (2007). *Leadership Research Findings, Practice, and Skills* (Fifth Edition). New York: Houghton Mifflin.

Emanuel, E. J. (2008). *Healthcare, Guaranteed: A Simple, Secure Solution for America*. Philadelphia: Perseus Books.

The Endocrine Society. (2009). Obesity-Related Diseases. www.obesityinamerica.org/under standingObesity/diseases.cfm.

Enthoven, A. C. (1978). Shattuck Lecture—Cutting Cost Without Cutting the Quality of Care. *New England Journal of Medicine 298*(22), 1229–1238.

Fairchild, A. L., Rosner, D., Colgrove, J., Bayer, R., and Fried, L. (2010). The Exodus of Public Health: What History Can Tell Us About the Future. *American Journal of Public Health, 100*(1), 54–63.

Family Violence Prevention Fund. (n.d.). *The Facts on Health Care and Domestic Violence*. http://endabuse.org/userfiles/file/Children_and_Families/HealthCare.pdf.

Family Violence Prevention Fund. (n.d.). *The Facts on Immigrant Women and Domestic Violence*. http://endabuse.org/userfiles/file/Children_and_Families/Immigrant.pdf.

Feldstein, P. J. (2005). *Health Economics*. Clifton Park, NY: Thomson Delmar Learning.

Feldstein, P. J. (2007). *Health Policy Issues: An Economic Perspective*. Chicago: Health Administration Press.

Fleming, S. T. (2008). *Managerial Epidemiology Concepts and Cases*. Chicago: Health Administration Press.

Florida Charts. (n.d.). Florida Population Estimates. www.floridacharts.com/charts/popquery.aspx.

Florida Department of Health, Bureau of Chronic Disease and Health Promotion. (2010). http://www.doh.state.fl.us/family/chronicdisease/.

Florida Department of Health. (2005). NPHP Local Public Health System Assessment Results. http://www.doh.state.fl.us/compass/Resources/FieldGuide/5LocalPHSystem/StateReportNPHPSP.pdf.

Fottler, M., Ford, R., and Heaton, C. (2010). *Achieving Service Excellence: Strategies for Healthcare* (Second Edition). Chicago: Health Administration Press.

Freudenberg, N., and Ruglis, J. (2007). Reframing School Dropout as a Public Health Issue. *Preventing Chronic Disease, 4*(4), 1–11.

Frieden, T. R. (2004). Asleep at the Switch: Local Public Health and Chronic Disease. *American Journal of Public Health, 94*(12), 2059–2061.

Friedman. T. (2008). *Hot, Flat, and Crowded: Why We Need a Green Revolution—and How It Can Renew America*. New York: Farrar, Straus and Giroux.

Frumkin, H., Hess, J., Luber, G., Malilay, J., and McGeehin, M. (2008). Climate Change: The Public Health Response. *American Journal of Public Health, 98*(3), 435–445.

Fuchs, V. R. (1998). *Who Shall Live? Health, Economics, and Social Choice*. River Edge, NJ: World Scientific.

Fuchs, V. R. (2008). Three "Inconvenient Truths" About Health Care. *New England Journal of Medicine, 359*(17), 1749–1751.

Gale Reference Team. (2007, August). Leadership Institutes Help Public Health Workers Advance Careers. *Nation's Health, 37*(6), 25.

Gallo, C. (2011). *The Innovation Secrets of Steve Jobs: Insanely Different Principles for Breakthrough Success*. New York: McGraw-Hill.

Geronimus, A. T. (2001). Understanding and Eliminating Racial Inequalities in Women's Health in the United States: The Role of the Weathering Conceptual Framework. *Journal of the American Medical Women's Association, 56*(4), 133–136, 149–150.

Gladwell, M. (2000). *The Tipping Point: How Little Things Can Make a Big Difference.* Boston: Little, Brown.

Goetzel, R. Z. (2009). Do Prevention or Treatment Services Save Money? The Wrong Debate. *Health Affairs, 28*(1), 37–41.

Grainger, C., and Griffiths, R. (1998). Public Health Leadership—Do We Have It? Do We Need It? *Journal of Public Health Medicine, 20*(4), 375–376.

Gray, M. (2009). Public Health Leadership: Creating the Culture for the Twenty-First Century. *Journal of Public Health, 31*(2), 208–209.

Greenleaf, R. K., and Spears, L. (2002). *Servant Leadership: A Journey into the Legitimate Power and Greatness* (Twenty-Fifth Anniversary Edition). New York: Paulist Press.

Griffiths, J. (2006). Mini-Symposium: Health and Environment Sustainability. The Convergence of Public Health and Sustainable Development. *Journal of the Royal Institute of Public Health, 120,* 581–584.

Haines, A., Kovats, R. S., Campbell-Lendrum, D., and Corvalan, C. (2006). Climate Change and Human Health: Impacts, Vulnerability and Public Health. *Public Health, 120*(7), 585–596.

Halliday, J., Asthana, S.N.M., and Richardson, S. (2004). Evaluating Partnership: The Role of Formal Assessment Tools. *Evaluation, 10*(3), 285–303.

Halvorson, G. C. (2009). *Health Care Will Not Reform Itself.* New York: CRC Press.

Hammer, M. (2007). The Process Audit. *Harvard Business Review, 85*(4), 111–123.

Hancock, T. (2000). Healthy Communities Must Also Be Sustainable Communities. *Public Health Reports, 115*(2-3), 151–156.

Harmon, K. (2010). Deadly Pandemic. *Scientific American, 302*(6), 48.

Healey, B. J., and Walker, K. (2009). *Introduction to Occupational Health in Public Health Practice.* San Francisco: Jossey-Bass.

Healey, B. J., and Zimmerman, R. S. (2010). *The New World of Health Promotion: New Program Development, Implementation and Evaluation.* Sudbury, MA: Jones & Bartlett Learning.

Health Services Agency/Public Health Community Assessment, Planning and Evaluation Unit. (2010). *Stanislaus County Community Health Improvement Plan (CHIP) 2010 Draft.*

Heath, S., Soep, E., and Roach, A. (1998). Living the Arts Through Language and Learning: A Report on Community-Based Youth Organizations. *Americans for the Arts MONOGRAPHS, 2*(7). www.americansforthearts.org/NAPD/files/9603/Living%20the%20Arts%20 Through%20Language%20and%20Learning%20%28November%20%2798%29.pdf.

Heifetz, R. (2006). Anchoring Leadership in the Work of Adaptive Process. In F. Hesselbein and M. Goldsmith (Eds.), *The Leader of the Future 2: Visions, Strategies, and Practices for the New Era* (pp. 73–85). San Francisco: Jossey-Bass.

Hemenway. D. (2010). Why We Don't Spend Enough on Public Health. *New England Journal of Medicine, 362*(18), 1657–1658.

Henderson, J. W. (2009). *Health Economics and Policy.* Mason, OH: South-Western Cengage Learning.

Herbold, R. J. (2007). *Seduced by Success: How the Best Companies Survive the Nine Traps of Winning.* New York: McGraw-Hill.

Herzlinger, R. (2007). *Who Killed Health Care?* New York: McGraw-Hill.

Hesselbein, F. (2008). *The Key to Cultural Transformation.* San Francisco: Jossey-Bass.

Hickman, G. R. (1998). *Leading Organizations: Perspectives for a New Era.* Thousand Oaks, CA: Sage.

Holmes, L. (2009). *Basics of Public Health Core Competencies*. Sudbury, MA: Jones & Bartlett Learning.

Honoré, P. A. (2009, November). *Quality in the Public Health System*. Presentation at the 137th annual American Public Health Association Meeting, Philadelphia, PA.

Hossain, P., Kawar, B., and El Nahas, M. (2007). Obesity and Diabetes in the Developing World—A Growing Challenge. *New England Journal of Medicine, 356*(3), 213–215.

House Committee on Government Reform. (2004, February 2). *A Review of This Year's Flu Season: Does Our Public Health System Need a Shot in the Arm?* 108th Congress, 2nd session.

House, J. S., and Williams, D. R. (2000). Paper Contribution B: Understanding and Reducing Socioeconomic and Racial/Ethnic Disparities in Health. In *Promoting Health: Intervention Strategies from Social and Behavioral Research* (pp. 81–124). Washington DC: Institute of Medicine.

How, S.K.H., Shih, A., Lau, J., and Schoen, C. (2008, August). *Public Views on U.S. Health System Organization: A Call for New Directions*. The Commonwealth Fund. http://www .commonwealthfund.org/~/media/Files/Surveys/2008/The%20Commonwealth %20Fund%20Survey%20of%20Public%20Views%20of%20the%20U%20S%20 %20Health%20Care%20System%20%202008/Public_Views_SurveyPg_8%204%2008 %20pdf.pdf.

Improving Chronic Illness Care. (n.d.). The Chronic Care Model. www.improvingchroniccare .org/index.php?p=The_Chronic_Care_Model&s=2.

Institute for Healthcare Improvement (IHI). (2003). The Breakthrough Series: IHI's Collaborative Model for Achieving Breakthrough Improvement (IHI Innovation Series White Paper). Boston: Institute for Healthcare Improvement. www.ihi.org/IHI/Results/WhitePapers/ TheBreakthroughSeriesIHIsCollaborativeModelforAchieving+ BreakthroughImprovement.htm.

Institute for Healthcare Improvement (IHI). (n.d.). Changes. www.ihi.org/IHI/Topics/ HealthcareAssociatedInfections/InfectionsGeneral/Changes/.

Institute of Medicine (IOM). (1988). *The Future of Public Health*. Washington DC: National Academies Press.

Institute of Medicine (IOM). (1996). *Using Performance Monitoring to Improve Community Health*. Washington DC: National Academies Press.

Institute of Medicine (IOM). (1997). *Improving Health in a Community*. Washington DC: National Academies Press.

Institute of Medicine (IOM). (1999). *To Err Is Human*. Washington DC: National Academies Press.

Institute of Medicine (IOM). (2000a). A Social Environmental Approach to Health and Health Interventions. In *Promoting Health: Intervention Strategies from Social and Behavioral Research*. Washington DC: Institute of Medicine.

Institute of Medicine (IOM). (2001). *Crossing the Quality Chasm: A New Health System for the 21st Century*. Washington DC: National Academies Press

Institute of Medicine (IOM). (2002). *The Future of the Public's Health in the 21st Century*. Washington D.C. National Academies Press.

Institute of Medicine (IOM). (2010a, April). *Bridging the Evidence Gap in Obesity Prevention: A Framework to Inform Decision Making* (Report brief). www.iom.edu/~/media/Files/Report %20Files/2010/Bridging-the-Evidence-Gap-in-Obesity-Prevention/Bridging%20the%20 Evidence%20Gap%202010%20%20Report%20Brief.ashx.

Institute of Medicine (IOM). (2010b). *A Population-Based Policy and System Change Approach to Prevent and Control Hypertension*. Washington DC: National Academies Press.

Institute of Medicine (IOM). (n.d.). Crossing the Quality Chasm: The IOM Health Care Quality Initiative. www.iom.edu/Global/News%20Announcements/Crossing-the-Quality-Chasm-The-IOM-Health-Care-Quality-Initiative.aspx.

Internal Revenue Service. (1983). Rev. Rule 83.157, 1983-2 C.B. 94. www.irs.gov/pub/irs-tege/rr83-157.pdf.

Jackson, R. J., and Kochtitzky, C. (2009). *Creating a Healthy Environment: The Impact of the Built Environment on Public Health*. Centers for Disease Control and Prevention. www.sprawlwatch.org.

James, P. T., Rigby, N., Leach, R., and International Obesity Task Force. (2004, February). The Obesity Epidemic, Metabolic Syndrome, and Prevention Strategies. *European Journal of Cardiovascular Prevention & Rehabilitation*, *11*(1), 3–8.

Jenkins, P., and Phillips, B. (2009). *Katrina Women Report, Tulane University*. www.tulane.edu/~wc/katrinawomenreportfeb2009/NCCROWreport08-chapter8.pdf.

Johnson, K., Grossman, W., and Cassidy, A. (Eds.). (1996). *Collaborating to Improve Community Health*. San Francisco: Jossey-Bass.

Johnson, T. D. (2008). Shortage of U.S. Public Health Workers Projected to Worsen. *Nation's Health*, *38*(4), p. 1.

Juran, J. M. (1988). *Juran's Quality Control Handbook* (Fifth Edition). New York: McGraw-Hill.

Kaplan, R. S., and Norton, D. P. (2001). *The Strategy-Focused Organization: How Balanced Scorecard Companies Thrive in the New Business Environment*. Boston: Harvard Business School Press.

Keyton, J. (2005). *Communication and Organizational Culture*. Thousand Oaks, CA: Sage.

Kindig, D., and Stoddart, D. (2003). What Is Population Health? *American Journal of Public Health*, *93*(3), 380–383.

Kinner, K., and Pelligrini, C. (2009). Expenditures for Public Health: Assessing Historical and Prospective Trends. *American Journal of Public Health*, *99*(10), 1780–1791.

Koh, H. (2010). A 2020 vision for healthy people. *New England Journal of Medicine*, *362*(8).

Koh, H. K., and Sebelius, K. G. (2010). Promoting Prevention Through the Affordable Care Act. *New England Journal of Medicine*, *363*(14). http://healthpolicyandreform.nejm.org/?p=12171&query=TOC.

Kotter, J. P. (1995, March-April). Leading Change: Why Transformation Efforts Fail. *Harvard Business Review*, *12*(1), pp. 59–67.

Kotter, J. P., and Heskett, J. L. (1992). *Corporate Culture and Performance*. New York: Free Press.

Kouzes, J. M., and Posner, B. Z. (1995). *The Leadership Challenge: How to Keep Getting Extraordinary Things Done in Organizations*. San Francisco: Jossey-Bass.

Kouzes, J. M., and Posner, B. Z. (2009). *The Truth About Leadership: The No-Fads, Heart-Of-The-Matter Facts You Need To Know*. San Francisco: Jossey-Bass.

Lantz P. M., House, J. S., Lepkowski, J. M., Williams, D. R., Mero, R. P., and Chen, J. (1998). Socioeconomic Factors, Health Behaviors, and Mortality. *Journal of the American Medical Association*, *279*(21), 1703–1708.

Larson, N., Story, M., and Nelson, M. (2009). Neighborhood Environments: Disparities in Access to Healthy Foods in the U.S. *American Journal of Preventive Medicine*, *36*(1), 74–81.

Lasker, R., Weiss, E., and Miller, R. (2001). Partnership Synergy: A Practical Framework for Studying and Strengthening the Collaborative Advantage. *Milbank Quarterly*, *79*(2), 179–205.

Ledlow, G., and Coppola. M. (2011) *Leadership for the Health Professional: Theory, Skills and Applications.* Sudbury, MA: Jones & Bartlett Learning.

Lee, T. H., and Mongan, J. J. (2009). *Chaos and Organization in Health Care.* Cambridge, MA: MIT Press.

Lenihan, P., Welter, C., Chang, C., and Gorenflo, G. (2007). The Operational Definition of a Functional Local Public Health Agency: The Next Strategic Step in the Quest for Identity and Relevance. *Journal of Public Health Management and Practice, 13*(4), 357–363.

Leonard, L. G. (1998). Primary Health Care and Partnerships: Collaboration of a Community Agency, Health Department, and University Nursing Program. *Journal of Nursing Education, 37*(3), 144–151.

Levi, J. L., Cohen, L., and Segal, L. M. (2008, October). Prevention for a Healthier *California: Investments in Disease Prevention Yield Significant Savings, Stronger Communities.* Trust for America's Health. http://tcenews.calendow.org/pr/tce/document/TFAHCAROI2008RptFnl.pdf.

Levy, B., and Sidel, V. (2008). *War and Public Health* (Second Edition). New York: Oxford University Press.

Lewin Group. (2002). *Community Participation Can Improve America's Public Health System.* http://ww2.wkkf.org/DesktopModules/WKF.00_DmaSupport/ViewDoc.aspx?LanguageID=0&CID=8&ListID=28&ItemID=83713&fld=PDFFile.

Lighter, D. E. (2009). *Advanced Performance Improvement In Health Care: Principles and Methods.* Sudbury, MA: Jones & Bartlett Learning.

Lleras-Muney, A. (2005). The Relationship Between Education and Adult Mortality in the United States. *Review of Economics Studies, 72*, 189–221.

Lussier, R. N., and Achua, C. F. (2004). *Leadership: Theory, Application, Skill Development* (Second Edition). Mason, OH: Thomson South-Western.

Maciariello, J. A. (2006). Peter F. Drucker on Executive Leadership and Effectiveness. In F. Hesselbein and M. Goldsmith (Eds.), *The Leader of the Future 2: Visions, Strategies, and Practices for the New Era* (pp. 3–27). San Francisco: Jossey-Bass.

Maciosek, M., Coffield, A., Flottemesch, T., Edwards, N., and Solberg, L. (2010). Greater Use of Preventive Services in U.S. Health Care Could Save Lives at Little or No Cost. *Health Affairs, 29*(9), 1656–1660.

Manning, G., and Curtis, K. (2007). *The Art of Leadership* (Second Edition). Boston: McGraw-Hill Irwin.

Mays, G. P., Halverson, P. K., Baker, E. L., Stevens, R., and Vann, J. J. (2004). Availability and Perceived Effectiveness of Public Health Activities in the Nation's Most Populous Communities. *American Journal of Public Health, 94*(6), 1019–1026.

Mays, G. P., McHugh, M. C., Shim, K., Perry, N., Lenaway, D., Halverson, P. K., and Moonesinghe, R. (2006). Institutional and Economic Determinants of Public Health System Performance. *American Journal of Public Health, 96*(3), 523–531.

Mays, G. P., Miller, C. A., and Halverson, P. K. (2000). *Local Public Health Practice: Trends and Models.* Washington DC: American Public Health Association.

Mays, G. P., Smith, S. A., Ingram, R. C., Racster, L. J., Lamberth, C. D., and Lovely, E. S. (2009). Public Health Delivery Systems: Evidence, Uncertainty, and Emerging Research Needs. *American Journal of Preventive Medicine, 36*(3), 256–265.

Mays, V. M., Cochran, S. D., and Barnes, N. W. (2007). Race, Race-Based Discrimination, and Health Outcomes Among African Americans. *Annual Review of Psychology, 58*, 201–225.

McGinnis, J. M. (2006). Can Public Health and Medicine Partner in the Public Interest? *Health Affairs, 25*(4), 1044–1052.

McGinnis J., and Foege, W. (1993). Actual Causes of Death in the United States. *Journal of the American Medical Association*, *270*(18), 2207–2212.

McGinnis, J. M., Williams-Russo, P., and Knickman, J. R. (2002). The Case for More Active Policy Attention to Health Promotion. *Health Affairs*, *21*(2), 78–93.

McKelvey, B. (2008). Emergent Strategy via Complexity Leadership: Using Complexity Science and Adaptive Tension to Build Distributed Intelligence. In M. Uhl-Bien and R. Marion (Eds.), *Complexity Leadership: Part I, Conceptual Foundations* (pp. 225–268). Charlotte, NC: Information Age.

McKenzie, J. F., Neiger, B. L., and Thackeray, R. (2009). *Planning, Implementing and Evaluating Health Promotion Programs: A Primer*. San Francisco: Benjamin Cummings.

McKenzie, J. F., Pinger, R. R., and Kotecki, J. E. (2005). *An Introduction to Community Health* (Fifth Edition). Sudbury, MA: Jones & Bartlett Learning.

McLaughlin, C. P., and McLaughlin, C. D. (2008). *Health Policy Analysis: An Interdisciplinary Approach*. Sudbury, MA: Jones & Bartlett Learning.

Mead, P. S., Slutsker, L., Dietz, V., McCaig, L. F., Bresee, J. S., Shapiro, C., Griffin, P. M., and Tauxe, R. V. (2010). Food-Related Illness and Death in the United States. Centers for Disease Control and Prevention. www.cdc.gov/ncidod/eid/vol5no5/mead.htm.

Mensah, G. (2005). *Eliminating Disparities in Cardiovascular Health: Six Strategic Imperatives and a Framework for Action*. http://circ.ahajournals.org/cgi/reprint/111/10/1332.

Merrill, R., and Timmreck, T. (2006). *Introduction to Epidemiology* (Fourth Edition). Sudbury, MA: Jones & Bartlett Learning.

Miller, A., Moore, K., McKaig, T., and Richards, C. (1994). A Screening Survey to Assess Public Health Performance. *Public Health Reports*, *109*(5), 659–664.

Miller, C. C. (2008, November 19). The Doctor Will See You Now—Online. *The New York Times*. http://bits.blogs.nytimes.com/2008/11/19/the-doctor-will-see-you-now-online/.

Miniño, A., Arias, E., Kochanek, K. D., Murphy, S. L., and Smith, B. L. (2002, September 16). Deaths: Final Data for 2000. *National Vital Statistics Reports*, *50*(15), 1–119. www.cdc.gov/nchs/data/nvsr/nvsr50/nvsr50_15.pdf.

Moen, R. A. (2002). *A Guide to Idealized Design*. Cambridge, MA: Institute for Healthcare Improvement.

Mokdad, A. H., Marks, J. S., Stroup, D. F., and Gerberding, J. L. (2004). Actual Causes of Death in the United States, 2000. *Journal of the American Medical Association*, *291*(10), 1238–1245.

Morewitz, S. J. (2006). *Chronic Diseases and Health Care*. New York: Springer.

Morland, K., Wing, S., Roux, A. D., and Poole, C. (2002). Neighborhood Characteristics Associated with the Location of Food Stores and Food Service Places. *American Journal of Preventive Medicine*, *22*(1), 23–29.

Morrow, J., and Breen, B. (2001, September). *Pennsylvania Health Risk Profile*. Commonwealth of Pennsylvania, Office of Mental Retardation.

Mukherjee, A. S. (2009). *The Spider's Strategy: Creating Networks to Avert Crisis, Create Change, and Really Get Ahead*. Upper Saddle River, NJ: Pearson.

Murray, C.J.L., and Frenk, J. (2010). Ranking 37th—Measuring the Performance of the U.S. Health Care System. *New England Journal of Medicine*, *362*(2), 98–99.

Mushlin, A. I., and Ghomrawi, H. (2010). Health Care Reform and the Need for Comparative-Effectiveness Research. *New England Journal of Medicine*, *10*(1058), 1–3.

National Association of County and City Health Officials (NACCHO). (2005a). *National Profile of Local Health Departments*. www.naccho.org/topics/infrastructure/profile/upload/NACCHO_report_final_000.pdf.

National Association of County and City Health Officials (NACCHO). (2005b). *Operational Definition of a Functional Local Health Department*. www.naccho.org/topics/infrastructure/ accreditation/upload/OperationalDefinitionBrochure-2.pdf.

National Association of County and City Health Officials (NACCHO). (2008). *The 2008 National Profile of Local Health Departments*. www.naccho.org/topics/infrastructure/profile/resources/ 2008report/upload/profilebrochure2009-10-17_COMBINED_post-to-web.pdf.

National Association of County and City Health Officials (NACCHO). (2009). *The Multi-State Learning Collaborative: Fostering Multi-Sector Collaborations Around Quality Improvement and Processes*. www.naccho.org/events/nacchoannual2009/upload/Montgomery-Robusky-Tabbott-Multi-State-Learning-Collaborative.pdf.

National Association of County and City Health Officers. (2010). *Trends in Local Health Departments Finance, Workforce, and Activities*. Washington, DC: NACCHO.

National Association of County and City Health Officials (NACCHO). (2011). Mobilizing for Action through Planning and Partnerships (MAPP). www.naccho.org/topics/ infrastructure/MAPP/index.cfm.

National Center for Health Statistics. (2007). *Health, United States, 2007 with Chartbook on Trends in the Health of Americans*. Centers for Disease Control and Prevention. www.cdc.gov/nchs/ data/hus/hus07.pdf.

National Center for Health Statistics. (n.d.). 1900–1940 Tables Ranked in National Office of Vital Statistics, December 1947. In *Leading Causes of Death, 1900–1998*. www.cdc.gov/nchs/data/dvs/lead1900_98.pdf.

National Committee on Quality Assurance. (2008). *U.S. Health Care Quality: Stuck in Neutral Slowdown Has Implications for Reform*. www.ncqa.org/tabid/1077/Default.aspx.

National Highway Traffic Safety Administration. (2004). *Sixth Report to Congress, Fourth Report to the President: The National Initiative for Increasing Safety Belt Use*.

National Institutes of Health. (2002). *NIH's Strategic Research Plan and Budget to Reduce and Ultimately Eliminate Health Disparities Volume 1: Fiscal Years 2002–2006*. www.nimhd.nih.gov/ our_programs/strategic/pubs/VolumeI_031003EDrev.pdf.

National Institutes of Health. (n.d.). NIH Home: Health Information. www.nih.gov/.

National Minority Health Month Foundation. (2007). *Study of Vital Statistics by ZIP Code Shows Health Disparities Affecting Minorities in the Treatment of Kidney and Cardiovascular Diseases*. www.rwjf.org/publichealth/product.jsp?id=18669.

National Network of Public Health Institutes. (2010). *Ready, Set, Go: Costing the Prerequisites*. http://ebookbrowse.com/using-qi-to-meet-accreditation-pre-requisites-84675-ppt-d110985231.

Neumann, P. J., Jacobson, P. D., and Palmer, J. A. (2008). Measuring the Value of Public Health Systems: The Disconnect Between Health Economists and Public Health Practitioners. *American Journal of Public Health*, *98*(12), 2173–2180.

Northern New England Cardiovascular Disease Study Group. (2009). Published Literature. www.nnecdsg.org/pub_lit_2.htm.

Northouse, P. G. (2007). *Leadership Theory and Practice* (Fourth Edition). Thousand Oaks, CA: Sage.

Northouse, P. G. (2009). *Introduction to Leadership Concepts and Practice*. Thousand Oaks, CA: Sage.

Novick, L. F., Morrow, C. B., and Mays, G. P. (2008). *Public Health Administration: Principles for Population-Based Management* (Second Edition). Sudbury, MA: Jones & Bartlett Learning.

Nussbaum, A., Tirrell, M., Wechsler, P., and Randall, T. (2010, March 24). Obamacare's Cost Scalpel. *BusinessWeek*, pp. 64–66.

Occupational Safety and Health Administration. (2009). *2009 Special Report: Impact and Funding of State Occupational Health Programs*. www.osha.gov/dcsp/osp/oshspa/oshspa_2009_report .html.

Olshanksy, S. J., Douglas, J. P., Hershow, R., Layden, J., Carnes, B., Brody, J., Hayflick, L., Butler, R., Allison, D., and Ludwig, D. (2005). A Potential Decline in Life Expectancy in the U.S. in the 21st Century. *New England Journal of Medicine, 352*(11), 1138–1145.

Organisation for Economic Co-operation and Development. (2007). *OECD Health Data 2007*.

Padgett, S. M., Bekemeier, B., and Berkowitz, B. (2004). Collaborative Partnerships at the State Level: Promoting Systems Changes in Public Health Infrastructure. *Journal of Public Health Management and Practice, 10*(3), 251–257.

Paez, K. A., Zhao, L., and Hwang, W. (2009). Rising Out-Of-Pocket Spending For Chronic Conditions: A Ten Year Trend. *Health Affairs, 28*(1), 15–25.

Pear, R. (2008, July 9). Report Links Dead Doctors to Payments by Medicare. *The New York Times*. www.nytimes.com/2008/07/09/washington/09fraud.html?_r=1 &pagewanted=print.

Peters, D., and Phillips, T. (2004). Mectizan Donation Program: Evaluation of a Public-Private Partnership. *Tropical Medicine and International Health, 9*(4), A4–A15.

Pierce, J. L., and Newstrom, J. W. (2006). *Leaders and the Leadership Process: Readings, Self-Assessments and Applications* (Fourth Edition.). Boston: McGraw-Hill Higher Education

Pincus, T., Esther, R., DeWalt, D. A., and Callahan, L. F. (1998). Social Conditions and Self-Management Are More Powerful Determinants of Health Than Access to Care. *Annals of Internal Medicine, 129*(5), 406–411.

Plowman, D. A., and Duchon, D. (2008). Dispelling the Myths About Leadership: From Cybernetics to Emergence. In M. Uhl-Bien and R. Marion (Eds.), *Complexity Leadership: Part I, Conceptual Foundations* (pp. 129–153). Charlotte, NC: Information Age.

PolicyLink. (2001). Community Mapping. www.policylink.org/site/c.lkIXLbMNJrE/ b.5136917/k.AB67/Community_Mapping.htm.

PolicyLink. (2002). *Reducing Health Disparities Through a Focus on Communities*. www.policylink .org/atf/cf/%7B97c6d565-bb43-406d-a6d5-eca3bbf35af0%7D/REDUCINGHEALTH DISPARITIES_FINAL.PDF.

Pothukuchi, K. (2005). Attracting Supermarkets to Inner-City Neighborhoods: Economic Development Outside the Box. *Economic Development Quarterly, 19*(3), 232–244.

Poverty and Race Research and Action Council. (2005). *Analysis of the U.S. Census Data with the Assistance of Nancy A. Denton and Bridget J. Anderson*.

Prevention Institute. (2004). THRIVE (Tool for Health and Resilience in Vulnerable Environments. http://thrive.preventioninstitute.org/thrive.html.

Prevention Institute. (2007). *Good Health Counts: A 21st Century Approach to Health and Community for California*. www.preventioninstitute.org/component/jlibrary/article/id-85/127.html.

Prevention Institute. (2008). *Key Informant Interviews* (Unpublished).

Prevention Institute, Harvard School of Public Health, and Southern California Injury Prevention Research Center, UCLA School of Public Health Prevention Institute. (2008). UNITY RoadMap: A Framework for Effectiveness and Sustainability. www.preventioninstitute .org/index.php?option=com_jlibrary&view=article&id=30&Itemid=127.

Public Health Accreditation Board (PHAB). (2009). *Proposed Local Standards and Measures*. www.phaboard.org/assets/documents/PHABLocalJuly2009-finaleditforbeta.pdf.

Public Health Accreditation Board (PHAB). (2010). Public Health Accreditation Board: About Accreditation. www.phaboard.org/index.php/accreditation/.

Public Health Leadership Society (PHLS). (2002). *Principles of the Ethical Practice of Public Health* (Version 2.2). http://phls.org/CMSuploads/Principles-of-the-Ethical-Practice-of-PH-Version-2.2-68496.pdf.

Q&A with Surgeon General Benjamin: "Transform Our Sick Care System into a Wellness System": Benjamin to Health Workers: "We Must Continue to Stay the Course." (2010, April). *Nation's Health, 40*, 5.

RAND. (2006). U.S. Health Compared with Health in Other Countries. www.randcompare.org/us-health-care-today/health#u.s.-health-compared-with-health-in-other-countries.

Rashid, J. R., Spengler, R. F., Wagner, R. W., Melanson, C., Skillen, E. L., Mays, R. A., Heurtin-Roberts S., and Long, J. A. (2009). Eliminating Health Disparities Through Transdisciplinary Research, Cross-Agency Collaboration, and Public Participation. *American Journal of Public Health, 99*(11), 1955–1961.

Reeves, M., Katten, A., and Guzman, M. (2002). *Fields of Poison 2002: California Farm Workers and Pesticides.* Pesticide Action Network and Californians for Pesticide Reform. www.panna.org/resources/gpc/gpc_200304.13.1.07.dv.html.

Rice, C. (2007). Four Priorities Build Bonds with Stakeholders. *Leadership Excellence, 24*(3).

Ringel, J. S., Trentacost, E., and Lurie, N. (2009). *How Well Did Health Departments Communicate About Risk at the Start of the Swine Flu Epidemic in 2009?* http://content.healthaffairs.org/cgi/content/abstract/hlthaff.28.4.w743v1.

Roberts, E., Friedman, S., Brady, J., Pouget, E., Tempalski, B., and Galea, S. (2010). Environmental Conditions, Political Economy, and Rates of Injection Drug Use in Large US Metropolitan Areas 1992–2002. *Drug and Alcohol Dependence, 106*(2-3), 142–153.

Robert Wood Johnson Foundation. (2009). *Building the Evidence for Quality Improvement Initiatives in Public Health Practice.* www.rwjf.org/publichealth/product.jsp?id=47048.

Robert Wood Johnson Foundation, (2010). Session Recap: Public Health Accreditation Implications for Public Health Administrators. http://rwjfapha.com/2010/11/session-recap-public-health-accreditation-implications-for-public-health-administrators/.

Rogow, F., Adelman, L., Poulain, R., and Cheng, J. (2008). Unnatural Causes Discussion Guide. www.unnaturalcauses.org/discussion_guides.php.

Roper, W., and Mays, G. (2000). Performance Measures in Public Health: Conceptual and Methodological Issues. *Journal of Public Health Management and Practice, 6*(5), 66–77.

Ross, C. E., and Mirowsky, J. (1999). Refining the Association Between Education and Health: The Effects of Quantity, Credential, and Selectivity. *Demography, 36*(4), 445–460.

Rothman, K. J., and Greenland, S. (2005). Causation and Causal Inference in Epidemiology. *American Journal of Public Health, 95*(Supplement 1), S144–S150.

Rowitz, L. (2006). *Public Health for the 21st Century: The Prepared Leader.* Sudbury, MA: Jones & Bartlett Learning.

RTI International. (2009, July). Obesity in America, Recent Studies. www.rti.org/news.cfm?nav=721&objectid=329246AF-5056-B172-B829FC032B70D8DE.

Russell, L. B. (2009). Preventing Chronic Disease: An Important Investment, but Don't Count on Cost Savings. *Health Affairs, 28*(1), 42–45.

Russo, P. (2007). Accreditation of Public Health Agencies: A Means, Not an End. *Journal of Public Health Management and Practice, 13*(4), 329–331.

Salber, P. R., and Taliaferro, E. (2006). The Physician's Guide to Intimate Partner Violence and Abuse: A Reference for All Health Care Professionals. pp. 89–99.

Sampson, R. J., Raudenbush, S. W., and Earls, F. (1997). Neighborhoods and Violent Crime: A Multilevel Study of Collective Efficacy. *American Association for the Advancement of Science, 277*(5328), 918–924.

Sanders, I. (2003). *What Is Complexity?* www.complexsys.org/pdf/what_is_complexity.pdf.

Satcher, D. (2006). The Prevention Challenge and Opportunity. *Health Affairs, 25*(4), 1009–1011.

Schmid, T. L., Pratt, M., and Howze, E. (1995). Policy as Intervention: Environmental and Policy Approaches to the Prevention of Cardiovascular Disease. *American Journal of Public Health, 85*(9), 1207–1211.

Schneider, M. J. (2006). *Introduction to Public Health* (Second Edition). Sudbury, MA: Jones & Bartlett Learning.

Scutchfield, F. D., and Keck, C. W. (2009). *Principles of Public Health.* Clifton Park, NY: Delmar.

Sensenig, A. L. (2007). Refining Estimates of Public Health Spending as Measured in the National Health Expenditures Accounts: The U.S. Experience. *Journal of Public Health Management and Practice, 13*(2), 103–14.

Shenson, D., Adams, M., and Bolen, J. (2008). Delivery of Preventive Services to Adults Ages 50–64: Monitoring Performance Using a Composite Measure, 1997–2004. *Journal of General Internal Medicine, 23*(6), 733–740.

Shewhart, W. A. (1986). *Statistical Method from the Viewpoint of Quality Control.* Mineola, NY: Dover.

Shi, L., and Singh, D. A. (2008). *Delivering Health Care in America: A Systems Approach.* Sudbury, MA: Jones & Bartlett Learning.

Shi, L., and Singh, D. A. (2010). *Essentials of the U.S. Health Care System* (Second Edition). Sudbury, MA: Jones & Bartlett Learning.

Shortell, S. (2010). Challenges and Opportunities for Population Health Partnerships. *Preventing Chronic Disease, 7*(6). www.cdc.gov/pcd/issues/2010/nov/10_0110.htm.

Shortell, S., Zukoski, A., Alexander, J., Bazzoli, G., Conrad, D., Hasnain-Wynia, R., Sofaer, S., Chan, B., Casey, E., and Margolin, F. (2002). Evaluating Partnerships for Community Health Improvement: Tracking the Footprints. *Journal of Health Politics, Policy, and Law, 27*(1), 49–91.

Siegel, B., Bretsch J., Sears, V., Regenstein, M., and Wilson, M. (2007). Assumed Equity: Early Observations from the First Hospital Disparities Collaborative. *Journal for Healthcare Quality, 29*(5), 11–15.

Siegel, M., and Lotenberg, L. D. (2006). *Marketing Public Health: Strategies to Promote Social Change* (Second Edition). Sudbury, MA: Jones & Bartlett Learning.

Simon, P. A., and Fielding, J. E. (2006). Public Health and Business: A Partnership That Makes Cents. *Health Affairs, 25*(4), 1029–1039.

Six Sigma Online (n.d.). www.sixsigmaonline.org/index.html.

Skogan, W. G., Hartnett, S. M., Bump, N., and Dubois, J. (2008). *Evaluation of CeaseFire-Chicago.*

Sloan, F. A., and Kasper, H. (2008). *Incentives and Choice in Health Care.* Cambridge, MA: MIT Press.

Sloane, D. C., Diamant, A. L., Lewis, L. B., Yancey, A. K., Flynn, G., Nascimento, L. M., McCarthy, W. J., Guinyard, J. J., and Cousineau, M. R., and REACH Coalition of the African American Building a Legacy of Health Project. (2003). Improving the Nutritional Resource Environment for Healthy Living Through Community-Based Participatory Research. *Journal of General Internal Medicine, 18*(7), 568–575.

Smedley, B. (2008). Moving Beyond Access: Achieving Equity in State Health Care Reform. *Health Affairs, 27*(2), 447–455.

Smedley, B., Jeffries, M., Adelman, L., and Cheng, J. (2008). *Race, Racial Inequity and Health Inequities: Separating Myth from Fact.* www.unnaturalcauses.org/assets/uploads/file/Race_Racial_Inequality_Health.pdf.

Smedley, B., Stith, A., and Nelson, A. (Eds.). (2003). *Unequal Treatment: Confronting Racial and Ethnic Disparities in Health Care.* Washington DC: Institute of Medicine.

Smircich, L., and Morgan, G. (2006). *Leadership: The Management of Meaning.* Boston: McGraw-Hill Irwin.

Smith, K. E., Bambra, C., Joyce, K. E., Perkins, N., Hunter, D. J., and Blenkinsopp, E. A. (2009). Partners in Health? A Systematic Review of the Impact of Organizational Partnerships on Public Health Outcomes in England Between 1997 and 2008. *Journal of Public Health* (Oxford), *31*(2), 210–221.

Smith, T. A., Minyard, K., Parker, C., Van Valkenburg, R., and Shoemaker, J. (2007). From Theory to Practice: What Drives the Core Business of Public Health? *Journal of Public Health Management and Practice*, *13*(2), 169–172.

Spear, S. (2009). *Chasing the Rabbit: How Market Leaders Outdistance the Competition and How Great Companies Can Catch Up and Win.* New York: McGraw-Hill.

Spitzer, D. (2008). *Leader to Leader: Enduring Insights on Leadership.* San Francisco: Jossey-Bass.

Stadler, C. (2007, July-August). The Four Principles of Enduring Success. *Harvard Business Review,* pp. 62–72. http://74.125.155.132/scholar?q=cache:adG7xfoWe9EJ:scholar.google.com/+stadler+the+four+principles+of+enduring+success&hl=en&as_sdt=0,39&as_vis=1.

Stallworth, J., and Lennon, J. (2003). An Interview with Dr. Lester Breslow. *American Journal of Public Health*, *93*(11), 1803–1805.

Stanislaus County. (n.d.). Healthy Birth Outcomes (HBO). www.schsa.org/publichealth/programs/pages/healthybirthoutcomes.html.

Starfield, B., Shi, L., Grover, A., and Macinko, J. (2005). The Effects of Specialist Supply on Populations' Health: Assessing the Evidence. *Health Affairs*, pp. 97–107.

Stern, M. J., and Seifert, S. C. (2000). *Working Paper #13 — Cultural Participation and Communities: The Role of Individual and Neighborhood Effects.* Social Impact of the Arts Project, University of Pennsylvania.

Stover, G. N., and Bassett, M. T. (2003, November). Practice Is the Purpose of Public Health. *American Journal of Public Health*, *93*(11), 1799–1801.

Studnicki, J., Steverson, B., Blais, H., Golely, E., Richards, T., and Thornton, J. (1994). Analyzing Organizational Practices in Public Health Departments. *Public Health Reports*, *109*(4), 485–490.

Sultz, H., and Young, K. (2009). *Health Care USA: Understanding Its Organization and Delivery.* Sudbury, MA: Jones & Bartlett Learning.

Taipale, I. (2002). *War or Health?* Cambridge, MA: IPPNW.

Tennyson, R. (2003). *The Partnering Toolbook.* London: International Business Leaders Forum, The Partnering Initiative.

Teutsch, S., and Churchill, R. E. (2000). *Principles and Practices of Public Health Surveillance.* New York: Oxford University Press.

Thomas, R. K. (2010). *Marketing Health Services* (Second Edition). Chicago: Health Administration Press.

Thorpe, K. E. (2006). Factors Accounting for the Rise in Health-Care Spending in the United States: The Role of Rising Disease Prevalence and Treatment Intensity. *Public Health*, *120*(11), 1002–1007.

Tichy, N. M. (1997). *The Leadership Engine: How Winning Companies Build Leaders at Every Level.* New York: HarperCollins.

Tilson, H., and Berkowitz, B. (2006). The Public Health Enterprise: Examining Our Twenty-First Century Policy Challenges. *Health Affairs, 25*(4), 900–910.

Trivedi, A., Gibbs, B., Nsiah-Jefferson, L., Ayanian, J. Z., and Prothrom-Stith, D. (2005). Creating a State Minority Health Policy Report Card. *Health Affairs, 24*(2), 388–396.

Trompenaars, F., and Voerman, E. (2010). *Servant Leadership Across Cultures.* New York: McGraw-Hill.

Trust for America's Health (TFAH). (2009). *Shortchanging America's Health.* Washington DC. http://healthyamericans.org/assets/files/shortchanging09.pdf.

Trust for America's Health (TFAH). (2010a). F as in Fat: How Obesity Threatens America's Future 2010. http://healthyamericans.org/reports/obesity2010/.

Trust for America's Health (TFAH). (2010b). Recognizing the Relationship Between Health and U.S. Economic Competitiveness. http://healthyamericans.org/assets/files/TFAH%202010Top10PrioritiesEconomy.pdf.

Trust for America's Health (TFAH), Prevention Institute (PI), The Urban Institute (UI), and New York Academy of Medicine (NYAM). (2008). *Prevention for a Healthier America: Investments in Disease Prevention Yield Significant Savings, Stronger Communities.* http://healthyamericans.org/reports/prevention08/Prevention08.pdf.

Turnock, B. J. (2007). *Essentials of Public Health.* Sudbury, MA: Jones & Bartlett Learning.

Turnock, B. J. (2009). *Public Health: What It Is and How It Works* (Fourth Edition). Sudbury, MA: Jones & Bartlett Learning.

Turnock, B. J., and Handler, A. S. (1997). From Measuring to Improving Public Health Practice. *Annual Review of Public Health, 18*, 261–282.

Turnock, B. J., Handler, A., Dyal, W. W., Christenson, G., Vaugh, E. H., Rowitz, L., Munson, J. W., Balderson, T., and Richards, T. B. (1994). Implementing and Assessing Organizational Practices in Local Health Departments. *Public Health Reports, 109*(4), 478–484.

Uhl-Bien, M., and Marion, R. (2008). Complexity Leadership—A Framework for Leadership in the Twenty-First Century. In M. Uhl-Bien and R. Marion (Eds.), *Complexity Leadership: Part I, Conceptual Foundations* (pp. xi–xxiv). Charlotte, NC: Information Age.

Uhl-Bien, M., Marion, R., and McKelvey, B. (2008). Complexity Leadership Theory: Shifting Leadership from the Industrial Age to the Knowledge Era. In M. Uhl-Bien and R. Marion (Eds.), *Complexity Leadership: Part I, Conceptual Foundations* (pp. 185–224). Charlotte, NC: Information Age.

Union for International Cancer Control. (2010). Campaign: "Cancer Can Be Prevented Too." www.uicc.org/programmes/campaign-cancer-can-be-prevented-too.

United Health Foundation. (2009). *Unhealthy Behaviors: Our Nation's Legacy.* www.americashealthrankings.org/2009/highlights.aspx.

United Nations General Assembly. (2010a). *Follow-Up to the Outcomes of the Millennium Summit.* www.un.org/en/mdg/summit2010/pdf/mdg%20outcome%20document.pdf.

United Nations General Assembly. (2010b). Millennium Development Goals Summary Matrix. www.un.org/en/mdg/summit2010/pdf/MDGSummit_Matrix_12Nov2010_rev2_REV%20DZ.pdf.

United States Breastfeeding Committee. (2002). *Workplace Breastfeeding Support.* Raleigh, NC: United States Breastfeeding Committee.

Urban Institute. (2009). *Bending the Cost Curve.* http://healthyamericans.org/assets/files/ BendingCostCurve.pdf.

U.S. Department of Health and Human Services (HHS). (1999). *Mental Health: A Report of the Surgeon General.* P. 38. Rockville, MD.

U.S. Department of Health and Human Services (HHS). (2007). *Community Health Worker National Workforce Study.* http://bhpr.hrsa.gov/healthworkforce/chw/ communityhealthworkers.pdf.

U.S. Department of Health and Human Services (HHS). (2007). Centers for Medicare and Medicaid Services. http://www.cms.hhs.gov/NationalHealthExpendData.

U.S. Department of Health and Human Services (HHS). (2008, August). Consensus Statement on Quality in the Public Health System. www.hhs.gov/ash/initiatives/quality/quality/ phqf-consensus-statement.html.

U.S. Department of Health and Human Services (HHS). (2010a). *Healthy People 2010 — Understanding and Improving Health* (Second Edition). Washington DC: U.S. Government Printing Office.

U.S. Department of Health and Human Services (HHS). (2010b). *Priority Areas for Improvement of Quality in Public Health.* www.hhs.gov/ash/initiatives/quality/quality/ improvequality2010.pdf.

U.S. Department of Health and Human Services Centers for Disease Control and Prevention (CDC). (2010). *Principles of Epidemiology in Public Health Practice: An Introduction to Applied Epidemiology and Biostatistics, Third Edition.* Office of Workforce and Career Development. Atlanta, GA. http://www.cdc.gov/training/products/ss1000/ss1000-od.pdf.

U.S. Department of Health and Human Services (HHS). (2011). Determinants of Health. www .healthypeople.gov/2020/about/DOHAbout.aspx.

U.S. Department of Transportation, (2006). *Race and Ethnicity in Fatal Motor Vehicle Traffic Crashes 1999–2004.* National Highway Traffic Safety Administration. www.watchtheroad.org/809956.pdf.

Van Velsor. E. (2008) A complexity perspective on leadership development. In M. Uhl-Bien and R. Mariona (Eds.), *Complexity leadership, Part I: Conceptual foundations* (pp. 333–346). Charlotte, NC: Information Age.

Vaughan. E., and Tinker, T. (2009) Effective Health Risk Communication About Pandemic Influenza for Vulnerable Populations. *American Journal of Public Health, 99*(52), 5324–5332.

Vetter, N., and Matthews, I. (1999). *Epidemiology and Public Health Medicine.* New York: Elsevier.

Voelker, R. (2008). Decades of Work to Reduce Disparities in Health Care Produce Limited Success. *Journal of the American Medical Association, 299*(12), 1411–1413.

Wandersman, A., and Nation, M. (1998). Urban Neighborhoods and Mental Health: Psychological Contributions to Understanding Toxicity, Resilience, and Interventions. *American Psychologist, 53*(6), 647–656.

Watson, J., Speller, V., Markwell, S., and Platt, S. (2000). The Verona Benchmark—Applying Evidence to Improve the Quality of Partnership. *Promotion and Education, 7*(2), 16–23.

Webb, P., Bain, C., and Pirozzo, S. (2005). *Essential Epidemiology: An Introduction for Students and Health Professionals.* New York: Cambridge University Press.

Weinstein, M., and Skinner, J. (2010). Comparative Effectiveness and Health Care Spending—Implications for Reform. *New England Journal of Medicine, 362*(5), 460–465.

Weiss, B. (2008). *An Assessment of Youth Violence Prevention Activities in USA Cities.* Urban Networks to Increase Thriving Youth (UNITY) Through Violence Prevention. Southern California Injury Prevention Research Center, UCLA School of Public Health, Los Angeles.

Whitehead, M. (1990). *The Concepts and Principles of Equity and Health*. http://whqlibdoc.who.int/euro/-1993/EUR_ICP RPD_414.pdf.

Wholey, D. R., White, K. M., and Kader, H. (2009). Accreditation and Accountability for Local Health Departments: Is the Cart Before the Horse? *American Journal of Public Health, 100*(1), pp. 4–5. http://ajph.aphapublications.org/cgi/eletters/99/9/1545.

Wilcox, D. (2000). Successful Partnership. www.partnerships.org.uk/AZP/part.html#anchor 3396283.

Wilkenson, R. (1999). Income Inequality, Social Cohesion, and Health: Clarifying the Theory—A Reply to Muntaner and Lynch. *International Journal of Health Services, 29*(3), 525–545.

Williams, S., and Torrens, P. (2008) *Introduction to Health Services*. Clifton Park, NY: Delmar.

Wilson, S., Seal, J., McManigal, L., Lovins, L., Cureton, M., and Browning, W. (1998). *Green Development: Integrating Ecology and Real Estate*. New York: Wiley.

World Health Organization (WHO). (1947). Constitution of the World Health Organization. *Chronicles of the World Health Organization, 1*, 29–43. Geneva, Switzerland: World Health Organization.

World Health Organization (WHO). (1998). *Health Promotion Glossary*. www.who.int/hpr/NPH/docs/hp_glossary_en.pdf.

World Health Organization (WHO). (2000). *The World Health Report 2000: Health Systems: Improving Performance*. Geneva, Switzerland: World Health Organization.

World Health Organization (WHO). (2007). *The World Health Report 2007—A Safer Future: Global Public Health Security in the 21st Century*. www.who.int/whr/2007/en/index.html.

World Health Organization (WHO). (2009, November). Diabetes. www.who.int/mediacentre/factsheets/fs312/en/.

World Health Organization (WHO). (2010). Climate Change and Health. www.who.int/mediacentre/fachsheets/fs266/en/print.html.

Yang W., Lu, J., Weng, J., Jia, W., Ji, L., Xiao, J., Shan, Z., Liu, J., Tian, H., Ji, Q., Zhu, D., Ge, J., Lin, L., Chen, L., Guo, X., Zhao, Z., Li, Q., Zhou, Z., Shan, G., and He, J. (2010). Prevalence of Diabetes Among Men and Women in China. *New England Journal of Medicine, 362*(12), 1090–1101.

Yin, R., Kaftarian, S., Yu, P., and Jansen, M. (1997). Outcomes from CSAP's Community Partnership Program: Findings from the National Cross-Site Evaluation. *Evaluation and Program Planning, 20*(3), 345–355.

Yukl, G. (2010). *Leadership in Organizations*. Upper Saddle River, NJ: Pearson Education.

Zenger, J. H., Folkman, J. R., and Edinger, S. K. (2009). *The Inspiring Leader: Unlocking the Secrets of How Extraordinary Leaders Motivate*. New York: McGraw-Hill.

INDEX

Page references followed by *fig* indicate an illustrated figure; followed by *t* indicate a table; followed by *e* indicate an exhibit.

Q